Polycystic Ovary Syndrome

CONTEMPORARY ENDOCRINOLOGY

P. Michael Conn, SERIES EDITOR

Polycystic Ovary Syndrome

Current Controversies, from the Ovary to the Pancreas

Edited by

Andrea Dunaif, MD

Division of Endocrinology, Metabolism and Molecular Medicine,
Northwestern University, Chicago, IL

R. Jeffrey Chang, MD

Department of Reproductive Medicine,
University of California, San Diego School of Medicine, La Jolla, CA

Stephen Franks, MD, FMEDSCI

Institute of Reproductive and Developmental Biology,
Imperial College London, London, UK

Richard S. Legro, MD

Department of Ob/Gyn, Penn State College of Medicine, Hershey, PA

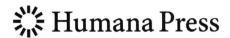 Humana Press

Editors

Andrea Dunaif, MD
Division of Endocrinology, Metabolism
and Molecular Medicine,
Northwestern University
Chicago, IL

R. Jeffrey Chang, MD
Department of Reproductive Medicine,
University of California, San Diego
School of Medicine,
La Jolla, CA

Stephen Franks, MD, FMedSci
Institute of Reproductive and
Developmental Biology,
Imperial College London,
London, UK

Richard S. Legro, MD
Department of Ob/Gyn,
Penn State College of Medicine,
Hershey, PA

Series Editor
P. Michael Conn
Oregon Health & Science University,
Beaverton, OR

ISBN: 978-1-58829-831-7   e-ISBN: 978-1-59745-108-6

Library of Congress Control Number: 2007933472

Cover illustration: Figure 1, Chapter 21, "Impact of Diagnostic Criteria: NICHD Versus Rotterdam," by Bulent O.
Yildiz.

Printed on acid-free paper

9 8 7 6 5 4 3 2 1

springer.com

This book is dedicated to the memory of Samuel S. C. Yen, MD, DSc, one of the preeminent reproductive endocrinologists of the latter half of the 20th century and a founding member of the Peacocks. Among his many contributions to the field were his pioneering studies on the pathogenesis and treatment of PCOS. We will miss not only his keen intellect but also his joie de vivre.

PREFACE

This volume is based on the proceedings of the first annual Peacocks polycystic ovary syndrome (PCOS) Forum on Disease Mechanisms and Therapeutic Strategies, October 6–9, 2005, Chateau de Vault de Lugny, Avallon, France. The Peacocks was founded by R. Jeffrey Chang, Andrea Dunaif, Stephen Franks, Richard S. Legro, and Samuel S. C. Yen. The name is based on PCOS when it is pronounced as a word "pcos" rather than as individual letters. The purpose of the Peacocks is to organize biannual meetings of experts to review the latest developments in the field. The second annual Peacocks meeting was held September 27–30, 2007, Castello di Spaltenna, Spaltenna, Italy.

It has become increasingly clear over the past several years that PCOS is a complex genetic disease resulting from the interaction of susceptibility genes and environmental factors. The insight that prenatal exposure to androgens can reproduce most of the features of the human syndrome in primates has led to a paradigm shift in concepts about the pathogenesis of the disorder. The evidence for the fetal origins of PCOS will be reviewed in animal models as well as in human studies. The novel mechanisms by which androgens may play a major role in the pathogenesis of the disorder will be presented. Other emerging areas of PCOS will also be discussed, such as prepubertal precursors of PCOS and the association between PCOS, epilepsy, and antiseizure medications. State-of-the-art treatment of the reproductive and metabolic consequences of the disorder will be reviewed. Finally, the impact of the differing diagnostic criteria for PCOS will be reviewed.

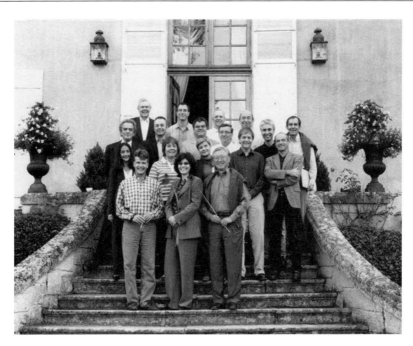

Participants' First Annual Peacock Forum. First row, from left to right: Richard S. Legro, Andrea Dunaif, and R. Jeffrey Chang. Second row, from left to right: Silva A. Arslanian, Eva Dahlgren, Evanthia Diamanti-Kandarakis, David H. Abbott, and Antoni J. Duleba. Third row, from left to right: Renato Pasquali, Bulent O. Yildiz, Ricardo Azziz, Enrico Carmina, Daniel A. Dumesic, and Michel Pugeat. Fourth row, from left to right: John C. Marshall, Adam Balen, Juha S. Tapanainen, and Roy Homburg. Not present: Stephen Franks, Didier Dewailly, and Robert J. Norman. Photograph by Antoni J. Duleba with permission.

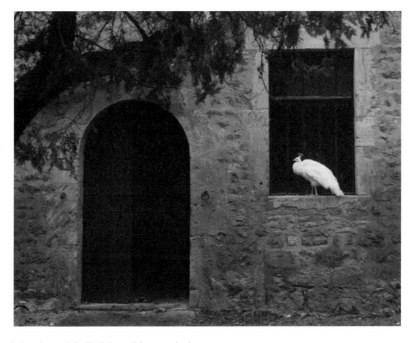

Photograph by Antoni J. Duleba with permission.

CONTENTS

ix

CONTRIBUTORS

DAVID H. ABBOTT, PHD, National Primate Research Center and Department of
Obstetrics and Gynecology, University of Wisconsin, Madison, WI

YVES ARDAENS, MD, Department of Radiology, Hopital Jeanne de Flandre, Centre
Hospitalier et Universitaire de Lille, France

SILVA A. ARSLANIAN, MD, Division of Pediatric Endocrinology, Metabolism and
Diabetes Mellitus, Children's Hospital of Pittsburgh, Pittsburgh, PA

RICARDO AZZIZ, MD, MPH, Department of Obstetrics and Gynecology, Cedars-Sinai
Medical Center, Los Angeles, CA, and Departments of Obstetrics and Gynecology
and Medicine, The David Geffen School of Medicine, UCLA, Los Angeles, CA

ADAM BALEN, MD, FRCOG, Reproductive Medicine and Surgery, Leeds Teaching
Hospitals, Clarendon Wing, Leeds General Infirmary, Leeds, UK

DEBORAH K. BARNETT, PHD, National Primate Research Center, University of
Wisconsin, Madison, WI, and Department of Biology, University of
Alaska-Southeast, Sitka, Alaska

SUSAN K. BLANK, MD, Center for Research in Reproduction, University of Virginia
Health System, Charlottesville, VA

CRISTIN M. BRUNS, MD, National Primate Research Center and Department of
Medicine, University of Wisconsin, Madison, WI

ENRICO CARMINA, MD, Endocrine Unit, Department of Clinical Medicine, University
of Palermo, Palermo, Italy

R. JEFFREY CHANG, MD, Department of Reproductive Medicine, University of
California, San Diego School of Medicine, La Jolla, CA

WENDY Y. CHANG, MD, Department of Obstetrics and Gynecology, Cedars-Sinai
Medical Center, Los Angeles, CA, and Department of Obstetrics and Gynecology,
The David Geffen School of Medicine, UCLA, Los Angeles, CA

EVA DAHLGREN, MD, PHD, Department of Obstetrics and Gynecology, Institute of
Clinical Sciences, The Sahlgrenska Academy, Göteborg University, Göteborg,
Sweden

DIDIER DEWAILLY, MD, Department of Endocrine Gynaecology and Reproductive
Medecine, Hopital Jeanne de Flandre, Centre Hospitalier et Universitaire de Lille,
Lille, France

EVANTHIA DIAMANTI-KANDARAKIS, MD, Medical School, University of Athens,
Athens, Greece

ANTONI J. DULEBA, MD, Department of Obstetrics/Gynecology, Yale University
School of Medicine, New Haven, CT

DANIEL A. DUMESIC, MD, National Primate Research Center, University of Wisconsin,
Madison, WI, and Reproductive Medicine & Infertility Associates, Woodbury, MN

ANDREA DUNAIF, MD, Division of Endocrinology, Metabolism and Molecular
Medicine, Northwestern University, Chicago, IL

STEPHEN FRANKS, MD, FMEDSCI, Institute of Reproductive and Developmental Biology, Imperial College London, London, UK

ALESSANDRA GAMBINERI, MD, Department of Internal Medicine, Division of Endocrinology, University Alma Mater Studiorum, S. Orsola-Malpighi Hospital, Bologna, Italy

KATE HARDY, PHD, Institute of Reproductive and Developmental Biology, Imperial College London, Hammersmith Hospital, London, UK

SARAH M. HOFFMANN, MD, National Primate Research Center, University of Wisconsin, Madison, WI

ROY HOMBURG, FRCOG, VU University Medical Centre, The Netherlands and IVF, Department of Obstetrics and Gynecology, Barzilai Medical Center, Ashkelon, Israel

SOPHIE JONARD, MD, Department of Endocrine Gynaecology and Reproductive Medecine, Hopital Jeanne de Flandre, Centre Hospitalier et Universitaire de Lille, Lille, France

NISRIN KADDAR, PHD, Federation of Endocrinology and Diabetology, East Center, Lyon Hospital Board, Lyon, and INSERM Unit-M 0322, Lyon, France

PINAR H. KODAMAN, MD, PHD, Department of Obstetrics/Gynecology, Yale University School of Medicine, New Haven, CT

RICHARD S. LEGRO, MD, Department of Ob/Gyn, Penn State College of Medicine, Hershey, PA

JON E. LEVINE, MD, Departments of Neurobiology and Physiology, Northwestern University, Evanston, IL

JOHN C. MARSHALL, MD, PHD, Center for Research in Reproduction, University of Virginia Health System, Charlottesville, VA

CHRISTOPHER R. MCCARTNEY, MD, Center for Research in Reproduction, University of Virginia Health System, Charlottesville, VA

LISA J. MORAN, PHD, Research Centre for Reproductive Health, Discipline of Obstetrics & Gynaecology, University of Adelaide, The Queen Elizabeth Hospital, Woodville, South Australia, Australia

LAURE MORIN-PAPUNEN, MD, PHD, Department of Obstetrics and Gynecology, Oulu University Hospital, University of Oulu, Oulu, Finland

PER OLOF JANSON, MD, PHD, Department of Obstetrics and Gynecology, Institute of Clinical Sciences, The Sahlgrenska Academy, Göteborg University, Göteborg, Sweden

QUIRINE LAMBERTS OKONKWO, MD, Center for Research in Reproduction, University of Virginia Health System, Charlottesville, VA

ROBERT J. NORMAN, MD, PHD, Research Centre for Reproductive Health, Discipline of Obstetrics & Gynaecology, University of Adelaide, The Queen Elizabeth Hospital, Woodville, South Australia, Australia

RENATO PASQUALI, MD, Department of Internal Medicine, Division of Endocrinology, University Alma Mater Studiorum, S. Orsola-Malpighi Hospital, Bologna, Italy

MICHEL PUGEAT, MD, PHD, Federation of Endocrinology and Diabetology, East Center, Lyon Hospital Board, Lyon, and INSERM Unit-M 0322, Lyon, France

VÉRONIQUE RAVEROT, PHD, Federation of Endocrinology and Diabetology, East Center, Lyon Hospital Board, Lyon, and INSERM Unit-M 0322, Lyon, France

YANN ROBERT, MD, Department of Radiology, Hopital Jeanne de Flandre, Centre
Hospitalier et Universitaire de Lille, Lille, France

REBECCA L. ROBKER, PHD, Research Centre for Reproductive Health, Discipline of
Obstetrics & Gynaecology, University of Adelaide, The Queen Elizabeth Hospital,
Woodville, South Australia, Australia

ANNELOES E. RUIFROK, Medical Student, Universitair Medisch Centrum Groningen
(UMCG), Discipline of Obstrics & Gynaecology, Groningen, the Netherlands

JUHA S. TAPANAINEN, MD, PHD, Department of Obstetrics and Gynecology, Oulu
University Hospital, University of Oulu, Oulu, Finland

ALICE F. TARANTAL, PHD, Departments of Pediatrics, Cell Biology and Human
Anatomy, California National Primate Research Center, University of California,
Davis, CA

MARGRIT URBANEK, PHD, Division of Endocrinology, Metabolism and Molecular
Medicine, Northwestern University Medical School, Chicago, IL

JULIA WARREN-ULANCH, MD, Division of Weight Management and Wellness,
Children's Hospital of Pittsburgh, Pittsburgh, PA

ELIZABETH A. WINANS, PHARMD, BCPP, College of Pharmacy, University of Illinois
at Chicago, Chicago, IL, and The Psychiatric Clinical Research Center, Rush
University Medical Center, Chicago, IL

BULENT O. YILDIZ, MD, Department of Internal Medicine, Endocrinology and
Metabolism Unit, Hacettepe University Faculty of Medicine, Ankara, Turkey

RAO ZHOU, MD, National Primate Research Center and Endocrinology-Reproductive
Physiology Program, University of Wisconsin, Madison, WI

List of Color Plates

The images listed below appear in the color insert that follows page 184.

1

Folliculogenesis in Polycystic Ovaries

Stephen Franks, MD, FMEDSCI,
and Kate Hardy, PHD

Summary

Polycystic ovary syndrome (PCOS) is the commonest cause of anovulatory infertility. Anovulation in PCOS is characterized by arrested growth of antral follicles. Although arrested antral follicle growth probably reflects the abnormal endocrine environment in PCOS (and, particularly the effect of hyperinsulinemia), there is increasing evidence of abnormalities of follicle development from the very earliest, gonadotropin-independent stages. The underlying molecular basis of this fundamental ovarian abnormality remains to be determined.

Key Words: Polycystic ovary syndrome; anovulation; luteinizing hormone; insulin; granulosa cells; preantral follicles; anti-Müllerian hormone.

1. INTRODUCTION

Polycystic ovary syndrome (PCOS) is the commonest cause of anovulatory infertility *(1,2)*, but the mechanism of anovulation remains uncertain. The typical gross morphology of anovulatory polycystic ovaries is the presence of multiple antral follicles 2–8 mm in diameter, which signifies arrest of follicle development prior to the preovulatory phase *(3)*. Ovulation can be induced in most cases by treatment which increases serum concentrations of follicle-stimulating hormone (FSH) *(4,5)*, but while serum levels of FSH are slightly lower than in the early follicular phase of the normal cycle, FSH deficiency is unlikely to be the primary abnormality in PCOS *(6)*.

From: *Contemporary Endocrinology: Polycystic Ovary Syndrome*
Edited by: A. Dunaif, R. J. Chang, S. Franks, and R. S. Legro © Humana Press, Totowa, NJ

2. ANTRAL FOLLICLE FUNCTION IN POLYCYSTIC OVARIES

Despite arrested follicle development, granulosa cells of follicles from anovulatory women with PCOS remain steroidogenically competent and indeed show evidence of both increased estradiol and progesterone production when compared with follicles of similar size from ovulatory women with either normal or polycystic ovaries (7–9). Estradiol production by granulosa cells of medium-sized antral follicles is typically increased in anovulatory women with polycystic ovaries but not in subjects with polycystic ovaries who have regular menses (8,9). Steroidogenesis by theca cells is, by contrast, abnormal in both anovulatory and ovulatory subjects with polycystic ovaries. After measurement of steroids in theca-conditioned medium, we observed that concentrations of androstenedione (20-fold), 17-α-hydroxyprogesterone (10-fold) and progesterone (fivefold) were significantly greater in cultures from polycystic ovaries compared with control cultures, regardless of menstrual cycle history (10). Similar results have been recorded in studies of passaged theca cell cultures from normal and polycystic ovaries, suggesting an intrinsic abnormality of theca cell steroidogenesis in the polycystic ovary (11). In summary, follicular cells in antral follicles from ovulatory subjects with PCO hypersecrete androgen but not estrogen, whereas cells from anovulatory women with PCO are characterized by excessive production of both androgen and estrogen. As increased androgen production is common to both ovulatory and anovulatory women with polycystic ovaries, it is unlikely that hyperandrogenism is the major cause of anovulation. It is possible, however, that excessive androgen production may contribute to the etiology of anovulation by adding to the accumulation of cyclic AMP (cAMP) in granulosa cells, as discussed below.

3. MECHANISMS OF ARRESTED ANTRAL FOLLICLE GROWTH IN PCOS

The explanation for the apparent disparity between arrested follicle growth and enhanced steroidogenesis almost certainly lies in the effect of the abnormal endocrine environment on follicle maturation. The endocrine environment in women with PCOS is characterized by hypersecretion of luteinizing hormone (LH), insulin and androgens. These factors may interact to produce supra-physiological intracellular concentrations of cyclic cAMP in the granulosa cell of the maturing antral follicle. In the normal menstrual cycle, granulosa cells in the dominant follicle (and the dominant follicle alone) acquire LH receptors (and responsiveness to LH) only in the mid-follicular phase. LH stimulates steroidogenesis by granulosa cells but also triggers terminal differentiation and arrest of follicle growth in the normal mature, preovulatory follicle (12). The switch from growth to terminal differentiation of granulosa cells in the preovulatory follicle is thought to be activated by exceeding a notional "ceiling" level of intracellular cAMP and is normally triggered by the onset of the mid-cycle LH surge (12). PCOS is characterized by hypersecretion of LH, and it is possible that this alone may promote premature arrest of follicular growth. However, many patients have normal serum concentrations of LH (5,13,14). In these subjects (as well as in those with elevated serum LH concentrations), the gonadotropic action of insulin may be a crucial factor in the mechanism of disordered follicular function.

In human granulosa cells of both normal and polycystic ovaries, insulin, in the absence of gonadotropins, stimulates estradiol and progesterone secretion *(15)*. Significantly, it has also been shown to augment, synergistically, LH-induced steroidogenesis by isolated granulosa cells *(15)*. Thus, elevated tonic levels of LH and/or amplification of LH action on the follicle by hyperinsulinemia could account for arrest of follicle growth but enhancement of estradiol and progesterone production *(16)*. Although there is little evidence that insulin has any direct effect on cAMP production, it is likely that the mechanism whereby insulin amplifies LH action involves an increase in the number of LH receptors on the maturing granulosa cells *(17)*. PCOS is characterized by peripheral insulin resistance *(18)*, but there appears to be no evidence for differences in insulin-stimulated steroidogenesis between normal and polycystic ovaries *(15,19)*. Furthermore, insulin appears to exert its action by binding to its own receptor rather than by "cross-talk" with the type-I IGF receptor *(20)*. Why then does the ovary retain apparently normal steroidogenesis in response to insulin in the face of peripheral insulin resistance? Data from studies in cultured granulosa-lutein cells may provide the answer. There is evidence for impaired insulin-mediated glucose uptake *(19)* and lactate production *(19,21,22)* but without significant impairment of progesterone production *(19)* (Fig. 1), suggesting a post-receptor defect affecting metabolic, but not steroidogenic, signaling pathways.

It is conceivable that androgens may also contribute to the disordered folliculogenesis of PCOS. In granulosa cell cultures, androgens augment gonadotropin-induced cAMP production *(23)*, and it is therefore possible that the hypersecretion of ovarian androgens, which is typical of the polycystic ovary, can by the same common intracellular mechanism, add to the effects of LH and insulin on follicle maturation.

There is direct evidence for premature responsiveness to LH in antral follicles of anovulatory women with polycystic ovaries. Granulosa cells from follicles of normal

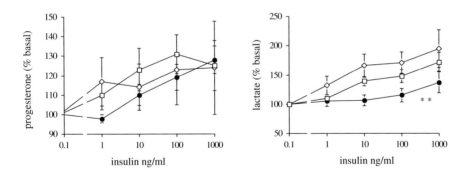

Fig. 1. Production of progesterone and lactate (expressed a percentage of baseline values) by cultured granulosa-lutein cells after 48 h of incubation in response to insulin (1–1000 ng/ml) or luteinizing hormone (LH) (1–5 ng/ml) in seven women with normal ovaries (open squares), six with ovulatory polycystic ovary (PCO) (open diamonds), and seven with anovulatory PCO (closed circles). Individual data points indicate mean ± SEM. There were significant differences in the dose–response curves between the groups with respect to insulin-stimulated lactate accumulation ($p \leq 0.0001$ ANOVA**) but not progesterone production. Note the different scales for progesterone and lactate production. Adapted from *(19)*.

ovaries (or from polycystic ovaries from ovulatory women) only secrete estradiol in response to LH when the follicle has reached 9–10 mm in diameter. By contrast, in cells derived from anovulatory women with polycystic ovaries, LH stimulated secretion of estradiol and progesterone in granulosa cells from follicles as small as 4 mm *(9)*. Furthermore, antral follicles around 6–8 mm in diameter produced levels of estradiol and progesterone that were similar to those found in the normal, preovulatory follicle. The mechanism of this "premature" response to LH remains to be determined; it could represent an effect of endogenous hyperinsulinemia (with or without the influence of hyperandrogenism) but may also reflect an intrinsic abnormality of the control of follicle development (see below). Inappropriate steroidogenesis by prematurely advanced antral follicles may also help explain the slightly but significantly lower levels of serum FSH in anovulatory women with PCOS. Using mathematical modeling, it can be predicted that enhanced estradiol production by a proportion of small antral follicles in a "cohort" would—by a negative feedback effect—suppress FSH and prevent further development of "healthy" follicles within that cohort *(24)*. This would also explain why low-dose FSH—presumably by promoting growth of the healthy follicles—leads to normal development of a dominant follicle in women with PCOS.

4. EARLY FOLLICULAR DEVELOPMENT IN PCOS

The abnormalities of antral follicle number and function are now well documented, but the question remains whether there is also an underlying and perhaps more fundamental abnormality of folliculogenesis originating in the preantral (and therefore largely endocrine independent) stages of development. There is indeed evidence that disordered folliculogenesis also involves the smaller, preantral follicles *(25)*. The observations by Hughesdon (made in archived ovarian tissue sections) that the numbers of primary and secondary follicles in the polycystic ovary are about twice those observed in the normal ovary *(25)* prompted us to further investigate early follicle development in women with PCOS. Using small cortical ovarian biopsies obtained from women undergoing routine laparoscopy, we performed follicle counts in tissue from normal and polycystic ovaries. We included a group of subjects with PCO but with a history of regular cycles. The density of small preantral follicles was significantly higher in cortex from women with polycystic ovaries and anovulatory cycles (or amenorrhea) than in cortical biopsies from normal ovaries *(26)*. Preantral follicle density in polycystic ovarian tissue obtained from regularly cycling women was intermediate between values in normal and anovulatory PCOS ovaries (Fig. 2a). In this study and in a subsequent report from the laboratory of Dr Gregory Erickson, the principal reason for the increased density of follicles in PCOS was an accumulation at the primary follicle stage (Fig. 2a) *(26,27)*. There were also significant differences between polycystic and normal ovaries in the proportion of primordial (resting) and growing follicles (i.e., primary and beyond) (Fig. 2b) *(26)*. In this case, polycystic ovaries from both ovulatory and anovulatory women showed a similar pattern. The mechanism of abnormal folliculogenesis in polycystic ovaries is not yet known.

Development of preantral follicles is not primarily under endocrine control, but it is not yet clear which of the many candidates among the paracrine and autocrine factors that have been identified in small follicles are the most important for early follicular growth *(28,29)*. There is evidence that AMH, a growth factor in the transforming

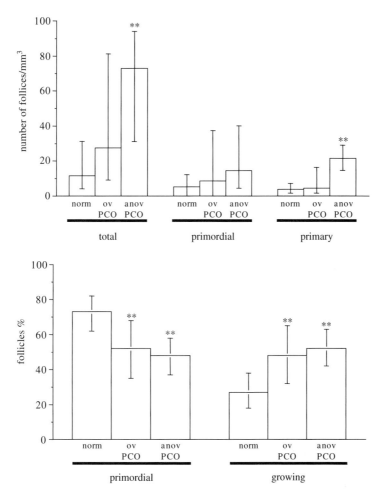

Fig. 2. (**a**) Density of preantral follicles (median and 95% CI) in cortical biopsies from normal or polycystic ovary (PCO). There were significant differences (**) between anovulatory PCO and normal in total preantral follicle density ($p = 0.009$) and primary follicle density ($p = 0.006$). (**b**) Proportion of primordial and growing follicles (mean and 95% CI) in normal and PCO ovaries. There was an increased proportion of growing follicles compared with normal in both ovulatory PCO ($p = 0.03$) and anovulatory PCO ($p = 0.001$). Adapted from (26).

growth factor beta (TGF-β) superfamily, plays an important role in *inhibiting* the initiation of follicle growth. AMH null mice show enhanced recruitment of growing follicles, and addition of AMH to mouse ovary cultures inhibits entry of follicles into the growing phase (30,31). In collaboration with Axel Themmen and co-workers in Rotterdam, we have recently demonstrated that AMH protein expression is significantly lower in primordial and transitional follicles in polycystic ovaries from anovulatory women than in normal ovaries (32). This suggests that AMH deficiency contributes to abnormal preantral follicle development in PCOS. Although this finding certainly does not preclude the involvement of other factors involved in initiation and maintenance of early follicle growth, it does illustrate that abnormalities of folliculogenesis in polycystic ovaries have their origin in the very earliest, gonadotropin-independent stages development and suggests a primary ovarian cause of PCOS.

REFERENCES

1. Hull, M.G. (1987) Epidemiology of infertility and polycystic ovarian disease: endocrinological and demographic studies. *Gynecol Endocrinol*, **1**, 235–45.

2. Kousta, E., White, D.M., Cela, E., McCarthy, M.I. and Franks, S. (1999) The prevalence of polycystic ovaries in women with infertility. *Hum Reprod*, **14**, 2720–3.

3. Franks, S., Mason, H.D., Polson, D.W., Winston, R.M., Margara, R. and Reed, M.J. (1988) Mechanism and management of ovulatory failure in women with polycystic ovary syndrome. *Hum Reprod*, **3**, 531–4.

4. Kousta, E., White, D.M. and Franks, S. (1997) Modern use of clomiphene citrate in induction of ovulation. *Hum Reprod Update*, **3**, 359–65.

5. White, D.M., Polson, D.W., Kiddy, D., Sagle, P., Watson, H., Gilling-Smith, C., Hamilton-Fairley, D. and Franks, S. (1996) Induction of ovulation with low-dose gonadotropins in polycystic ovary syndrome: an analysis of 109 pregnancies in 225 women. *J Clin Endocrinol Metab*, **81**, 3821–4.

6. Franks, S., Mason, H. and Willis, D. (2000) Follicular dynamics in the polycystic ovary syndrome. *Mol Cell Endocrinol*, **163**, 49–52.

7. Erickson, G.F., Magoffin, D.A., Garzo, V.G., Cheung, A.P. and Chang, R.J. (1992) Granulosa cells of polycystic ovaries: are they normal or abnormal? *Hum Reprod*, **7**, 293–9.

8. Mason, H.D., Willis, D.S., Beard, R.W., Winston, R.M., Margara, R. and Franks, S. (1994) Estradiol production by granulosa cells of normal and polycystic ovaries: relationship to menstrual cycle history and concentrations of gonadotropins and sex steroids in follicular fluid. *J Clin Endocrinol Metab*, **79**, 1355–60.

9. Willis, D.S., Watson, H., Mason, H.D., Galea, R., Brincat, M. and Franks, S. (1998) Premature response to luteinizing hormone of granulosa cells from anovulatory women with polycystic ovary syndrome: relevance to mechanism of anovulation. *J Clin Endocrinol Metab*, **83**, 3984–91.

10. Gilling-Smith, C., Willis, D.S., Beard, R.W. and Franks, S. (1994) Hypersecretion of androstenedione by isolated thecal cells from polycystic ovaries. *J Clin Endocrinol Metab*, **79**, 1158–65.

11. Nelson, V.L., Legro, R.S., Strauss, J.F., 3rd and McAllister, J.M. (1999) Augmented androgen production is a stable steroidogenic phenotype of propagated theca cells from polycystic ovaries. *Mol Endocrinol*, **13**, 946–57.

12. Hillier, S.G. (1996) Roles of follicle stimulating hormone and luteinizing hormone in controlled ovarian hyperstimulation. *Hum Reprod*, **11**(Suppl 3), 113–21.

13. Conway, G.S., Honour, J.W. and Jacobs, H.S. (1989) Heterogeneity of the polycystic ovary syndrome: clinical, endocrine and ultrasound features in 556 patients. *Clin Endocrinol (Oxf)*, **30**, 459–70.

14. Franks, S. (1989) Polycystic ovary syndrome: a changing perspective. *Clin Endocrinol (Oxf)*, **31**, 87–120.

15. Willis, D., Mason, H., Gilling-Smith, C. and Franks, S. (1996) Modulation by insulin of follicle-stimulating hormone and luteinizing hormone actions in human granulosa cells of normal and polycystic ovaries. *J Clin Endocrinol Metab*, **81**, 302–9.

16. Franks, S., Robinson, S. and Willis, D.S. (1996) Nutrition, insulin and polycystic ovary syndrome. *Rev Reprod*, **1**, 47–53.

17. Hattori, M. and Horiuchi, R. (1992) Biphasic effects of exogenous ganglioside GM3 on follicle-stimulating hormone-dependent expression of luteinizing hormone receptor in cultured granulosa cells. *Mol Cell Endocrinol*, **88**, 47–54.

18. Dunaif, A. (1997) Insulin resistance and the polycystic ovary syndrome: mechanism and implications for pathogenesis. *Endocr Rev*, **18**, 774–800.

19. Rice, S., Christoforidis, N., Gadd, C., Nikolaou, D., Seyani, L., Donaldson, A., Margara, R., Hardy, K. and Franks, S. (2005) Impaired insulin-dependent glucose metabolism in granulosa-lutein cells from anovulatory women with polycystic ovaries. *Hum Reprod*, **20**, 373–81.

20. Willis, D. and Franks, S. (1995) Insulin action in human granulosa cells from normal and polycystic ovaries is mediated by the insulin receptor and not the type-I insulin-like growth factor receptor. *J Clin Endocrinol Metab*, **80**, 3788–90.

21. Lin, Y., Fridstrom, M. and Hillensjo, T. (1997) Insulin stimulation of lactate accumulation in isolated human granulosa-luteal cells: a comparison between normal and polycystic ovaries. *Hum Reprod*, **12**, 2469–72.

22. Fedorcsak, P., Storeng, R., Dale, P.O., Tanbo, T. and Abyholm, T. (2000) Impaired insulin action on granulosa-lutein cells in women with polycystic ovary syndrome and insulin resistance. *Gynecol Endocrinol*, **14**, 327–36.

23. Harlow, C.R., Winston, R.M., Margara, R.A. and Hillier, S.G. (1987) Gonadotrophic control of human granulosa cell glycolysis. *Hum Reprod*, **2**, 649–53.

24. Chavez-Ross, A., Franks, S., Mason, H.D., Hardy, K. and Stark, J. (1997) Modelling the control of ovulation and polycystic ovary syndrome. *J Math Biol*, **36**, 95–118.

25. Hughesdon, P.E. (1982 Feb) Morphology and morphogenesis of the Stein-Leventhal ovary and of so-called 'hyperthecosis'. *Obstet Gynecol Surv*, **37**, 59–77.

26. Webber, L.J., Stubbs, S., Stark, J., Trew, G.H., Margara, R., Hardy, K. and Franks, S. (2003) Formation and early development of follicles in the polycystic ovary. *Lancet*, **362**, 1017–21.

27. Maciel, G.A., Baracat, E.C., Benda, J.A., Markham, S.M., Hensinger, K., Chang, R.J. and Erickson, G.F. (2004) Stockpiling of transitional and classic primary follicles in ovaries of women with polycystic ovary syndrome. *J Clin Endocrinol Metab*, **89**, 5321–7.

28. McNatty, K.P., Heath, D.A., Lundy, T., Fidler, A.E., Quirke, L., O'Connell, A., Smith, P., Groome, N. and Tisdall, D.J. (1999) Control of early ovarian follicular development. *J Reprod Fertil Suppl*, **54**, 3–16.

29. Elvin, J.A., Yan, C. and Matzuk, M.M. (2000) Oocyte-expressed TGF-beta superfamily members in female fertility. *Mol Cell Endocrinol*, **159**, 1–5.

30. Durlinger, A.L., Kramer, P., Karels, B., de Jong, F.H., Uilenbroek, J.T., Grootegoed, J.A. and Themmen, A.P. (1999) Control of primordial follicle recruitment by anti-Mullerian hormone in the mouse ovary. *Endocrinology*, **140**, 5789–96.

31. Durlinger, A.L., Gruijters, M.J., Kramer, P., Karels, B., Ingraham, H.A., Nachtigal, M.W., Uilenbroek, J.T., Grootegoed, J.A. and Themmen, A.P. (2002 Mar) Anti-Mullerian hormone inhibits initiation of primordial follicle growth in the mouse ovary. *Endocrinology*, **143**, 1076–84.

32. Stubbs, S.A., Hardy, K., Da Silva-Buttkus, P., Stark, J., Webber, L.J., Flanagan, A.M., Themmen, A.P., Visser, J.A., Groome, N.P. and Franks, S. (2005) Anti-mullerian hormone protein expression is reduced during the initial stages of follicle development in human polycystic ovaries. *J Clin Endocrinol Metab*, **90**, 5536–43.

2 Accounting for the Follicle Population in the Polycystic Ovary

Daniel A. Dumesic, MD,
and David H. Abbott, PhD

CONTENTS

Summary

Recruitment of primordial follicles through selection of the dominant follicle and its eventual ovulation requires complex interactions between reproductive and metabolic functions, as well as intraovarian paracrine signals to coordinate granulosa cell proliferation, theca cell differentiation, and oocyte maturation. Early follicle development to an initial antral stage is relatively independent of gonadotropins and relies mostly on mesenchymal–epithelial cell interactions, intraovarian paracrine signals, and oocyte-secreted factors. Beyond this stage, cyclic follicle development depends upon circulating gonadotropins in combination with these locally derived regulators. Recruitment, growth, and subsequent selection of the dominant follicle are perturbed in women with polycystic ovaries (PCO). Ovarian hyperandrogenism, hyperinsulinemia from insulin resistance, and altered intrafollicular paracrine signaling contribute to the accumulation of small antral follicles within the periphery of the ovary, giving it a polycystic morphology. Prenatal androgen excess also entrains multiple organ systems in utero and demonstrates that the hormonal environment of intrauterine life may program the morphology of the ovary in adulthood.

Key Words: Polycystic ovaries; androgens; insulin; kit ligand; inhibin; anti-Mullerian hormone; growth differentiation factor-9.

1. INTRODUCTION

Initiation of primordial follicle recruitment, selection of the dominant follicle, and ovulation of a single mature oocyte require a constellation of reproductive, metabolic, and intraovarian events that coordinate granulosa cell proliferation and

From: *Contemporary Endocrinology: Polycystic Ovary Syndrome*
Edited by: A. Dunaif, R. J. Chang, S. Franks, and R. S. Legro © Humana Press, Totowa, NJ

differentiation, theca cell function, and oocyte maturation. Relatively independent of gonadotropins, preantral and early antral follicle development depends mostly on mesenchymal–epithelial cell interactions, intraovarian paracrine signals, and oocyte-secreted factors. Beyond these stages, cyclic follicle development depends upon circulating gonadotropins as well as intraovarian paracrine signals so that a dominant follicle is selected for eventual ovulation, while subordinate follicles undergo atresia.

Any of these mechanisms can be perturbed in women with polycystic ovaries (PCO), leading to the accumulation of small antral follicles within the periphery of the ovary, giving it a polycystic morphology. Ovarian hyperandrogenism, hyperinsulinemia from insulin resistance, and altered intraovarian paracrine signaling can disrupt normal folliculogenesis by enhancing follicle recruitment, impairing follicle growth, or both. In animal models, prenatal androgen excess also entrains multiple organ systems in utero, demonstrating that the hormonal environment of intrauterine life can theoretically program the morphology of the ovary in adulthood. This chapter addresses crucial metabolic, endocrine, and intraovarian mechanisms governing normal follicular development and discusses how abnormalities in the regulation of these processes initiate a cascade of events predisposing to PCO by increased follicle recruitment and/or by impairing follicle growth.

2. NORMAL FOLLICULAR GROWTH

As an essential element of female reproduction, human follicle development is an ordered process, in which primordial follicles are recruited into a cohort of growing follicles, from which one antral follicle is selected to ovulate, while the others undergo atresia. At the beginning of this process, the primordial follicle consists of an oocyte arrested at the diplotene stage of prophase one and surrounded by squamous granulosa cells. When the primordial follicle initiates growth, its oocyte begins to synthesize ribonucleic acid (RNA), and its squamous granulosa cells enlarge into a single layer of mixed squamous and cuboidal granulosa cells (i.e., intermediate follicle) or of cuboidal granulosa cells entirely (i.e., primary follicle) *(1,2)*. With continued granulosa cell proliferation into two or more layers, the secondary follicle is formed. Theca cells are recruited from surrounding stromal stem cells and are organized into distinct theca cell layers around the follicle, establishing mesenchymal–epithelial cell interactions that promote development of the follicle and its oocyte.

Initiation of primordial follicle growth is only minimally follicle-stimulating hormone (FSH) dependent *(2)*. Instead, growth of primordial follicles is influenced primarily by paracrine/endocrine factors as FSH receptor messenger ribonucleic acid (mRNA) expression does not occur in human primordial follicles and is poorly coupled with the adenylate cyclase second messenger system in intermediate and primary follicles *(3,4)*. Granulosa cell-derived paracrine factors can activate resting primordial follicles [e.g., kit ligand (KL), transforming growth factor alpha (TGF-α), and epidermal growth factor (EGF)] or can inhibit them and may originate locally or from neighboring growing follicles responsive to FSH *(2,5)*. In mammals, expression of granulosa cell-derived KL and its receptor c-kit on oocytes and theca cells of growing follicles is particularly important for initiating early folliculogenesis, inducing mesenchymal–epithelial cell signaling, and developing the oocyte *(1,2)*. In rodents, for example, KL initiates primordial follicle development and oocyte growth *(6,7)*. It also acts as a putative "granulosa cell-derived theca cell organizer" (with TGF-α and EGF) to attract stromal cells around the developing preantral follicle and to stimulate their differentiation into theca cells expressing luteinizing hormone (LH) receptors and steroidogenic enzymes necessary for androgen synthesis *(2,8)*. These KL actions, along with those of other local factors, cause secondary follicles to develop over several months; to acquire FSH, estrogen, and androgen receptors; and to become physiologically coupled by gap junctions *(2,9)*.

Recruitment ends with the formation of the antral or tertiary follicle, characterized by slower oocyte growth (reaching a maximum diameter of 140 μm), formation of extracellular fluid, and differentiation of granulosa cell layers into mural and cumulus cell subpopulations *(1,2)*. The human antral follicle that is 2–5 mm in size becomes primarily responsive to FSH. Each month one such follicle normally becomes dominant and eventually ovulates *(2,9)*. In reproductive-aged women, hundreds of primordial follicles initiate growth, 10–20 selectable antral follicles remain at the beginning of the normal cycle, but just one normally proceeds to ovulation *(1)*. The entire process of follicular growth from primordial to preovulatory stage takes approximately 6 months, with the final 2 weeks of follicular development dependent on cyclical changes in circulating gonadotropin levels *(10)*.

3. INCREASED FOLLICLE RECRUITMENT

Several morphological findings implicate increased recruitment of growing follicles from the primordial follicle pool as a contributing factor in the development of the PCO. In one of three studies, histological examination of ovarian tissue with PCO morphology shows an increased proportion of primary follicles and a reciprocally decreased proportion of primordial follicles, independent of ovulatory status or atresia *(11–13)* (Fig. 1).

New sonographic studies add further evidence of abnormal early follicular development causing PCO formation. Originally defined by the presence of ≥10 cysts measuring 2–8 mm in diameter, arranged peripherally around a dense core of stroma, or scattered throughout an increased amount of stroma *(14)*, recent Rotterdam criteria for PCOS (using transvaginal ultrasonography) redefine PCO as the presence of 12 or

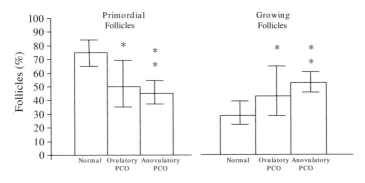

Fig. 1. Mean proportion of follicles at the primordial and growing primary stages in normal and polycystic ovaries. Data presented are means and 95% confidence intervals. *$p < 0.05$, **$p < 0.005$ compared with control values. Reproduced with permission *(12)*.

more follicles in each ovary [i.e., follicle number per ovary (FNPO)] measuring 2–9 mm in diameter and/or increased ovarian volume (>10 mL) *(15)*. Using these PCO criteria, important pathophysiological correlations exist between follicle number and hyperandrogenism as well as insulin resistance. In PCOS patients, an increased cohort size of 2–5 mm follicles positively correlates with serum androgen levels, whereas a normal cohort size of 6–9 mm follicles negatively correlates with fasting serum insulin and testosterone levels, as well as BMI *(16)*. These findings suggest that ovarian hyperandrogenism promotes excessive early follicular growth, which does not progress to the dominant stage because of hyperinsulinemia and/or androgen excess.

3.1. Hyperandrogenism

Androgens promote early follicle growth in primates. Testosterone administration to adult female rhesus monkeys increases the number of primary, growing preantral and small antral follicles and the proliferation of granulosa cells within them by acting through its own receptor *(17,18)* (Fig. 2). Androgen treatment in such monkeys also increases mRNA expression of FSH receptor, insulin-like growth factor I (IGF-I) receptor, and IGF-I in granulosa cells *(19,20)* while enhancing IGF-I and IGF-I receptor mRNA expression in primordial follicle oocytes *(21)*.

The ability of androgens to initiate follicle growth corresponds with observations that follicular fluid androstenedione levels are elevated in ovulatory women with PCO and that androstenedione production by cultured theca cells from women with PCO is increased *(22,23)*. Moreover, in vitro studies of PCOS theca cells show intrinsically increased androgen biosynthesis and augmented expression of several steroidogenic enzymes, including cytochrome P450 cholesterol side chain cleavage, 17α-hydroxylase/17–20 lyase (P450$_{c17}$), and 3β-hydroxysteroid dehydrogenase *(24,25)*. The clinical relevance of these in vitro data is that serum androstenedione levels in normal and PCOS women correlate with antral follicle number *(16,26)* and in normal women predict the number of oocytes retrieved following gonadotropin stimulation for in vitro fertilization (IVF) *(26)*. Conversely, anti-androgen therapy to PCOS patients improves PCO morphology *(27)*.

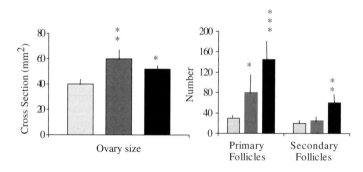

Fig. 2. Number of ovarian follicles in adult female rhesus monkeys treated with subcutaneous testosterone pellets for 3 or 10 days. Data presented are means ± SEM for *n* = 4–6 monkeys in each group. *$p < 0.05$, **$p < 0.005$, ***$p < 0.0005$ compared with control values. White, control; gray, testosterone pellets for 3 days; black, testosterone pellets for 10 days. Reproduced with permission *(17)*.

Androgen effects on early follicle growth also can be induced by reprogramming adult ovarian morphology during prenatal development *(28)*. Female rhesus monkeys *(29)*, sheep *(30)*, mice *(31)*, and rats *(32)* exposed prenatally to excessive levels of testosterone or its non-aromatizable metabolite, dihydrotestosterone (DHT), exhibit ovulatory dysfunction in adulthood. Ovaries are enlarged and polyfollicular in prenatally androgenized monkeys and sheep and also are hyperandrogenic in prenatally androgenized monkeys and mice *(31,33,34)*.

A PCOS-like phenotype can be produced by injecting pregnant rhesus monkeys carrying female fetuses with 10–15 mg testosterone propionate (TP) for 15–35 days starting on either days 40–60 (early treated) or days 100–115 (late treated) postconception (total gestation, 165 days), which elevates circulating testosterone levels in fetal females to those normally found in fetal males *(35,36)*. These prenatal androgen treatments coincide with gonadal differentiation, pancreatic organogenesis, and the beginning of neuroendocrine development in early-treated females and with ovarian follicle development and functional acquisition of hypothalamic sensitivity to hormone negative feedback in late-treated females. Prenatally androgenized females exhibit ovarian dysfunction beginning at puberty *(37–39)* and have a 10-fold increase in the risk of anovulation as adults, with 40% of these females (vs. 14% of controls) having enlarged multifollicular ovaries resembling PCO *(33)*.

Prenatal exposure of sheep to TP from days 30–90 of gestation also induces multifollicular ovarian development *(34)*. The ability of prenatal androgen excess to decrease the relative proportion of primordial follicles, while increasing that of growing follicles (primary, preantral, and antral follicles combined), emphasizes increased follicular recruitment as a cause for the multifollicular phenotype *(40)*. Furthermore, total follicle number is diminished, and growing follicles contain larger oocytes at an early preantral stage *(40)*, suggesting that prenatal androgen exposure enhances intraovarian paracrine signaling during early follicular development. In this regard, testosterone plus FSH upregulate KL mRNA expression in cultured murine granulosa cells *(41)*, whereas androgens augment the mitogenic effects of oocyte-secreted factors, including growth differentiation factor-9 (GDF-9) on IGF-I-stimulated porcine granulosa cells *(42)*.

3.2. Hyperinsulinemia

Insulin acts primarily on its own receptors to induce tyrosine phosphorylation of insulin–receptor substrates that initiate glucose uptake, protein synthesis, and steroidogenesis *(43,44)*. As insulin receptors are located on theca cells, surrounding stroma, granulosa cells, and oocytes *(45,46)*, insulin acting alone or as a co-gonadotropin stimulates theca cell androgen production *(47,48)* and amplifies LH-stimulated granulosa cell E_2 and P4 production *(49)*.

Insulin sensitivity in PCOS patients, however, is intrinsically impaired from abnormal postreceptor signal transduction. Increased serine, rather than tyrosine, phosphorylation of insulin–receptor substrates in some PCOS patients reduces insulin-mediated glucose uptake *(50)* without affecting steroidogenesis *(44,51)*. Consequently, PCOS patients have insulin resistance that is independent of and additive to that of obesity, with combined PCOS and obesity synergistically impairing glucose–insulin homeostasis and contributing to frequent hyperandrogenic symptoms in obese PCOS patients *(49)*. The resulting hyperinsulinemia promotes ovarian hyperandrogenism by stimulating theca cell 17α-hydroxylase activity *(52)*, amplifying LH- and IGF-I-stimulated androgen production *(47)*, elevating serum-free T levels through decreased hepatic sex hormone-binding globulin (SHBG) production, and enhancing serum IGF-I bioactivity through suppressed IGF-binding protein production *(44)*.

Acting directly or indirectly through androgens, insulin promotes follicle recruitment in rat organ culture *(53)*. Hyperinsulinemia from insulin resistance in PCOS patients is positively associated with the degree of multifollicular ovarian development, with hyperinsulinemic PCOS patients undergoing gonadotropin therapy developing a larger number of follicles between 12 and 16 mm in diameter and having a greater risk of ovarian hyperstimulation syndrome than normoinsulinemic women *(54,55)*. Moreover, the insulin response to oral glucose tolerance testing in women undergoing gonadotropin therapy is positively correlated with ovarian volume *(56)*. While still investigational, the insulin sensitizer metformin has been administered to PCOS patients receiving gonadotropin therapy for IVF to determine whether it improves hyperinsulinemia and ovarian hyperandrogenism and if so whether it lowers the risks of exaggerated multifollicular recruitment and ovarian hyperstimulation syndrome. In one of two prospective, randomized, double-blind studies, pretreatment of PCOS patients with metformin preceding GnRH analog/rhFSH therapy for IVF did not affect ovarian responsiveness to FSH therapy nor pregnancy outcome *(57)*. In the other, metformin therapy to PCOS women lowered serum fasting insulin, total and free T as well as E$_2$ levels at oocyte retrieval, enhanced clinical pregnancy and livebirth rates, and diminished the risk of severe ovarian hyperstimulation syndrome *(58)*.

3.3. Anti-Mullerian Hormone Deficiency

The TGF-β superfamily consists of several functionally diverse proteins, including TGF-β, anti-Mullerian hormone (AMH), inhibins, activins, bone morphogenic proteins (BMPs), and GDFs. As one of its members, AMH is normally produced by granulosa cells of growing follicles *(59,60)* so that low AMH levels occur in primordial and primary follicles, increase to maximal levels in large preantral and small antral stages, and then decline during final follicular maturation *(60–63)*. As a serum marker of growing follicles, serum AMH levels in normal women positively correlate with number of antral follicles, serum androgen concentrations, and oocytes retrieved and negatively correlate with amount of rhFSH administered *(62,64)*. Serum AMH levels are elevated in normoandrogenic women with PCO and are further increased in hyperandrogenic women with PCO, independent of antral follicle number *(63)*. Serum AMH levels in PCOS patients are elevated two to threefold, are positively correlated with antral follicle number and serum androgen levels, and are reduced in parallel with antral follicle number by metformin therapy *(64)*.

In vitro rodent studies show that AMH inhibits primordial follicle growth *(65)*. Its deficiency increases the proportion of growing follicles arising from the primordial follicle pool *(66)*, suggesting that AMH produced by growing follicles normally inhibits growth of adjacent primordial follicles *(60,67)*. Although such a phenomenon in humans remains uncertain, histological examination of human ovaries shows reduced AMH levels in primordial and transitional follicles of anovulatory women with PCO versus regularly

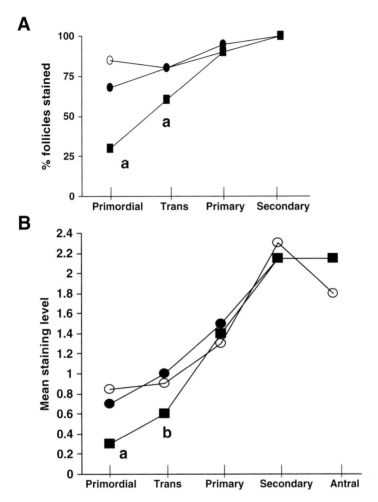

Fig. 3. (**A**) Percent of follicles staining positive for anti-mullerian hormone (AMH) and (**B**) mean intensity of AMH staining based on follicle stage and ovary type. a, $p < 0.005$; b, <0.05 versus normal ovaries and ovulatory polycystic ovaries (pco). o, normal; ● ovucatory pco; ■, anovulatory pco. Copyright 2005, The Endocrine Society.

cycling women (with or without PCO), implicating relative AMH deficiency with increased primordial follicle growth under some conditions *(60)* (Fig. 3).

4. FOLLICULAR ARREST

In follicles of 6–8 mm in size, granulosa cells begin to express cytochrome P450 aromatase *(68)*, allowing androgens produced by LH-stimulated theca cells to undergo aromatization to estrogens by FSH-stimulated granulosa cells. This steroidogenic mechanism exists because $P450_{c17}$, a rate-limiting step in androgen synthesis, occurs in theca cells but not granulosa cells while aromatase and FSH receptors are expressed in granulosa cells. During follicle development, LH-stimulated thecal cell androstenedione production through $P450_{c17}$ activity is enhanced by granulosa cell-derived paracrine factors *(69)*, with inhibins and IGF-I-stimulating thecal cell androgen production, and follistatin binding activin and inhibiting its androgen-suppressing effect *(8)*. Within the preovulatory follicle, granulosa cells acquire LH receptors *(70)* and shift steroidogenesis from androgen and estrogen to progesterone production after the LH surge during final oocyte maturation *(71)*.

4.1. Elevated 5a-Reduced Androgens

Follicular arrest in PCOS occurs at the stage when granulosa cells normally begin to express aromatase and secrete E_2 *(10,68)*. An endogenous inhibitor of estrogen synthesis may exist, as small PCOS follicles are estrogen deplete despite having sufficient bioactive FSH and aromatizable androgens, whereas granulosa cells from such follicles have an exaggerated E_2 responsiveness to FSH in vitro *(23,72)*.

Small PCOS follicles also have elevated 5α-reductase activity, which increases 5α-reduced androgen levels to concentrations capable of inhibiting granulosa cell aromatase activity in vitro *(73,74)* (Fig. 4). Increased 5α-reductase and decreased aromatase activities also occur in E_2-deficient follicles of early prenatally androgenized female rhesus monkeys receiving rhFSH therapy *(75)*, agreeing with the ability of DHT to impair gonadotropin-stimulated E2 secretion in a separate study of normal female rhesus monkeys *(76)* and to inhibit proliferation of cultured rat granulosa cells *(77)*.

4.2. Premature Follicle Luteinization

Hyperinsulinemia from adiposity-related insulin resistance plays a key role in the follicular arrest of PCOS *(49)*. Anovulatory PCOS patients have a greater BMI than their ovulatory sisters despite both siblings having ovarian hyperandrogenism *(78)*, whereas weight loss in obese PCOS patients induces ovulation and reverses anovulatory infertility *(79,80)*. In addition, the number of 6–9 mm follicles visible by sonography in ovaries of PCOS patients is negatively correlated with fasting serum insulin levels and BMI, with fewer such follicles observed in obese compared to lean individuals

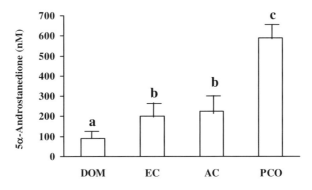

Fig. 4. 5α-Androstane-3,17-dione concentrations in normal and polycystic ovary syndrome (PCOS) follicles. DOM, dominant follicles from regularly cycling women ($n = 15$); EC, estrogenic cohort follicles, 6- to 8-mm cohort follicles from regularly cycling women with an $A4/E_2$ ratio ≤ 4 ($n = 4$); AC, androgenic cohort follicles, 5- to 8-mm cohort follicles from regularly cycling women with an $A4/E_2$ ratio > 4 ($n = 10$); PCO, 4- to 7-mm follicles from PCOS patients ($n = 26$). Data presented are means ± SEM. Bars with different letters are significantly different ($p < 0.01$). Reproduced with permission *(74)*. Copyright 1996, The Endocrine Society.

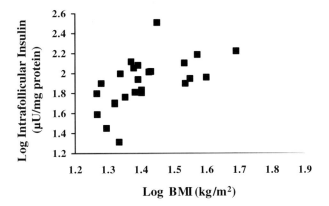

Fig. 5. Correlation between body mass index (BMI) and intrafollicular insulin levels in women undergoing GnRHanalog/rhFSH therapy for in vitro fertilization (IVF). Data modified from *(46)*.

(16). Furthermore, the amount of insulin present in the human follicle is positively correlated with BMI and fasting serum insulin levels and is highest in those women with impaired glucose tolerance *(46)* (Fig. 5).

Normally, insulin enhances FSH-induced upregulation of LH receptors in granulosa cells during differentiation and increases their ability to produce P4 in response to LH *(43,81,82)*. Hyperinsulinemia is associated with premature follicle luteinization, which arrests cell proliferation and subsequent follicle growth. Evidence for premature follicle luteinization in PCOS is found in the premature response of cultured granulosa cells from small PCOS follicles to LH: they exhibit P4 hypersecretion and overexpress LH receptors *(83,84)*, causing an exaggerated steroidogenic shift from E_2 to progesterone production in small PCOS follicles *(85)*. Similarly, premature follicle differentiation occurs in early prenatally androgenized female rhesus monkeys undergoing rhFSH stimulation followed by hCG administration, in which LH hypersecretion and relative insulin excess from increased abdominal adiposity is associated with an exaggerated shift in intrafollicular steroidogenesis from androgen and E_2 to progesterone *(86)*.

4.3. Inhibins, Activins, and Follistatin

Granulosa cell-derived inhibins and activins are dimeric glycoproteins belonging to the TGF-β superfamily. Inhibins consist of an α-subunit covalently joined by disulfide links to either a βA-subunit (inhibin A) or a βB-subunit (inhibin B) and suppress FSH synthesis. Dimerization of β-subunits produces three forms of activin [activin A (βA-βA), activin AB (βA-βB). and activin B (βB-βB)] that enhance FSH secretion *(87)*. Follistatin, a glycoprotein structurally unrelated to the TGF-β superfamily, binds activin with high affinity to inhibit its action *(87)*. In vitro studies show that activin promotes follicle development by stimulating granulosa cell proliferation while delaying luteinization, by increasing granulosa cell FSH receptor expression and E_2 synthesis and by decreasing androgen production *(87)*.

Inhibin A is detectable in follicles as small as 6.5 mm and increases in parallel with α- and βA-subunit mRNA expression as the antral follicle grows *(88,89,90)*. The ability of inhibin A to increase LH-stimulated aromatizable androgenic substrate for E_2 synthesis *(91)* indicates its important role in promoting follicular development.

In contrast, intrafollicular inhibin B levels do not necessarily increase nor does its βB-subunit mRNA expression vary, by follicle size, indicating that inhibin B regulation is independent of follicular development *(88,90)*. Therefore, activins produced by small follicles appear to promote follicular development by enhancing granulosa cell responsiveness to FSH and by suppressing androgen synthesis, whereas inhibins produced by the dominant follicle stimulate theca cell androgen production for E_2 synthesis *(69,87,88,90)*.

Inhibin α- and βA-subunit mRNA levels are reduced in PCOS granulosa cells *(89)*. Inhibin A and B concentrations also are decreased in some, but not all, small PCOS follicles despite normal amounts of activin and follistatin unbound to activin *(90,92)*. Although exogenous FSH stimulates growth of PCOS follicles, intrafollicular inhibin A levels in PCOS patients receiving GnRH analog/gonadotropin therapy for IVF remain reduced *(93)*. Moreover, exogenous hCG and endogenous insulin suppress serum inhibin B in PCOS patients *(94)*, linking defective inhibin biosynthesis with follicular arrest. High follistatin and low activin A levels also have been reported in the circulation of some PCOS patients, which may further contribute to follicle arrest *(95,96)*.

5. IMPAIRED FOLLICULAR GROWTH

Two histological studies of ovaries from PCOS patients show an increase in the number of primary, secondary, and antral follicles that cannot be completely explained by increased recruitment or decreased atresia *(11,13)*. Another explanation for these findings is impaired follicular growth. Follicle growth is influenced by the oocyte-secreted factor GDF-9, which in mice regulates KL and promotes granulosa cell proliferation and preantral growth *(97,98,99)*. Deficiency of GDF-9 in mice impairs granulosa cell proliferation and causes follicular arrest at the primary follicle stage *(100,101)*. In humans, GDF-9 expression normally begins in oocytes at the primordial-primary follicle transition and increases with preantral follicle growth *(102,103)*. GDF-9 also induces growth and development of human ovarian follicles in vitro *(104)*. The further observation that GDF-9 mRNA is reduced in PCOS oocytes from initiation of primordial follicle growth through the small antral follicle stage of development suggests that impaired oocyte signaling decreases granulosa cell proliferation and follicle growth, promoting accumulation of follicles with a PCO appearance *(13,103)*. Such a hypothesis agrees with sonographic evidence in prenatally androgenized sheep of persistent follicular cysts, suggesting that abnormal folliculogenesis during fetal development predisposes to the development of PCO in adulthood *(105)*.

ACKNOWLEDGMENTS

The authors thank Rebekah R. Herrmann for preparation of the figures and Richard Tasca for review of the manuscript. This work was supported in part by the National Institutes of Health Grants U01 HD044650-01 and R01 RR 013635, Mayo Clinical Research Grant 2123-01, Mayo Grant M01-RR-00585, Grant P51 RR 000167 to the National Primate Research Center, University of Wisconsin, Madison (a facility constructed with support from Research Facilities Improvement Program grant numbers RR15459-01 and RR020141-01), and Serono Pharmaceuticals. This work was partially supported by NIH as part of the NICHD National Cooperative Program on Female Health and Egg Quality under cooperative agreement U01 HD044650.

REFERENCES

1. Faddy MJ, Gosden RG. Modelling the dynamics of ovarian follicle utilization throughout life. In: Trounson AO, Gosden RG, eds. *Biology and Pathology of the Oocyte. Role in Fertility and Reproductive Medicine*. Cambridge: Cambridge University Press, 2003:44–52.

2. Gougeon A. The early stages of folliclar growth. In: Trounson AO, Gosden RG, eds. *Biology and Pathology of the Oocyte. Role in Fertility and Reproductive Medicine*. Cambridge: Cambridge University Press, 2003:29–43.

3. Oktay K, Briggs D, Gosden RG. Ontogeny of follicle-stimulating hormone receptor gene expression in isolated human ovarian follicles. *J Clin Endocrinol Metab* 1997;82:3748–3751.

4. Wandji SA, Fortier MA, Sirard MA. Differential response to gonadotropins and prostaglandins E_2 in ovarian tissue during prenatal and postnatal development in cattle. *Biol Reprod* 1992;46:1034–1341.

5. Horie K, Fujita J, Takakura K, Kanzaki H, Suginami H, Iwai M, Nakayama H, Mori T. The expression of c-kit protein in human adult and fetal tissues. *Hum Reprod* 1993;8:1955–1962.

6. Parrott JA, Skinner MK. Kit-ligand/stem cell factor induces primordial follicle development and initiates folliculogenesis. *Endocrinology* 1999;140:4262–4271.

7. Driancourt MA, Reynaud K, Cortvrindt R, Smitz J. Roles of KIT and KIT LIGAND in ovarian function. *Rev Reprod* 2000;5:143–152.

8. Zachow RJ, Magoffin DA. Ovarian androgen biosynthesis: paracrine/autocrine regulation. In: Azziz R, Nestler JE, and Dewailly D, eds. *Androgen Excess Disorders in Women*. Philadelphia, PA: Lippincott-Raven, 1997:13–22.

9. Adashi EY. The ovarian follicular apparatus. In: Adashi EY, Rock JA, Rosenwaks Z, eds. *Reproductive Endocrinology, Surgery, and Technology*. Philadelphia, PA: Lippincott-Raven, 1996:18–40.

10. Gougeon A. Regulation of ovarian follicular development in primates: facts and hypothesis. *Endocr Rev* 1996;17:121–155.

11. Hughesdon PE. Morphology and morphogenesis of the Stein-Leventhal ovary and of so-called "hyperthecosis." *Obstet Gynecol Surv* 1982;37:59–77.

12. Webber LJ, Stubbs S, Stark J, Trew GH, Margara R, Hardy K, Franks S. Formation and early development of follicles in the polycystic ovary. *Lancet* 2003;362:1017–1021.

13. Maciel GA, Baracat EC, Benda JA, Markham SM, Hensinger K, Chang RJ, Erickson GF. Stockpiling of transitional and classic prima0ry follicles in ovaries of women with polycystic ovary syndrome. *J Clin Endocrinol Metab* 2004;89:5321–5327.

14. Adams J, Polson DW, Franks, S. Prevalence of polycystic ovaries in women with anovulation and idiopathic hirsutism. *Br Med J* 1986;293:355–359.

15. The Rotterdam ESHRE/ASRM-sponsored PCOS consensus workshop group. Revised 2003 consensus on diagnostic criteria and long-term health risks related to polycystic ovary syndrome (PCOS). *Hum Reprod* 2004;19:41–47.

16. Jonard S, Robert Y, Cortet-Rudelli C, Pigny P, Decanter C, Dewailly D. Ultrasound examination of polycystic ovaries: is it worth counting the follicles? *Hum Reprod* 2003;18:598–603.

17. Vendola KA, Zhou J, Adesanya OO, Weil SJ, Bondy CA. Androgens stimulate early stages of follicle growth in the primate ovarian. *J Clin Invest* 1998;101:2622–2629.

18. Weil SJ, Vendola K, Zhou J, Adesanya OO, Wang J, Okafor J, Bondy CA. Androgen receptor gene expression in the primate ovary: cellular localization, regulation, and functional correlations. *J Clin Endocrinol Metab* 1998;83:2479–2485..

19. Weil S, Vendola K, Zhou J, Bondy CA. Androgen and follicle-stimulating hormone interactions in primate ovarian follicle development. *J Clin Endocrinol Metab* 1999;84:2951–2956.

20. Vendola K, Zhou J, Wang J, Bondy CA. Androgens promote insulin-like growth factor-I and insulin-like growth factor-I receptor gene expression in the primate ovary. *Hum Reprod* 1999;14:2328–2332.

21. Vendola K, Zhou J, Wang J, Famuyiwa OA, Bievre M, Bondy CA. Androgens promote oocyte insulin-like growth factor I expression and initiation of follicle development in the primate ovary. *Biol Reprod* 1999;61:353–357.

22. Gilling-Smith C, Willis DS, Beard RW, Franks S. Hypersecretion of androstenedione by isolated theca cells from polycystic ovaries. *J Clin Endocrinol Metab* 1994;79: 1158–1165.

23. Mason HD, Willis DS, Beard RW, Winston RM, Margara R, Franks S. Estradiol production by granulosa cells of normal and polycystic ovaries: relationship to menstrual cycle history and concentrations of gonadotropins and sex steroids in follicular fluid. *J Clin Endocrinol Metab* 1994;79: 1355–1360.

24. Nelson VL, Legro RS, Strauss JF III, McAllister JM. Augmented androgen production is a stable steroidogenic phenotype of propagated theca cells from polycysitc ovaries. *Mol Endocrinol* 1999;13:946–957.

25. Nelson VL, Qin K, Rosenfield RL, Wood JR, Penning TM, Legro RS, Strauss JF III, McAllister JM. The biochemical basis for increased testosterone production in theca cells propagated from patients with polycystic ovary syndrome. *J Clin Endocrinol Metab* 2001;86:5925–5933.

26. Dumesic DA, Damario MA, Session DR, Famuyide A, Lesnick TG, Thornhill AR, McNeilly AS. Ovarian Morphology and Serum Hormone Markers as Predictors of Ovarian Follicle Recruitment by Gonadotropins for In Vitro Fertilization. *J Clin Endocrinol Metab* 2001;86:2538–2543.

27. De Leo V, Lanzetta D, D'Antona D, la Marca A, Morgante G. Hormonal effects of flutamide in young women with polycystic ovary syndrome. *J Clin Endocrinol Metab* 1998;83:99–102.

28. Abbott DH, Barnett DK, Bruns CM, Dumesic DA. Androgen excess fetal programming of female reproduction: a developmental aetiology for polycystic ovary syndrome? *Hum Reprod Update* 2005;11:357–374.

29. Abbott DH, Dumesic DA, Eisner JR, Colman RJ, Kemnitz JW. Insights into the development of polycystic ovary syndrome (PCOS) from studies of prenatally androgenized female rhesus monkeys. *Trends Endocrinol Metab* 1998;9:62–67.

30. Birch RA, Padmanabhan V, Foster DL, Unsworth WP, Robinson JE. Prenatal programming of reproductive neuroendocrine function: fetal androgen exposure produces progressive disruption of reproductive cycles in sheep. *Endocrinology* 2003;144:1426–1434.

31. Sullivan SD and Moenter SM. Prenatal androgens alter GABAergic drive to gonadotropin-releasing hormone neurons: implications for a common fertility disorder. *Proc Natl Acad Sci USA* 2004;101: 7129–7134.

32. Foecking EM, Szabo M, Schwartz NB, Levine JF. Neuroendocrine consequences of prenatal androgen exposure in the female rat: absence of luteinizing hormone surges, suppression of progesterone receptor gene expression, and acceleration of the gonadotropin-releasing hormone pulse generator. *Biol Reprod* 2005;72:1475–1483.

33. Abbott DH, Dumesic DA, Eisner JR, Kemnitz JW, Goy RW. The prenatally androgenized female rhesus monkey as a model for PCOS. In: Azziz R, Nestler JE, Dewailly D, eds. *Androgen Excess Disorders in Women*. Philadelphia, PA: Lippincott-Raven, 1997:369–382.

34. West C, Foster DL, Evans NP, Robinson J, Padmanabhan V. Intra-follicular activin availability is altered in prenatally-androgenized lambs. *Mol Cell Endocrinol* 2001;185:51–59.

35. Resko JA, Ellinwood WE. Sexual differentiation of the brain of primates. In: Serio M, Motta M, Zanisi M, Martini L, eds. *Sexual Differentiation: Basic and Clinical Aspects*. New York: Raven Press, 1984:169–181.

36. Resko JA, Buhl AE, Phoenix CH. Treatment of pregnant rhesus macaques with testosterone propionate: observations on its fate in the fetus. *Biol Reprod* 1987;37:1185–1191.

37. Goy RW, Robinson JA. Prenatal exposure of rhesus monkeys to patent androgens: morphological, behavioral, and physiological consequences. *Banbury Report* 1982;11:355–378.

38. Goy RW, Kemnitz JW. Early, persistent and delayed effects of virilizing substances delivered transplacentally to female rhesus monkeys. In: Zbinden G, Cuomo V, Racagni G, Weiss B, eds. *Applications of Behavioral Pharmacology in Toxicology*. New York: Raven Press, 1983: 303–314.

39. Goy RW, Uno H, Sholl SA. Psychological and anatomical consequences of prenatal exposure to androgens in female rhesus. In: Mori T, Nagasawa H, eds. *Toxicity of Hormones in Perinatal Life*. Boca Raton, FL: CRC Press, 1988:127–142.

40. Steckler T, Wang J, Bartol FF, Roy SK, Padmanabhan V. Fetal programming: prenatal testosterone treatment causes intrauterine growth retardation, reduces ovarian reserve and increases ovarian follicular recruitment. *Endocrinology* 2005;146:3185–3193.

41. Joyce IM, Pendola FL, Wigglesworth K, Eppig JJ. Oocyte regulation of kit ligand expression in mouse ovarian follicles. *Dev Biol* 1999;214:342–353.

42. Hickey TE, Marrocco DL, Amato F, Ritter LJ, Norman RJ, Gilchrist RB, Armstrong DT. Androgens augment the mitogenic effects of oocyte-secreted factors and growth differentiation factor 9 on porcine granulosa cells. *Biol Reprod* 2005;73:825–832.

43. Willis D, Franks S. Insulin action in human granulosa cells from normal and polycystic ovaries is mediated by the insulin receptor and not the type-1 insulin-like growth factor receptor. *J Clin Endocrinol Metab* 1995;80:3788–3790.

44. Balen AH, Conway GS, Homburg R, Legro RS. *Polycystic Ovary Syndrome. A Guide to Clinical Management*. London: Taylor and Francis; 2005:47–67.

45. Samoto T, Maruo T, Ladines-llave C, Matsuo H, Deguchi J, Barnea E, Mochizuki M. Insulin receptor expression in the follicular and stroma compartments of the human ovary over the course of follicular growth, regression, and atresia. *Endocr J* 1993;40:715–726.

46. Phy JL, Conover CA, Abbott DH, Zschunke MA, Walker DL, Session DR, Tummon IS, Thornhill AR, Lesnick TG, Dumesic DA. Insulin and messenger ribonucleic acid expression of insulin receptor isoforms in ovarian follicles from nonhirsute ovulatory women and polycystic ovary syndrome patients. *J Clin Endocrinol Metab* 2004;89:3561–3566.

47. Bergh C, Carlsson B, Olsson JH, Selleskog H, Hillensjo T. Regulation of androgen production in cultured human theca cells by insulin-like growth factor-I and insulin. *Fertil Steril* 1993;59: 323–331.

48. McGee EA, Sawetawan C, Bird I, Rainey WE, Carr BR. The effect of insulin and insulin-like growth factors on the expression of steroidogenic enzymes in a human ovarian thecal-like tumor cell model. *Fertil Steril* 1996;65:87–93.

49. Franks S, Gilling-Smith C, Watson H, Willis D. Insulin action in the normal and polycystic ovary. *Endocrinol Metab Clin North Am* 1999;28:361–378.

50. Dunaif A. Insulin resistance and the polycystic ovarian syndrome: mechanism and implications for pathogenesis. *Endo Rev* 1997;18:774–800.

51. Baillargeon JP, Nestler JE. Commentary: polycystic ovary syndrome: a syndrome of ovarian hypersensitivity to insulin? *J Clin Endocrinol Metab* 2006;91:22–24.

52. Moghetti P, Castello R, Negri C, Tosi F, Perrone F, Caputo M, Zanolin E, Muggeo M. Metformin effects on clinical features, endocrine and metabolic profiles, and insulin sensitivity in polycystic ovary syndrome: a randomized, double-blind, placebo-controlled 6-month trial, followed by open, long-term clinical evaluation. *J Clin Endocrinol Metab* 2000;85:139–146.

53. Kezele PR, Nilsson EE, Skinner MK. Insulin but not insulin-like growth factor-I promotes the primordial to primary follicle transition. *Mol Cell Endocrinol* 2002;192:37–43.

54. Fulghesu AM, Villa P, Pavone V, Guido M, Apa R, Caruso A, Lanzone A, Rossodivita A, Mancuso S. The impact of insulin secretion on the ovarian response to exogenous gonadotropins in polycystic ovary syndrome. *J Clin Endocrinol Metab* 1997;82:644–648.

55. Navot D, Bergh P, Laufer N. The ovarian hyperstimulation syndrome. In: Adashi E, Rock J, Rosenwaks Z, eds. *Reproductive Endocrinology, Surgery, and Technology.* Philadelphia, PA: Lippincott-Raven, 1996: 2216–2232.

56. Filicori M, Flamigni C, Cognigni G, Dellai P, Michelacci L, Arnone R. Increased insulin secretion in patients with multifollicular and polycystic ovaries and its impact on ovulation induction. *Fertil Steril* 1994;62:279–285.

57. Kjotrod SB, During VV, Carlsen, SM. Metformin treatment before IVF/ICSI in women with polycystic ovary syndrome; a prospective, randomized, double blind study. *Hum Reprod* 2004;19:1315–1322.

58. Tang T, Glanville J, Orsi N, Barth JH, Balen AH. The use of metformin for women with PCOS undergoing IVF treatment. *Hum Reprod* 2006;21:1416–1425.

59. Knight PG, Glister C. Local roles of TGF-β superfamily members in the control of ovarian follicle development. *Anim Reprod Sci* 2003;78:165–183.

60. Stubbs SA, Hardy K, Da Silva-Buttkus P, Stark J, Webber LJ, Flanagan AM, Themmen APN, Visser JA, Groome NP, Franks S. Anti-Mullerian hormone protein expression is reduced during the initial stages of follicle development in human polycystic ovaries. *J Clin Endocrinol Metab* 2005;90: 5536–5543.

61. Weenen C, Laven JS, Von Bergh AR, Cranfield M, Groome NP, Visser JA, Kramer P, Fauser BC, Themmen AP. Anti-Mullerian hormone expression pattern in the human ovary: potential implications for initial and cyclic follicle recruitment. *Mol Hum Reprod* 2004;10:77–83.

62. Fanchin R, Louafi N, Lozano DHM, Frydman N, Frydman R, Taieb J. Per-follicle measurements indicate that anti-Mullerian hormone secretion is modulated by the extent of follicular development and luteinization and may reflect qualitatively the ovarian follicular status. *Fertil Steril* 2005;84:167–173.

63. Eldar-Geva T, Margalioth EJ, Gal M, Ben-Chetrit A, Algur N, Zylber-Haran E, Brooks B, Huerta M, Spitz IM. Serum anti-Mullerian hormone levels during controlled ovarian hyperstimulation in women with polycystic ovaries with and without hyperandrogenism. *Hum Reprod* 2005;20:1814–1819.

64. Piltonen T, Morin-Papunen L, Koivunen R, Perheentupa A, Ruokonen A, Tapanainen JS. Serum anti-Mullerian hormone levels remain high until late reproductive age and decrease during metformin therapy in women with polycystic ovary syndrome. *Hum Reprod* 2005;20:1820–1826.

65. Durlinger ALL, Gruijters MJ, Kramer P, Karels B, Ingraham HA, Nachtigal MW, Uilenbroek JT, Grootegoed JA, Themmen AP. Anti-Mullerian hormone inhibits initiation of primordial follicle growth in the mouse ovary. *Endocrinology* 2002;143:1076–1084.

66. Durlinger AL, Kramer P, Karels B, de Jong FH, Uilenbroek JTJ, Grootegoed JA, Themmen APN. Control of primordial follicle recruitment by anti-Mullerian hormone in the mouse ovary. *Endocrinology* 1999;140:5789–5798.

67. Fortune JE. The early stages of follicular development: activation of primordial follicles and growth of preantral follicles. *Anim Reprod Sci* 2003;78:135–163.

68. Jakimiuk AJ, Weitsman SR, Brzechffa PR, Magoffin DA. Aromatase mRNA expression in individual follicles from polycystic ovaries. *Mol Hum Reprod* 1998;4:1–8.

69. Hillier SG, Whitelaw PF, Smyth CD. Follicular oestrogen synthesis: the 'two-cell, two-gonadotropin' model revisited. *Mol Cell Endocrinol* 1994;100:51–54.

70. Shima K, Kitayama S, Nakano R. Gonadotropin binding sites in human ovarian follicles and corpora lutea during the menstrual cycle. *Obstet Gynecol* 1987;69:800–806.

71. Chaffin CL, Hess DL, Stouffer RL. Dynamics of periovulatory steroidogenesis in the rhesus monkey follicle after ovarian stimulation. *Hum Reprod* 1999;14:642–649.

72. Erickson GF, Magoffin DA, Garzo VG, Cheung AP, Chang RJ. Granulosa cells of polycystic ovaries: are they normal or abnormal? *Hum Reprod* 1992;7:293–299.

73. Jakimiuk AJ, Weitsman SR, Magoffin DA. 5a-Reductase activity in women with polycystic ovary syndrome. *J Clin Endocrinol Metab* 1999;84:2414–2418.

74. Agarwal SK, Judd HL, Magoffin DA. A mechanism for the suppression of estrogen production in polycystic ovary syndrome. *J Clin Endocrinol Metab* 1996;81:3686–3691.

75. Dumesic DA, Schramm RD, Bird IM, Peterson E, Paprocki AM, Zhou R, Abbott DH. Reduced intrafollicular androstenedione and estradiol levels in early-treated prenatally androgenized female rhesus monkeys receiving FSH therapy for in vitro fertilization. *Biol Reprod* 2003;69:1213–1219.

76. Zeleznik AJ, Little-Ihrig L, Ramasawamy S. Administration of dihydrotestosterone to rhesus monkeys inhibits gonadotropin-stimulated ovarian steroidogenesis. *J Clin Endocrinol Metab* 2004;89:860 866.

77. Pradeep PK, Li X, Peegel H, Menon KMJ. Dihydrotestosterone inhibits granulosa cell proliferation by decreasing the cyclin D2 mRNA expression and cell cycle arrest at G1 phase. *Endocrinology* 2002;143:2930–2935.

78. Legro RS, Bentley-Lewis R, Driscoll D, Wang SC, Dunaif A. Insulin resistance in the sisters of women with polycystic ovary syndrome: association with hyperandrogenemia rather than menstrual irregularity. *J Clin Endocrinol Metab* 2002;87:2128–2133.

79. Clark AM, Thornley B, Tomlinson L, Galletley C, Norman RJ. Weight loss in obese infertile women results in improvement in reproductive outcome for all forms of fertility treatment. *Hum Reprod* 1998;13:1502–1505.

80. Kiddy DS, Hamilton-Fairley D, Bush A, Short F, Anyaoku V, Reed MJ, Franks S. Improvement in endocrine and ovarian function during dietary treatment of obese women with polycystic ovary syndrome. *Clin Endocrinol (Oxf)* 1992;36:105–111.

81. Eppig, J.J., O'Brien, M.J., Pendola, F.L., and Watanabe, S. Factors affecting the developmental competence of mouse oocytes grown in vitro: follicle stimulating hormone and insulin. *Biol Reprod* 1998;59:1445–53.

82. Willis D, Mason H, Gilling-Smith C, Franks, S. Modulation by insulin of follicle-stimulating hormone and luteinizing hormone actions in human granulosa cells of normal and polycystic ovaries. *J Clin Endocrinol Metab* 1996;81:302–309.

83. Willis D, Watson H, Mason H, Galea R, Brincat M, Franks S. Premature response to LH of granulosa cells from anovulatory women with polycystic ovaries: relevance to mechanism of anovulation. *J Clin Endocrinol Metab* 1998;83:3984–3991.

84. Jakimiuk AJ, Weitsman SR, Navab A, Magoffin DA. Luteinizing hormone receptor, steroidogenesis acute regulatory protein, and steroidogenic enzyme messenger ribonucleic acids are overproduced in thecal and granulosa cells from polycystic ovaries. *J Clin Endocrinol Metab* 2001;86:1318–1323.

85. Franks S, Mason H, Willis D. Follicular dynamics in the polycystic ovary syndrome. *Mol Cell Endocrinol* 2000;163:49–52.

86. Dumesic DA, Schramm RD, Peterson E, Paprocki AM, Zhou R, Abbott DH. Impaired developmental competence of oocytes in adult prenatally androgenized female rhesus monkeys undergoing gonadotropin stimulation for *in vitro* fertilization. *J Clin Endocrinol Metab* 2002;87:1111–1119.

87. Knight PG, Glister C. Potential local regulatory functions of inhibins, activins and follistatin in the ovary. *Reproduction* 2001;121:503–512.

88. Schneyer AL, Fujiwara T, Fox J, Welt CK, Adams J, Messerlian GM, Taylor AE. Dynamic changes in the intrafollicular inhibin/activin/follistatin axis during human follicular development: relationship to circulating hormone levels. *J Clin Endocrinol Metab* 2000;85:3319–3330.

89. Fujiwara T, Sidis Y, Welt CK, Lambert-Messerlian G, Fox J, Taylor AE, Schneyer A. Dynamics of inhibin subunit and follistatin mRNA during development of normal and PCOS follicles. *J Clin Endocrinol Metab* 2001;86:4206–4215.

90. Magoffin DA, Jakimiuk AJ. Inhibin A, inhibin B and activin concentrations in follicular fluid from women with polycystic ovary syndrome. *Hum Reprod* 1998;13:2693–2698.

91. Smyth CD, Miro F, Whitelaw PF, Howles CM, Hillier SG. Ovarian thecal/interstitial androgen synthesis is enhanced by a follicle-stimulating hormone-stimulated paracrine mechanism. *Endocrinology* 1993;133: 1532–1538.

92. Welt CK, Taylor AE, Fox J, Messerlian GM, Adams JM, Schneyer AL. Follicular arrest in polycystic ovary syndrome is associated with deficient inhibin A and B biosynthesis. *J Clin Endocrinol Metab* 2005;90:5582–5587.

93. Lambert-Messerlian G, Taylor A, Leykin L, Isaacson K, Toth T, Chang Y, Schneyer A. Characterization of intrafollicular steroid hormones, inhibin, and follistatin in women with and without polycystic ovarian syndrome following gonadotropin stimulation. *Biol Reprod* 1997;57:1211–1216.

94. Welt CK, Taylor AE, Martin KA, Hall JE. Serum inhibin B in polycystic ovary syndrome: regulation by insulin and luteinizing hormone. *J Clin Endocrinol Metab* 2002;87:5559–5565.

95. Norman RJ, Milner CR, Groome NP, Robertson DM. Circulating follistatin concentrations are higher and activin levels are lower in polycystic ovarian syndrome. *Hum Reprod* 2001;16:668–672.

96. Eldar-Geva T, Spitz IM, Groome NP, Margalioth EJ, Homberg R. Follistatin and activin A serum concentrations in obese and non-obese patients with polycystic ovary syndrome. *Hum Reprod* 2001;16:2552–2556.

97. Elvin JA, Clark AT, Wang P, Wolfman NM, Matzuk MM. Paracrine actions of growth differentiation factor-9 in the mammalian ovary. *Mol Endocrinol* 1999B;13:1035–1048.

98. Hayashi M, McGee EA, Min G, Klein C, Rose UM, van Duin M, Hsueh AJW. Recombinant growth differentiation factor-9 (GDF-9) enhances growth and differentiation of cultured early ovarian follicles. *Endocrinology* 1999;140:1236–1244.

99. Vitt UA, Hayashi M, Klein C, Hsueh AJW. Growth differentiation factor-9 stimulates proliferation but suppresses the follicle-stimulating hormone-induced differentiation of cultured granulosa cells from small antral and preovulatory rat follicles. *Biol Reprod* 2000;62:370–377.

100. Dong J, Albertini DF, Nishimori K, Kumar TR, Lu N, Matzuk MM. Growth differentiation factor-9 is required during early ovarian folliculogenesis. *Nature* 1996;383:531–535.

101. Elvin JA, Yan C, Wang P, Nishimori K, Matzuk MM. Molecular characterization of the follicle defects in the growth differentiation factor 9-deficient ovary. *Mol Endocrinol* 1999;13:1018–1034.

102. Aaltonen J, Laitinen MP, Vuojolainen K, Jaatinen R, Horelli-Kuitunen N, Seppa L, Louhio H, Tuuri T, Sjoberg J, Butzow R, Hovatta O, Dale L, Ritvos O. Human growth differentiation factor 9 (GDF-9) and its novel homolog GDF-9B are expressed in oocytes during early folliculogenesis. *J Clin Endocrinol Metab* 1999;84:2744–2750.

103. Filho FLT, Baracat EC, Lee TH, Suh CS, Matsui M, Chang RJ, Shimasaki S, Erickson GF. Aberrant expression of growth differentiation factor-9 in oocytes of women with polycystic ovary syndrome. *J Clin Endocrinol Metab* 2002;87:1337–1344.

104. Hreinsson JG, Scott JE, Rasmussen C, Swahn ML, Hsueh AJW, Hovatta O. Growth differentiation factor-9 promotes the growth, development, and survival of human ovarian follicles in organ culture. *J Clin Endocrinol Metab* 2002;87:316–321.

105. Manikkam M, Steckler TL, Welch KB, Inskeep EK, Padmanabhan V. Fetal programming: prenatal testosterone treatment leads to follicular persistence/luteal defects. Partial restoration of ovarian function by cyclic progesterone treatment. *Endocrinology* 2006;147:1997–2007.

3

What Is the Appropriate Imaging of the Polycystic Ovary

Sophie Jonard, MD, Yann Robert, MD,
Yves Ardaens, MD, and Didier Dewailly, MD

CONTENTS

Summary

The need for a calibrated imaging of polycystic ovaries (PCO) is now stronger than ever since the recent consensus conference held in Rotterdam, May 1–3, 2003. However, imaging PCO is not an easy procedure, and it requires a thorough technical and medical background. The two-dimensional (2-D) ultrasonography (U/S) remains the standard for imaging PCO and the current consensus definition of PCO determined at the joint ASRM/ESHRE consensus meeting on PCOS rests on this technique: either 12 or more follicles measuring 2–9 mm in diameter and/or increased ovarian volume (>10 cm^3). The other techniques such as Doppler, 3-D U/S, and magnetic resonance imaging (MRI) can help for the diagnosis but are so far only second-line techniques.

Key Words: Polycystic ovary; two-dimensional ultrasonography; Doppler; three-dimensional ultrasonography; magnetic resonance imaging; ovarian volume; ovarian area; follicle number.

1. INTRODUCTION

The need for a calibrated imaging of polycystic ovaries (PCO) is now stronger than ever since the recent consensus conference held in Rotterdam in 2003. Indeed, the subjective criteria that were proposed 20 years ago and still used until recently by the vast majority of authors are now replaced by a stringent definition using objective criteria *(1,2)*.

Imaging PCO is not an easy procedure. It requires a thorough technical and medical background. The goal of this chapter is to provide the reader with the main issues

From: *Contemporary Endocrinology: Polycystic Ovary Syndrome*
Edited by: A. Dunaif, R. J. Chang, S. Franks, and R. S. Legro © Humana Press, Totowa, NJ

ensuring a well-controlled imaging for the diagnosis of PCO. The two-dimensional (2-D) ultrasonography (U/S) will be first and extensively addressed as it remains the standard for imaging PCO. Other techniques such as Doppler, 3-D U/S, and magnetic resonance imaging (MRI) will be then more briefly described.

2. 2-D ULTRASONOGRAPHY

2.1. Technical Aspects and Recommendations

The transabdominal route should always be the first step of pelvic sonographic examination, followed by the transvaginal route, excepted in virgin or refusing patients. Of course, a full bladder is required for visualization of the ovaries. However, one should be cautious that an overfilled bladder can compress the ovaries, yielding a falsely increased length. The main advantage of this route is that it offers a panoramic view of the pelvic cavity. Therefore, it allows excluding associated uterine or ovarian abnormalities with an abdominal development. Indeed, lesions with cranial growth could be missed by the transvaginal approach exclusively.

With the transvaginal route, high-frequency probes (>6 MHz) with a better spatial resolution but a less examination depth can be used, because the ovaries are close to the vagina and/or the uterus and because the presence of fatty tissue is usually less disturbing (except when very abundant). With this technique, not only the size and the shape of ovaries are visualized but also their internal structure, namely follicles and stroma. It is now possible to get pictures that have a definition close to anatomical cuts. However, the evaluation of the ovarian size through the transvaginal approach is difficult. To be the most accurate, it requires choosing meticulously the picture where the ovary appears the longest and the widest. This picture must then be frozen. Two means can be proposed for calculating the ovarian area: either fitting an ellipse to the ovary in which the area is given by the machine or outlining by hand the ovary with automatic calculation of the outlined area. This last technique must be preferred in cases of a non-ellipsoid ovaries, as sometimes observed. The volume is the most complete approach. Traditionally, it can be estimated after the measurement of the length, width, and the thickness and use of the classical formula for a prolate ellipsoid: $L \times W \times T \times 0.523$ (3,4,5). However, the ovaries have to be studied in three orthogonal planes, a condition that is not always respected. The 3-D U/S is an attractive alternative for the accurate assessment of ovarian volume but this technique is not commonly available (see paragraph 3.1).

To count the total number of "cysts" (in fact, follicles) and to evaluate their size and position, each ovary should be scanned in longitudinal and/or transversal cross-section from the inner to outer margins.

2.2. The Consensus Definition of PCO

According to the literature review dealing with all available imaging systems and to the discussion at the joint ASRM/ESHRE consensus meeting on PCOS held in Rotterdam, May 1–3, 2003, the current consensus definition of PCO is the following: either 12 or more follicles measuring 2–9 mm in diameter in the whole ovary *and/or* increased ovarian volume (>10 cm³).

The priority was given to the ovarian volume and to the follicle number because both have the advantage of being physical entities that can be measured in real time conditions and because both are still considered as the key and consistent features of PCO.

2.2.1. THE INCREASED OVARIAN VOLUME

Many studies have reported an increased mean ovarian volume in series of patients with PCOS (4–9). However, the upper normal limit of the ovarian volume suffers from some variability in the literature (from 8 to 15.6 cm³). Such variability may be explained by the following:

- the small number of controls in some studies and/or
- differences in inclusion or exclusion criteria for control women and/or
- operator-dependent technical reasons: it is difficult indeed to obtain strictly longitudinal ovarian cuts, which is an absolute condition for accurate measures of the ovarian axis (length, width, and thickness).

The consensus volume threshold to discriminate a normal ovary from a PCO is 10 cm³ (1). It has been empirically retained by the expert panel for the Rotterdam consensus, as being the best compromise between the most complete studies (6,7). Indeed, no study published so far has used an appropriate statistical appraisal of sensitivity and specificity of the volume threshold. This prompted us to recently revisit this issue through a prospective study including 154 women with PCOS compared to 57 women with normal ovaries. The receiver operating characteristic (ROC) curves indicated that a threshold at 10 cm³ yielded a good specificity (98.2%) but a bad sensitivity (39%). Setting the threshold at 7 cm³ offered the best compromise between specificity (94.7%) and sensitivity (68.8%) (10). Thus, in our opinion, the threshold at 10 cm³ should be lowered to increase the sensitivity of the ultrasound PCO definition. In agreement with this proposal, Carmina et al. (11) have recently compared 326 women with PCOS to 50 age-matched and weight-matched ovulatory women and confirmed our results by considering that ovarian volumes larger than 7.5 cm³ were excessive.

2.2.2. THE INCREASED FOLLICLE NUMBER

The polyfollicular pattern (i.e., excessive number of small echoless regions less than 10 mm in diameter) is strongly suggestive of PCO. It is now broadly accepted that most of these cysts are in fact healthy oocyte-containing follicles and are not atretic.

The consensus definition for a PCO is one that contains 12 or more follicles of 2–9 mm diameter. Again, the expert panel for the Rotterdam consensus considered this threshold as being the best compromise between the most complete studies, including the one in which we compared 214 patients with PCOS to 112 women with normal ovaries (12). By ROC analysis, a follicle number per ovary (FNPO) of ≥12 follicles of 2–9 mm diameter yielded the best compromise between sensitivity (75%) and specificity (99%) for the diagnosis of PCO.

Since then, however, a recent study using 3-D U/S has disputed this threshold (13). These authors used appropriate statistical approach by ROC curves but their population samples were very small (29 normoandrogenic women and 10 PCOS patients). In addition, their patients had a severe PCOS with anovulation and obesity and did not represent therefore a "standard" PCOS population. Not surprisingly, they found a higher threshold for the FNPO (20) and for the ovarian volume (13 mL). Indeed, a FNPO set at 20 yielded 70% sensitivity and 100% specificity. However, if one looks closely at their data, setting the threshold lower would have improved the sensitivity without a substantial loss of specificity. Also, it is not known whether counting the follicles by 3-D U/S yields different values from those obtained by scanning the ovaries with conventional U/S.

It is also debated whether the FNPO should be counted in the whole ovary or in a single median sonographic plane. No study using appropriate statistical approach has compared the two techniques. Therefore, it is so far not possible to validate any threshold for the latter.

Finally, the Rotterdam consensus did not address the difficult issue about the presence of multi-follicular ovaries (MFO) in situations other than PCOS. Again, the terminology might be better annotated as multi-follicular rather than multi-cystic. There is no consensus definition for MFO although they have been described as ovaries in which there are multiple (≥ 6) follicles, usually 4–10 mm in diameter, with normal stromal echogenicity (4). No histological data about MFO are available. MFO are characteristically seen during puberty and in women recovering from hypothalamic amenorrhea—both situations being associated with follicular growth without consistent recruitment of a dominant follicle (14,15). Although the clinical pictures are theoretically different, there may be some overlap however, hence the confusion between PCO and MFO by inexperienced ultrasonographers. This issue stresses the need for considering carefully the other clinical and/or biological components of the consensus definition for PCOS. We recently revisited the ovarian follicular pattern in a group of women with hypothalamic amenorrhea. About one-third had a FNPO higher than 12 (unpublished personal data). As they were oligo-ovulatory, they could be considered as having PCOS if one applied the Rotterdam definition! This might be true in some of them if one supposes that the clinical and biological expression of their PCOS had been modified by the chronically suppressed LH levels due to their secondary hypothalamic dysfunction (16). In the others, however, such an overlap in the FNPO emphasizes the need for a wise and careful utilization of the Rotterdam criteria as well as for considering other ultrasound criteria for PCO in difficult situations.

2.3. Other Criteria and Other Definitions

2.3.1. External Morphological Signs of PCO

At its beginning in the 1970's, the weak resolution of U/S abdominal probes allowed only the external morphological ovarian features to be assessed. Thus, these features were used as the first criteria defining PCO:

1. the length, with an upper limit is 4 cm, is the simplest criterion, but this uni-dimensional approach may lead false positive results when a full bladder compresses the ovary (with the transabdominal route) or false negative results when the ovaries are spheric, with a relatively short length;
2. because of the increased ovarian size and the normal uterine width, the uterine width/ovarian length (U/O) ratio is decreased (<1) in PCO;

3. PCO often display a spherical shape in contrast to normal ovaries that are ellipsoid. This morphological change can be evaluated by the sphericity index (ovarian width/ovarian length), which is higher than 0.7 in PCO.

These parameters are less used nowadays because of their poor sensitivity *(17)*.

2.3.2. THE OVARIAN AREA

Ovarian area is less frequently used as a diagnostic criterion than the ovarian volume, and it was not retained in the consensus definition. However, in our recent study revisiting the ovarian volume *(10)*, the ovarian area (assessed by the ROC curves) had a slightly better diagnostic value than the ovarian volume (sensitivity, 77.6% and specificity, 94.7% for a threshold at 5 cm²/ ovary). We also observed that the measured ovarian area (by outlining by hand the ovary or by fitting an ellipse to the ovary) was more informative than the calculated ovarian area (by using the formula for an ellipse: length × width × π/4). Indeed, ovaries are not strictly ellipsoid, and this can explain why the diagnostic value of the former was better than the latter. We previously reported that the mean ovarian area was less than 5.5 cm² in a large group of normal women *(18,19)*. However, from our recent data, a threshold at 5 cm² seems to offer the best compromise between sensitivity and specificity. Beyond this threshold, the diagnosis of PCO can be suggested.

2.3.3. THE INCREASED STROMA

Stromal hypertrophy is characterized by an increased component of the ovarian central part, which seems to be rather hyperechoic (Fig. 1). In our *(17,18)* and in others' opinion *(8)*, the stromal hypertrophy and hyperechogenicity are specific for PCO and help

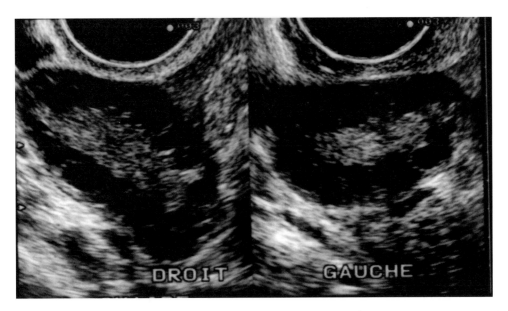

Fig. 1. Polycystic ovary (B mode). The ovarian outlined area (9.7 cm² at right and 8.9 cm² at left) is increased. The follicle number, with a diameter between 2 and 9 mm, is more than 12. The small follicles display a typical peripheral pattern, around the hyperechoic stroma.

distinguishing between PCO and MFO. However, the estimation of hyperechogenicity is considered as highly subjective, mainly because it depends on the settings of the ultrasound machine. Likewise, in the absence of a precise quantification, the stromal hypertrophy is also a subjective sign.

For standardizing the assessment of stromal hypertrophy, we designed a computerized quantification of ovarian stroma, allowing selective calculation of the stromal area by subtraction of the cyst area from the total ovarian area on a longitudinal ovarian cut *(18,19)*. By this means, we were able to set the upper normal limit of the stromal area (i.e., 95th percentile of a large control group of 48 normal women) at 380 mm^2 per ovary. However, providing a precise outlining of the ovarian shape on a strictly longitudinal cut of the ovaries, the diagnostic value of the total ovary equaled the one of stromal area since both were highly correlated.

Fulghesu et al. *(9)* proposed the ovarian stroma/total area ratio as a good criterion for the diagnosis of PCOS. The ovarian stromal area was evaluated by outlining with the caliper the peripheral profile of the stroma, identified by a central area slightly hyperechoic with respect to the other ovarian area. However, this evaluation might not be easy to reproduce in routine practice.

Others have used a semi-quantitative measure of stromal echogenicity, scored 1 if normal, 2 if moderately increased, or 3 if frankly increased *(20)*. In this study, this parameter correlated significantly to the total follicle number (both ovaries). Echogenicity has also been quantified by Al-Took et al. *(21)* as the sum of the product of each intensity level (ranging from 0–63 on the scanner) and the number of pixels for that intensity level divided by the total number of pixels in the measured area. By using the same formula, Buckett et al. *(22)* found no difference in the stromal echogenicity between women with PCOS and women with normal ovaries. They concluded that the subjective impression of increased stromal echogenicity was due to increased stromal volume but also to posterior echo reinforcement behind the follicles with reduced echogenicity.

In summary, ovarian volume or area correlates well with ovarian function and is both more easily and reliably measured in routine practice than ovarian stroma. Thus, in order to routinely define the polycystic ovary, neither qualitative or quantitative assessment of the ovarian stroma is required.

2.3.4. FOLLICLE DISTRIBUTION

In PCO, the follicle distribution is predominantly peripheral, with typically an echoless peripheral array, as initially described by Adams et al. *(4)* (Fig. 1). For some authors *(23)*, younger patients display more often this peripheral distribution while a more generalized pattern, with small cysts in the central part of the ovary, is noticed in older women. At the Rotterdam meeting, this subjective criterion was judged to be too inconstant and subjective to be retained for the consensus definition of PCO *(1)*.

3. OTHER TECHNIQUES FOR IMAGING PCO

3.1. 3-D Ultrasonography

To avoid the difficulties and pitfalls in outlining or measuring the ovarian shape, the 3-D U/S has been proposed using a dedicated volumic probe or a manual survey of the ovary *(24–26)*. From the stored data, the scanned ovarian volume is displayed on the screen in three adjustable orthogonal planes, allowing the three dimensions and subsequently the volume to be more accurately evaluated. In a study of Kyei-Mensah et al. *(27)*, three groups of patients were defined: (a) those with normal ovaries, (b) those with asymptomatic PCO, and (c) those with polycystic ovary syndrome The ovarian and stromal volumes were similar in groups b and c and both greater than group a. Stromal volume was positively correlated with serum androstenedione concentrations in group c only. The mean total volume of the follicles was similar in all groups, indicating that increased stromal volume is the main cause of ovarian enlargement in PCO.

Nardo et al. *(28)* found good correlations between 2-D and 3-D ultrasound measurements of ovarian volume and polycystic ovary morphology. However, in this prospective study, total ovarian volume, ovarian stromal volume, follicular volume and follicle number did not correlate with testosterone concentration.

Thus, 3-D imaging improves spatial awareness and stores information for later use. However, 3-D ultrasound requires an expensive equipment and an intensive training. Storage and analysis of data are time consuming. Therefore, its superiority over 2-D ultrasound for imaging PCO in clinical practice is so far not evident. In addition, no precise threshold for ovarian volume and FNPO has been proposed up to now with this technique, except in the aforementioned study of Allemand et al. *(13)* that needs to be validated in larger populations.

3.2. Doppler Ultrasonography

The assessment of uterine arteries will not be addressed in this chapter exclusively devoted to PCO imaging. Color (or power) Doppler allows detection of the vascularization network within the ovarian stroma. Power Doppler is more sensitive to the slow flows and shows more vascular signals within the ovaries, but it does not discriminate between arteries and veins. Moreover, the sensitivity of the machines differs from one to another. The pulsed Doppler focuses on the hilum or internal ovarian arteries and offers a more objective approach. Because of the slow flows, the pulse repetition frequency (PRF) is at minimum (400 Hz) with the lowest frequency filter (50 Hz).

The study of the ovarian vascularization by these techniques is still highly subjective. The blood flow is more frequently visualized in PCOS (88%) than in normal patients (50%) in early follicular phase and seems to be increased *(29)*. No significant difference was found between obese and lean women with PCO, but the stroma was less vascularized in patients displaying a general cystic pattern than in those with peripherical cysts. In the latter, the pulsatility index (PI) values were significantly lower and inversely correlated to the follicle-stimulating hormone/luteinizing hormone (FSH/LH) ratio *(30)*. In an other study *(31)*, the resistive index (RI) and PI were significantly lower in PCOS (RI = 0.55 + 0.01 and PI = 0.89 + 0.04) than in normal patients (RI = 0.78 + 0.06 and PI = 1.87 + 0.38), and the peak systolic velocity was greater in PCOS (11.9 + 3.2) than in normal women (9.6 + 2.1). No correlation was found with the number of follicles and the ovarian volume but there was a positive correlation between LH levels and increased peak systolic velocity. In Zaidi et al. *(32)* study, no significant difference in PI values was found between the normal and PCOS groups, whereas the ovarian flow, as reflected by the peak sytolic velocity, was increased in the former. Some data indicate that Doppler blood flow may have some value in predicting the risk for ovarian hyperstimulation during gonadotropin therapy *(33)*. Increased stromal blood flow has also been suggested as a more relevant predictor of ovarian response to hormonal stimulation than parameters such as ovarian or stromal volume *(22,34)*.

To summarize, the increased stroma component in PCO seems to be accompanied by an increased peak systolic velocity and a decreased PI at the ovarian Doppler study. However, in all studies, values in patients with PCO overlapped widely with the ones of the normal patients. No data support so far any diagnostic usefulness of Doppler in PCO.

3.3. Magnetic Resonance Imaging

Data about MRI for PCO are still scarce in the literature *(35–37)*. This technique allows a multiplanar approach of the pelvic cavity, which helps to localize the ovaries. Imaging quality is improved by the use of pelvic-dedicated phased-array coil receiver. The most useful planes are the transversal and coronal views. The T2-weighted sequence suits the best to the ovarian morphology. With this sequence, the follicular fluid displays an hypersignal (white) and the solid component (stroma) a low signal (black). T1-weighted sequences offer less information, but the gadolium injection allows studying the stromal vascularization. The fat saturation technique increases the contrast obtained after the medium uptake by the vascularized areas.

The external signs of PCO (see above) are easy to analyze on MRI transversal sections. In addition, the T2-weighted sequence displays the excessive number of follicles, but their detection and numbering are less easy than with U/S, because of the poor spatial resolution of MRI, unless high magnetic fields are used (1–1.5 Tesla). As with U/S, the stromal hypertrophy remains a subjective observation although obvious in many cases. After Gadolinium injection, there is a high uptake by the stroma, suggesting that it is highly vascularized in PCO.

In most cases in practice, MRI does not afford more information than U/S for imaging PCO *(36)*. It is only helpful in difficult situations such as a severe hyperandrogenism, when U/S is not possible or not contributive [virgin or obese patients, respectively, or both *(38)*]. Its main role is to exclude a virilizing ovarian tumor that should be suspected when the ovarian volume is not symmetrical and/or when there is a circumscribed signal abnormality, either before or after Gadolinium injection. PCO associated with an ovarian tumor might be a pitfall.

4. CONCLUSIONS AND FUTURE AVENUES OF INVESTIGATION

The U/S study of PCO has now left its era of artistic haziness. It must be viewed as a diagnostic tool that requires the same quality controls as a biological one, such as the plasma LH assay. This supposes that its results are expressed as quantitative variables rather than purely descriptive data. Also, stringent normative data have to be established with the use of appropriate statistical methods. Lastly, it can be used by the clinician only if the ultrasonographer is sufficiently trained and repro-ducible in his/her results. By its sensitivity (providing that sufficient specificity is guaranteed), U/S has widened the clinical spectrum of PCOS, and this has led to a reduction in the numbers of cases diagnosed with "idiopathic hirsutism" and "idiopathic anovulation."

The establishment of an international consensus definition for PCO was essential. However, one should keep in mind that the endovaginal U/S is an improving technique and becomes more and more accurate with time. Therefore, the thresholds of the currently used criteria are prone to change and new criteria defining PCO will probably appear in the future. Sooner or later, some new consensus criteria will probably be needed.

REFERENCES

1. Balen AH, Laven JSE, Tan SL, Dewailly D. Ultrasound assessment of the polycystic ovary: international consensus definitions. *Human Reprod Update* 2003;9: 505–514.
2. The Rotterdam ESHRE/ASRM-sponsored PCOS consensus workshop group. Revised 2003 consensus on diagnostic criteria and long-term health risks related to polycystic ovary syndrome (PCOS). *Human Reprod* 2004;19: 41–47.
3. Sample WF, Lippe BM, Gyepes MT. Grey-scale ultrasonography of the normal female pelvis. *Radiology* 1977;125: 477–483.
4. Adams JM, Polson DW, Abulwadi N, Morris DV, Franks S, Mason HD, Tucker M, Price J, Jacobs HS. Multifollicular ovaries: clinical and endocrine features and response to pulsatile gonadotropin-releasing hormone. *Lancet* 1985;2: 1375–1378.
5. Orsini LF, Venturoli S, Lorusso R. Ultrasonic findings in polycystic ovarian disease. *Fertil Steril* 1985;43: 709–714.
6. Yeh HC, Futterweit W, Thornton JC. Polycystic ovarian disease: US features in 104 patients. *Radiology* 1987;163: 111–116.
7. Van Santbrink EJP, Hop WC, Fauser BCJM. Classification of normogonadotropic infertility: polycystic ovaries diagnosed by ultrasound versus endocrine characteristics of polycystic ovary syndrome. *Fertil Steril* 1997;67: 452–458.
8. Pache TD, Wladimiroff JW, Hop WCJ, Fauser BCJM. How to descriminate between normal and polycystic ovaries: transvaginal US study. *Radiology* 1992;183: 421–423.
9. Fulghesu AM, Ciampelli M, Belosi C, Apa R, et al. A new ultrasound criterion for the diagnosis of polycystic ovary syndrome: the ovarian stroma/ total area ratio. *Fertil Steril* 2001;76: 326–331.
10. Jonard S, Robert Y, Dewailly D. Revisiting the ovarian volume as a diagnostic criterion for polycystic ovaries. *Hum Reprod* 2005;20:2893–2898.
11. Carmina E, Orio F, Palomba S, Longo RA, Lombardi G, Lobo RA. Ovarian size and blood flow in women with polycystic ovary syndrome and their correlations with endocrine parameters. *Fertil Steril* 2005;84:413–419.
12. Jonard S, Robert Y, Cortet-Rudelli C, Pigny P, Decanter C, Dewailly D. Ultrasound examination of polycystic ovaries: is it worth counting the follicles? *Human Reprod* 2003;18: 598–603.
13. Allemand MC, Tummon IS, Phy JL, Foong SC, Dumesic DA, Session DR. Diagnosis of polycystic ovaries by three-dimensional transvaginal ultrasound. *Fertil Steril* 2006;85:214–219.
14. Venturoli S, Porcu E, Fabbri R, Paradisi R, Orsini LF and Flamigni C. Ovaries and menstrual cycles in adolescence. *Gynecol Obstet Invest* 1983;17: 219–223.
15. Stanhope R, Adams J, Jacobs HS and Brook CG. Ovarian ultrasound assessment in normal children, idiopathic precocious puberty, and during low dose pulsatile gonadotrophin releasing hormone treatment of hypogonadotrophic hypogonadism. *Arch Dis Child* 1985; 60: 116–119.
16. Reyss AC, Merlen E, Demerle C, Dewailly D. Revelation of a polymicrocystic ovary syndrome after one month's treatment by pulsatile GnRH in a patient presenting with functional hypothalamic amenorrhea. *Gynecol Obstet Fertil* 2003;31: 1039–1042.
17. Ardaens Y, Robert Y, Lemaitre L, Fossati P, Dewailly D. Polycystic ovarian disease: contribution of vaginal endosonography and reassessment of ultrasonic diagnosis. *Fertil Steril* 1991;55: 1062–1068.

18. Dewailly D., Robert Y, Helin I, et al. Ovarian stromal hypertrophy in hyperandrogenic women. *Clinical Endocrinology* 1994;41: 557–562.

19. Robert Y, Dubrulle F, Gaillandre G et al. Ultrasound assessment of ovarian stroma hypertrophy in hyperandrogenism and ovulation disorders: visual analysis versus computerized quantification. *Fertil Steril* 1995;64: 307–312.

20. Pache TD, Hop WC, Wladimiroff JW, Schipper J and Fauser BCJM. Transvaginal sonography and abnormal ovarian appearance in menstrual cycle disturbances. *Ultrasound Med Biol* 1991;17: 589–593.

21. Al-Took S, Watkin K, Tulandi T, Tan SL. Ovarian stromal echogenicity in women with clomiphene citrate-sensitive and clomiphene citrate-resistant polycystic ovary syndrome. *Fertil Steril* 1999;71: 952–954.

22. Buckett WM, Bouzayen R, Watkin KL, Tulandi T, Tan SL. Ovarian stromal echogenicity in women with normal and polycystic ovaries. *Human Reprod* 1999;14: 618–621.

23. Battaglia C, Artini PG, Salvatori M, Giulini S, Petraglia F, Maxia N, Volpe A. Ultrasonographic pattern of polycystic ovaries: color Doppler and hormonal correlations. *Ultrasound Gynaecol Obstet* 1998;11: 332–336.

24. Wu M-H, Tang H-H, Hsu C-C, Wang S-T, Huang K-E. The role of three-dimensional ultrasono-graphic imaging in ovarian measurment. *Fertil Steril* 1998; 69:1152–1155.

25. Kyei-Mensah A, Maconochie N, Zaidi J, Pittrof R, Campbell S, Tan SL. Transvaginal three-dimensional ultrasound: accuracy of ovarian follicular volume measurements. *Fertil Steril* 1996;65:371–376.

26. Kyei-Mensah A, Zaidi J, Campbell S. Ultrasound diagnosis of polycystic ovary syndrome. *Baillieres Clin Endocrinol Metab* 1996;10:249–262.

27. Kyei-Mensah A, Tan SL, Zaidi J, Jacobs HS. Relationship of ovarian stromal volume to serum androgen concentrations in patients with polycystic ovary syndrome. *Human Reprod* 1998;13: 1437–1441.

28. Nardo LG, Buckett WM and Khullar V. Determination of the best-fitting ultrasound formulaic method for ovarian volume measurement in women with polycystic ovary syndrome. *Fertil Steril* 2003;79: 632–633.

29. Battaglia C, Artini PG, Genazzani AD, Sgherzi MR, Salvatori M, Giulini S, Volpe A. Color Doppler analysis in lean and obese women with polycystic ovaries. *Ultrasound Gynaecol Obstet* 1996;7: 342–346.

30. Battaglia C, Genazzani AD, Salvatori M, et al. Doppler, ultrasonographic and endocrinological environment with regard to the number of small subcapsular follicles in polycystic ovary syndrome. *Gynecol Endocrinol* 1999;13: 123–129.

31. Aleem FA, Predanic MP. Transvaginal color Doppler determination of the ovarian and uterine blood flow characteristics in polycystic ovary disease. *Fertil Steril* 1996;65:510–516.

32. Zaidi J, Campbell S, Pittrof R, Kyei-Mensah A, Shaker A, Jacobs HS, Tan SL. Ovarian stromal blood flow in women with polycystic ovaries: a possible new marker for diagnosis? *Human Reprod* 1995,10:1992–1996.

33. Agrawal R, Conway G, Sladkevicius P, Tan SL, Engmann L, Payne N, Bekir J, Campbell S, Jacobs H. Serum vascular endothelial growth factor and Doppler blood flow velocities in in vitro fertil-ization: relevance to ovarian hyperstimulation syndrome and polycystic ovaries. *Fertil Steril* 1998; 70:651–658.

34. Engmann L, Sladkevicius P, Agrawal LR, Bekir JS, Campbell S, Tan SL. Value of ovarian stromal blood flow velocity measurement after pituitary suppression in the prediction of ovarian respon-siveness and outcome of *in vitro* fertilization treatment. *Fertil Steril* 1999;71: 22–29.

35. Maubon A, Courtieu C, Vivens F, Tailland ML, Saucerotte H, Bringer J, Mares P, Rouanet JP. Magnetic resonance imaging of normal and polycystic ovaries. Preliminary results. *Ann N Y Acad Scie* 1993;687:224–229.

36. Kimura I, Togashi K, Kawakami S, Nakano Y, Takakura K, Mori T, Konishi J. Polycystic ovaries: implications of diagnosis with MR imaging. *Radiology* 1996;201:549–552.
37. Woodward PJ, Gilfeather M. Magnetic resonance imaging of the female pelvis. *Semin Ultrasound CT MR* 1998;19:90–103.
38. Yoo RY, Sirlin CB, Gottschalk M, Chang RJ. Ovarian imaging by magnetic resonance in obese adolescent girls with polycystic ovary syndrome: a pilot study. *Fertil Steril* 2005;84:985–995.

4 Polycystic Ovary Versus Polycystic Ovary Syndrome

A Necessary Distinction

Adam Balen, MD, FRCOG

Summary

The polycystic ovary syndrome (PCOS) is a heterogeneous condition. Polycystic ovaries are detected in 19–33% of the "general population," of whom approximately 80% have symptoms of PCOS, albeit for many such symptoms are usually mild. Thus, about 20% of women with polycystic ovaries are symptom free. It appears that ovarian dysfunction is expressed when the ovaries of women with polycystic ovaries alone are stressed, by either a gain in weight, a rise in circulating insulin levels, or stimulation with follicle-stimulating hormone (FSH) for assisted conception treatments. Longitudinal studies are required to better explore the evolution of signs and symptoms of the syndrome over time in women with polycystic ovaries and by comparison with those with normal ovaries.

Key Words: Polycystic ovary syndrome; polycystic ovaries; ultrasound; insulin resistance; oligomenorrhea; hyperandrogenism.

1. INTRODUCTION

The polycystic ovary (PCO) is the morphological ovarian phenotype in women with the polycystic ovary syndrome (PCOS). There are several extra-ovarian aspects to the pathophysiology of PCOS, yet ovarian dysfunction is central. The definition

From: *Contemporary Endocrinology: Polycystic Ovary Syndrome*
Edited by: A. Dunaif, R. J. Chang, S. Franks, and R. S. Legro © Humana Press, Totowa, NJ

of the syndrome has been much debated. In 2003, a joint ESHRE/ASRM consensus meeting produced a refined definition of PCOS: namely the presence of two out of the following three criteria: (1) oligo- and/or anovulation, (2) hyperandrogenism (clinical and/or biochemical), and (3) polycystic ovaries, with the exclusion of other etiologies *(1)*. The morphology of the PCO was redefined as an ovary with 12 or more follicles measuring 2–9 mm in diameter and/or increased ovarian volume (>10 cm^3) *(2)*.

Polycystic ovaries are commonly detected by ultrasound or other forms of pelvic imaging, with estimates of the prevalence in the general population being in the order of 20–33% *(3,4)*. However, not all women with polycystic ovaries demonstrate the clinical and biochemical features that define the PCOS *(2)*. There is considerable heterogeneity of symptoms and signs among women with PCOS, and for an individual, these may change over time although there is a paucity of longitudinal data *(5)*. For example, a gain in weight is associated with a worsening of symptoms due largely to the stimulatory effect of increased insulin levels on ovarian androgen production, which in turn may affect ovarian morphology and function. Also women with previously undetected polycystic ovaries may require ovarian stimulation in the context of in vitro fertilization (IVF) treatment. When stimulated with follicle-stimulating hormone (FSH), their ovaries exhibit a typical polycystic response with the production of significantly more follicles than women with normal ovaries *(6)*.

The biochemical features of the syndrome—namely elevated serum concentrations of testosterone, androstenedione, luteinizing hormone (LH) and insulin—may vary between individuals and change with time. There also appear to be national and racial differences in the expression of PCOS.

This chapter will discuss the particular relevance of having polycystic ovaries either alone or in the context of the syndrome.

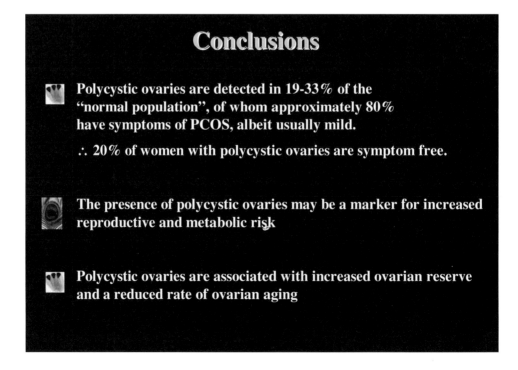

Conclusions

- Polycystic ovaries are detected in 19-33% of the "normal population", of whom approximately 80% have symptoms of PCOS, albeit usually mild.

  ∴ 20% of women with polycystic ovaries are symptom free.

- The presence of polycystic ovaries may be a marker for increased reproductive and metabolic risk

- Polycystic ovaries are associated with increased ovarian reserve and a reduced rate of ovarian aging

Conclusions

Ovarian dysfunction is expressed when the ovaries of women
with polycystic ovaries alone are stressed,
by either a gain in weight / rise in circulating insulin levels
or stimulation with FSH for assisted conception treatments.

Longitudinal studies are required to better explore the evolution
of signs and symptoms of the syndrome over time
in women with polycystic ovaries
and by comparison those with normal ovaries.

2. POLYCYSTIC OVARIES IN THE ABSENCE OF HYPERANDROGENISM

In a study of over 1871 women with PCOS, we found that one-third had an elevated serum total testosterone concentration and that the 95 percentile for total testosterone was 4.8 nmol/l (5). Women with the "classical" syndrome have the highest levels of androgens although even women with polycystic ovaries and mild or no symptoms have mean serum concentrations of testosterone that are higher than in those with normal ovaries (4,7). The bulk of evidence points to the ovary being the source of excess androgens, which appears to result from an abnormal regulation (dysregulation) of steroidogenesis (8), combined with an excess of external promoters, principally LH and insulin. There are undoubtedly women with PCOS who have an absence of overt clinical hyperandrogenism and normal serum androgen concentrations (5,9).

In the series of 1871 women with PCOS, 38% were overweight (BMI > 25 kg/m^2). Obesity was significantly associated with an increased risk of hirsutism, menstrual cycle disturbance, and an elevated serum testosterone concentration. Obesity was also associated with an increased rate of infertility and menstrual cycle disturbance. Many other groups have similarly reported heterogeneity in their populations with PCOS. Franks reported a series, also from England, of 300 women recruited from a specialist endocrine clinic (9). Some years earlier Goldzieher et al. (10) compiled a comprehensive review of 1079 cases of surgically proven polycystic ovaries. The features of these series are represented in Tables 1 and 2. The heterogeneity of the syndrome is clearly evident with a spectrum of symptoms and endocrine abnormalities, which may occur together or separately.

Table 1

Clinical Symptoms and Signs in Women with polycystic ovary syndrome (PCOS)

	Percentage frequency of symptom or sign			
	Balen et al. *(5)* (n = 1741) (%)	Franks *(9)* (n = 300) (%)	Goldzieher *(10)* (*n* = 1079) [*n* (%)] %	Number of cases[a]
Menstrual cycle disturbance				
Oligomenorrhea	47	52	29[b]	*n* = 547
Amenorrhea	19.2	28	51	*n* = 640
Hirsutism	66.2	64	69	*n* = 819
Obesity	38.4	35	41	*n* = 600
Acne	34.7	27	–	–
Alopecia	6	3	–	–
Acanthosis nigricans	2.5	<1	–	–
Infertility (primary/secondary)	20	42	74	*n* = 596

[a]In the Goldzieher study, clinical details were not available for the entire 1079 women, thus the number of cases that were used to determine the frequency of each symptom is stated.

[b]In this series, any abnormal pattern of uterine bleeding was included. –, Denotes feature not recorded.

Table 2

Biochemical Features of Women with polycystic ovary syndrome (PCOS)

	Percentage frequency	
	Balen et al. (5) (n = 1741) (%)	*Franks (9) (n = 300) (%)*
Elevated serum LH	39.8	51
Elevated serum testosterone	28.9	50
Elevated serum prolactin	11.8	7

3. POLYCYSTIC OVARIES IN THE ABSENCE OF MENSTRUAL DYSFUNCTION

In the series reported by Balen et al. *(5)*, approximately 20% were amenorrheic, 50% oligomenorrheic, and 30% had a regular menstrual cycle, whereas the series of Franks and Goldzieher each reported 20% with a regular menstrual cycle *(9,10)*.

Several studies have been performed to attempt to determine the prevalence of polycystic ovaries as detected by ultrasound alone in the general population and have found prevalence rates in the order of 17–33% *(4,11–16)* The study designs and results are summarized in Table 3. All of the studies used transabdominal ultrasound for the diagnosis of polycystic ovaries except for Cresswell et al. *(16)*, who converted to a transvaginal scan if the transabdominal picture was unclear.

Table 3
The Prevalence of Polycystic Ovaries in the General Population

Authors	Polson et al. (11)	Tayob et al. (12)	Clayton et al. (13)	Farquhar et al (14)	Botis et al. (15)	Cresswell et al. (16)	Michelmore et al. (4)
Study population	Volunteers recruited from clinical and secretarial staff at St. Mary's Hospital, London (n = 257)	Volunteers using a low dose combined OCP, recruited from routine clinics at the Margaret Pyke centre and the Royal Free Hospital, London (n = 120)	Volunteers born between 1952 and 1969 recruited from a list of a Group Practice in Harrow, London, by random postal invitation (n = 190)	Volunteers recruited from two electoral roles in Auckland, NZ, by random postal invitation (n = 183)	Volunteers recruited from women presenting to an outpatient clinic for routine Pap smear (n = 1078)	Volunteers born between 1952 and 1953 recruited from records of the Jessop Hospital, Sheffield, by invitation and personal interview (n = 235)	Volunteers from a University population and general practice in Oxford (n = 230)
Response rate	Unknown	Unknown	18%	16%	Unknown	68%	
Age range	18–36 years	18–30 years (mean = 24 years)	18–36 years	18–45 years (mean = 33 years)	17–40 years	40–42 years	17–25 years
Prevalence	22%	22%	22%	21%	17%	21%	33%
95% CI	17–27%	14–30%	16–28%	14–27%	14–19%	16–26%	27–39%

The study populations recruited by Polson et al. *(11)*, Tayob et al. *(12)*, and Botis et al. *(15)* were all subject to a degree of selection bias because of the fact that they recruited women from hospital-associated populations (both hospital workers and patients) and not from the general population. The low response rates achieved in the community-based studies by Clayton et al. *(13)* and Farquhar et al. *(14)* might reduce confidence in the validity of their estimates of prevalence, but reassuringly Cresswell et al. *(16)* who achieved a much higher response rate in their sample determined a very similar prevalence. However, in the absence of a large, cross-sectional population-based study, the prevalence rates detected above provide the best estimates of the occurrence of polycystic ovaries in the "normal" population. The pooled prevalence is 26.6%, indicating that polycystic ovaries (as defined by their ultrasound appearance) are extremely common.

In all of the studies, hirsutism was identified more commonly in women with polycystic ovaries. Menstrual cycle abnormalities were also found to be more common in the PCO groups, except in the study by Clayton et al. *(13)*, which detected no significant difference in menstrual patterns when comparing women with polycystic versus those with normal ovaries. Botis et al. *(15)* noted a greater tendency toward obesity in their group of women with polycystic ovaries, but significant differences in obesity were not identified in the other reports. All of these studies determined higher mean ovarian volumes in women with polycystic ovaries when compared with women with normal ovaries. The frequency of symptoms and signs identified in women with and without polycystic ovaries is summarized in Table 4.

The inconsistencies between these studies may be due in part to differences in the definitions used for each symptom or sign that was recorded. However, the method of recruitment may also be relevant as the community-based studies *(13,14,16)* show frequencies of menstrual cycle disturbances and of hirsutism that are much lower than those recorded in the larger studies of women with PCOS recruited from reproductive/endocrine clinics (Table 1). The studies by Botis and by Polson *(11,15)* record frequencies that resemble more closely those previously determined in the hospital-based studies, suggesting that their populations were subject to greater selection bias.

In a study of 224 normal female volunteers between the ages of 18 and 25 years, polycystic ovaries were identified using transabdominal ultrasound in 33% of participants *(4)*. Fifty percent of the participants were using some form of hormonal contraception, which is a common experience when studying young women, but the prevalence of polycystic ovaries in users and non-users of hormonal contraception was identical. Polycystic ovaries in the non-users of hormonal contraception were associated with irregular menstrual cycles and significantly higher serum testosterone concentrations when compared with women with normal ovaries; however, only a small proportion of women with polycystic ovaries (15%) had "elevated" serum testosterone concentrations outside the normal range. Interestingly, there were no significant differences in acne, hirsutism, body mass index (BMI), or body fat percentage between women with polycystic and normal ovaries, and hyperinsulinism and reduced insulin sensitivity were not associated with polycystic ovaries in this group. Also, no significant differences were identified for β-cell function between the groups, unlike other studies that have shown pancreatic β-cell dysfunction in women with PCOS when compared with controls *(17)*.

Table 4
Frequency of Clinical Symptoms and Signs in Women with and Without Polycystic Ovaries

	Polson et al. (11) (%)		Clayton et al. (13) (%)		Farquhar et al. (14) (%)		Botis et al. (15) (%)		Cresswell et al. (16) (%)		Michelmore et al. (4) (%)	
	PCO (n = 33[a])	Norm (n = 116[a])	PCO (n = 43)	Norm (n = 165)	PCO (n = 39)	Norm (n = 144)	PCO (n = 183)	Norm (n = 823)	PCO (n = 49)	Norm (n = 186)	PCO (n = 74)	Norm (n = 150)
Menstrual cycle disturbance	76	1	29[a]	27	46	20	80	–	41	27	65	45
Hirsutism	–	–	14	2	23	4	40	10	14	2	12	10
Obesity	–	–	33	29	23	19	41	10	35	48	26	22

[a]Value includes only non-OCP users with PCO.

In this study by Michelmore et al. *(4)*, the prevalence of PCOS was as low as 8% using the NIH consensus definition for PCOS *(17)* or as high as 26% if the broader "European criteria" *(1)* were applied. However, features included in the European criteria (menstrual irregularity, acne, hirsutism, BMI > 25 kgm^2, raised serum testosterone, or raised LH) were found to occur frequently in women without polycystic ovaries, and 75% of women with normal ovaries had one or more of these attributes. Sub-group analyses of women, according to the presence of normal ovaries, polycystic ovaries alone, or polycystic ovaries and features of PCOS, revealed greater mean BMI in women with PCOS but also indicated *lower* fasting insulin concentrations and *greater* insulin sensitivity in PCO and PCOS groups when compared with women with normal ovaries, which is in contrast to studies of older women *(18,19)*. These interesting findings were difficult to interpret in light of current understanding of PCOS but forced us to consider the possibility that this young, mainly non-overweight population might reflect women early in the natural history of the development of PCOS and that abnormalities of insulin metabolism might evolve following weight gain in later life.

Despite the problems of small sample populations and inconsistent methodology, the epidemiological studies indicate a high prevalence (27%) of polycystic ovaries in the "general" population. They have also shown that many of these women have symptoms and signs that may be attributable to PCOS but reinforce the observation that in some women with polycystic ovaries, no clinical or biochemical abnormalities are detected.

The question of whether polycystic ovaries alone are pathological or a normal variant of ovarian morphology is still debated. The consensus statement on defining the morphology of the PCO states that "A woman having PCO in the absence of an ovulation disorder or hyperandrogenism ("asymptomatic PCO") should not be considered as having PCOS, until more is known about this situation" *(2)*. While the spectrum of "normality" might include the presence of polycystic ovaries in the absence of signs or symptoms of PCOS, there is evidence that women with polycystic morphology alone show typical responses to stresses such as gonadotropin stimulation during IVF treatment or to weight gain, whether spontaneous or as stimulated by sodium valproate therapy *(5,20)*. The difficulty in answering this question lies in the fact that to date there are no large scale, longitudinal prospective studies of women with polycystic ovaries.

4. OVARIAN DYSFUNCTION IN PCOS

The distinct ovarian morphology is pathognemonic for the syndrome, its major marker being hyperandrogenemia arising from the theca cells. Follicular development is disturbed with antral follicles arrested at a diameter of 2–9 mm. It is thought that the abnormal endocrine environment adversely affects follicular maturation although it is uncertain whether there is in addition an intrinsic abnormality within the follicle of polycystic ovaries. The whole process of follicle development from primordial to preovulatory takes about 6 months, with only the final 2 weeks being gonadotropin dependent. Preantral follicle development is dependent on local growth factors that determine growth and survival of those follicles that escape death by atresia.

A study of follicle densities from normal and polycystic ovaries found that normal ovaries contained 11.4 small preantral follicles/m^3 (4–34) ovulatory polycystic ovaries had a density of 27.4 follicles/m^3 (9–81), whereas anovulatory polycystic ovaries had a density of 73.0 follicles/m^3 (31–94). This significant difference was also demonstrated for primary follicles *(21)*. Anovulatory polycystic ovaries had the highest overall density of follicles although there was no significant difference between those from anovulatory and ovulatory polycystic ovaries or between ovulatory polycystic ovaries and normal ovaries. Primordial follicle density was similar in all three groups although those from polycystic ovaries were less likely to be healthy. Thus, there appears to be a significantly higher density of small preantral follicles particularly in anovulatory polycystic ovaries. This is thought to be due to a higher rate of recruitment from the resting follicle pool in polycystic ovaries rather than a reduced rate of atresia (which if anything may be slightly increased). The observation that women with PCOS do not have an early menopause suggests that there may be a higher starting follicle pool although this is yet to be proven.

The presence of enlarged polycystic ovaries suggests that the ovary is the primary site of endocrine abnormality, particularly the hyperandrogenism. A number of studies have shown that the primary cause of excess androgen production by the PCO is not solely due to hypersecretion of LH, and the intrinsic defect was due to an ovarian theca-interstitial cell dysfunction or other stimulatory influences such as insulin or insulin-like growth factor (IGF)-1 *(2–25)*.

Inhibin is an FSH-inducible factor that is capable of interfering with the downregulation of steroidogenesis. Plasma inhibin and androstenedione concentrations correlate, and women with PCOS have elevated serum inhibin-B *(26)*. This helps to explain the relatively low serum concentrations of FSH compared with LH in anovulatory women with PCOS. As inhibin stimulates androgen production and androgens in turn stimulate inhibin secretion, there is a potential for the development of a vicious cycle within the ovary that would inhibit follicle development. Alternatively, a defect in the IGF system could cause an alteration of the set point for the response of the granulosa cell to FSH. It has been suggested that LH acts on granulosa cells in the presence of insulin, thereby leading to premature luteinization, maturational arrest, and excess androgen production *(25)*.

In summary, as a consequence of dysregulation of androgen synthesis within the ovary, women with PCOS have ovarian hyper-responsiveness to gonadotropins: that of thecal cells to LH explaining the excess androgens and that of granulosa cells to FSH leading to increased estrogens. A PCO functioning relatively "normally" may therefore behave in a more typically "polycystic" fashion when the balance is tipped by a change in either the gonadotropin or insulin/growth factor milieu.

5. EXPRESSION OF PCOS IN WOMEN WITH PCO

It has been found that some women with hypogonadotropic hypogonadism (HH) also have polycystic ovaries detected by pelvic ultrasound, and when these women were treated with pulsatile GnRH to induce ovulation, they had significantly higher serum LH concentrations than women with HH and normal ovaries *(27)*. Furthermore, the elevation in LH concentration was observed before serum estradiol concentrations rose. Thus, hypersecretion of LH occurred in these women when the hypothalamus was replaced by an artificial GnRH pulse generator (i.e., the GnRH pump), with a fixed GnRH pulse interval of 90 min (equivalent to the pulse interval in the early follicular phase). These results suggest that the cause of hypersecretion of LH involves a perturbation of ovarian–pituitary feedback rather than a primary disturbance of hypothalamic pulse regulation.

Polycystic ovaries with or without clinical symptoms are also a common finding in patients referred for IVF. For example, two studies have identified between 33 and 43.5% of patients presenting with previously undetected polycystic ovaries *(6,28)*.

It must be stressed that the first-line treatment for PCOS is not IVF. Occasionally, the IVF specialist will be presented with a patient with PCOS or polycystic ovaries alone, who either has never had induction of ovulation or assisted conception. Provided there is no other cause for their infertility, for example tubal damage, it then behooves the clinician to try induction of ovulation first. Infertility in patients with polycystic ovaries is caused either by PCOS (i.e., failure to ovulate at a normal rate and/or hypersecretion of LH) or by all the other causes of infertility or a combination of the two. Ovulation induction is appropriate for the first group (PCOS). IVF may be necessary in the second group (other causes) and in patients with PCOS who have failed to conceive despite at least six ovulatory cycles (i.e., those who have coexisting "unexplained" infertility).

The response of the PCO to stimulation in the context of ovulation induction aimed at the development of unifollicular ovulation is well documented and differs significantly from that of normal ovaries. The response tends to be slow initially but then with a danger of exceeding the threshold thereby presenting a significant risk of multiple follicle formation, multiple pregnancy, and ovarian hyperstimulation *(4,29–31)*. Conventional IVF currently depends on inducing multifollicular recruitment. It is thus to be expected that the response of the PCO within the context of an IVF program should also differ from the normal, with an 'explosive' nature of the ovarian response. There are several possible explanations for this 'explosive' response, which are beyond the scope of this chapter. Ovarian follicles, of which there are too many in polycystic ovaries, are increasingly sensitive to FSH (receptors for which are stimulated by high local concentrations of estrogen), and as a result, there is multiple follicular development associated with very high levels of circulating estrogen. In some cases, this may result in the ovarian hyperstimulation syndrome (OHSS), to which patients with polycystic ovaries are particularly prone *(32)*.

It is interesting also to note that the presence of polycystic ovaries is a marker for increased ovarian reserve and a reduced rate of ovarian aging *(33,34)*.

5.1. Insulin Resistance and Expression of PCOS

The cellular and molecular mechanisms of insulin resistance in PCOS have been extensively investigated, and it is evident that the major defect is a decrease in insulin sensitivity secondary to a post-binding abnormality in insulin receptor-mediated signal transduction, with a less substantial, but significant, decrease in insulin responsiveness *(35)*. It appears that decreased insulin sensitivity in PCOS is potentially an intrinsic defect in genetically susceptible women, as it is independent of obesity, metabolic abnormalities, body fat topography, and sex hormone levels. There may be genetic abnormalities in the regulation of insulin receptor phosphorylation, resulting in increased insulin-independent serine phosphorylation and decreased insulin-dependent tyrosine phosphorylation *(35)*.

Although the insulin resistance may occur irrespective of BMI, the common association of PCOS and obesity has a synergistic deleterious impact on glucose homeostasis and can worsen both hyperandrogenism and anovulation. Insulin acts through multiple sites to increase endogenous androgen levels. Increased peripheral insulin resistance results in a higher serum insulin concentration. Excess insulin binds to the IGF-1 receptors which enhances the theca cells androgen production in response to LH stimulation *(36)*. Hyperinsulinemia also decreases the synthesis of sex hormone-binding globulin (SHBG) by the liver. Therefore, there is an increase in serum-free testosterone (T) concentration and consequent peripheral androgen action. At the heart of the pathophysiology of PCOS for many is insulin resistance and hyperinsulinemia, and even if this is not the initiating cause in some, it is certainly an amplifier of hyperandrogenism in those that gain weight.

6. CONCLUSIONS

The presence of polycystic ovaries presents the possibility for a hyperandrogenic state and the expression of the PCOS in a facilitative environment, for example when stimulated by endogenous or exogenous gonadotropins or insulin. A counter argument may propose that the PCO is a secondary effect, whereby it is the exposure of a normal ovary to androgens (stimulated through insulin or LH) that makes it polycystic—although against this proposition is the observation that normalization of endocrinology does not appear to correct ovarian morphology.

There are likely to be many routes to the development of the PCOS, including a genetic predisposition, environmental factors, and disturbances of a number of endocrine pathways (e.g., the hypothalamic–pituitary–ovarian axis, feedback loops, hyperinsulinemia, and the metabolic syndrome). In some, the ovary may change as a secondary effect, whereas in others there may be an inherent defect originating in the ovary.

Polycystic ovaries are detected in about 27% of the general population, of whom approximately 80% have symptoms of PCOS, albeit usually mild. Thus, approximately 20% of women with polycystic ovaries are symptom free. The presence of polycystic ovaries, however, may be a marker for increased reproductive and metabolic risk. The presence of polycystic ovaries also appears to be associated with an increased ovarian reserve and a reduced rate of ovarian aging.

Ovarian dysfunction is expressed when the ovaries of women with polycystic ovaries alone are stressed, by either a gain in weight and rise in circulating insulin levels or stimulation with FSH for assisted conception treatments. Longitudinal studies are required to better explore the evolution of signs and symptoms of the syndrome over time in women with polycystic ovaries and by comparison with those with normal ovaries.

REFERENCES

1. Fauser B, Tarlatzis B, Chang J, Azziz R, Legro R, Dewailly D, Franks S, Balen AH, Bouchard P, Dahlgren E, Devoto, Diamanti E, Dunaif A, Filicori M, Homburg R, Ibanez L, Laven J, Magoffin D, Nestler J, Norman R, Pasquali R, Pugeat M, Strauss J, Tan SL, Taylor A, Wild R, Wild S. The Rotterdam ESHRE/ASRM-sponsored PCOS consensus workshop group. Revised 2003 consensus on

diagnostic criteria and long-term health risks related to polycystic ovary syndrome (PCOS). *Human Reprod* 2004; **19**:41–47.

2. Balen AH, Laven JSE, Tan SL, Dewailly D. Ultrasound assessment of the polycystic ovary: international consensus definitions. *Human Reprod Update* 2003; **9**:505–514.

3. Polson DW, Adams J, Wadsworth J, Franks S. Polycystic ovaries–a common finding in normal women. *Lancet* 1988;**1**:870–872.

4. Michelmore KF, Balen AH, Dunger DB, Vessey MP. Polycystic ovaries and associated clinical and biochemical features in young women. *Clin Endocrinol (Oxf)* 1999; **51**:779–786.

5. Balen AH, Conway GS, Kaltsas G, Techatraisak K, Manning PJ, West C, Jacobs HS. Polycystic ovary syndrome: the spectrum of the disorder in 1741 patients. *Human Reprod* 1995; **10**:2705–2712.

6. MacDougall MJ, Tan SL, Balen A, Jacobs HS. A controlled study comparing patients with and without polycystic ovaries undergoing in-vitro fertilization. *Hum Reprod* 1993; **8**:233–236.

7. Franks S, White D, Gilling-Smith C, Carey A, Waterworth D, Williamson R. Hypersecretion of androgens by polycystic ovaries: the role of genetic factors in the regulation of cytochrome P450c17α, *Ballieres Clin Endocrinol Metabol* 1996, **10**(2):193–203.

8. Rosenfield RL, Barnes RB, Cara JF, Lucky AW. Dysregulation of cytochrome P450c17α as the cause of polycystic ovarian syndrome. *Fertility Sterility* 1990, **53**(5):785–791.

9. Franks S. Polycystic ovary syndrome: a changing perspective. *Clin Endocrinol (Oxf)* 1989; **31**: 87–120.

10. Goldzieher JW. Polycystic ovarian disease. *Fertil Steril* 1981; **35**:371–394.

11. Polson DW, Adams J, Wadsworth J, Franks S. Polycystic ovaries–a common finding in normal women. *Lancet* 1988; **1**:870–872.

12. Tayob Y, Robinson G, Adams J, et al. Ultrasound appearance of the ovaries during the pill-free interval. *Br J Family Planning* 1990; **16**:94–96.

13. Clayton RN, Ogden V, Hodgkinson J, et al. How common are polycystic ovaries in normal women and what is their significance for the fertility of the population? [see comments]. *Clin Endocrinol (Oxf)* 1992; **37**:127–134.

14. Farquhar CM, Birdsall M, Manning P, Mitchell JM, France JT. The prevalence of polycystic ovaries on ultrasound scanning in a population of randomly selected women. *Aust N Z J Obstet Gynaecol* 1994; **34**:67–72.

15. Botsis D, Kassanos D, Pyrgiotis E, Zourlas PA. Sonographic incidence of polycystic ovaries in a gynecological population. *Ultrasound Obstet Gynecol* 1995; **6**:182–185.

16. Cresswell JL, Barker DJ, Osmond C, Egger P, Phillips DI, Fraser RB. Fetal growth, length of gestation, and polycystic ovaries in adult life. *Lancet* 1997; **350**:1131–1135.

17. Zawadski JK, Dunaif A Diagnostic criteria for polycystic ovary syndrome; towards a rational approach. In: *Polycystic Ovary Syndrome*. Dunaif A, Givens JR, Haseltine F, eds. Boston: Blackwell Scientific. 1992:377–384.

18. Dunaif A, Finegood DT. Beta-cell dysfunction independent of obesity and glucose intolerance in the polycystic ovary syndrome. *J Clin Endocrinol Metab* 1996; **81**:942–947.

19. Conway et al, 1993 Conway GS, Clark PM, Wong D. Hyperinsulinaemia in the polycystic ovary syndrome confirmed with a specific immunoradiometric assay for insulin. *Clin Endocrinol (Oxf)* 1993; **38**:219–222.

20. Isojarvi IT, Laatikainen T, Pakarinen AJ, Juntunen KTS, Myllyla VV. Polycystic ovaries and hyperandrogenism in women taking valporate for epilepsy. *N Engl J Med* 1993; **329**:1383–1388.

21. Webber LJ, Stubbs S, Stark J, Trew GH, Franks S. Formation and early development of follicles in the polycystic ovary. *Lancet* 2003; **362**:1017–1021.

22. White DW, Leigh A, Wilson C, et al. Gonadotrophin and gonadal steriod response to a single dose of a long-acting agonist of gonadotrophin-releasing hormone in ovulatory and anovulatory women with polycystic ovary syndrome. *Clin Endocrinol* 1995, **42**:475–481.

23. Barnes, RB, Rosenfield RL, Burstein S et al, Pituitary-ovarian response to nafarelin testing in the polycystic ovary syndrome. *N Engl J Med* 1989; **320**:559–563.

24. Erickson GF, Magoffin DA, Garza VG, et al., Granulosa cells of polycystic ovaries: are they normal or abnormal? *Hum Reprod* 1992 , **7**:293–299.

25. Mason HD, Willis DS, Beard RW, et al. Estradiol production by granulosa cells of normal and polycystic ovaries (PCO): relationship to menstrual cycle history and to concentrations of gonadotrophins and sex steroids in follicular fluid. *J Clin Endocrinol Metab* 1994, **79**:1355.

26. Anderson R, Groome N, Baird D. Inhibin A and inhibin B in women with polycystic ovarian syndrome during treatment with FSH to induce mono-ovulation. *Clin Endocrinol* 1998, **48**:577–582.

27. Schachter M, Balen AH, Patel A, Jacobs HS. Hypogonadotrophic patients with ultrasonographically diagnosed polycystic ovaries have aberrant gonadotropin secretion when treated with pulsatile gonadotrophin releasing hormone–a new insight into the pathophysiology of polycystic ovary syndrome. *Gynecol Endocrinol* 1996; **10**:327–335.

28. MacDougall JM, Tan SL, Hall V, Balen AH, Mason BA, Jacobs HS. Comparison of natural with clomiphene citrate-stimulated cycles in IVF: a prospective randomized trial. *Fertil Steril* 1994; **61**:1052–1057.

29. Balen AH, Braat DDM, West C, Patel A, Jacobs HS. Cumulative conception and live birth rates after the treatment of anovulatory infertility. An analysis of the safety and efficacy of ovulation induction in 200 patients. *Hum Reprod* 1994; **9**:1563–1570.

30. Smitz J, Camus M, Devroey P, Evard P, Wisanto A, Van Steirteghem AC. Incidence of severe ovarian hyperstimulation syndrome after gonadotropin releasing hormone agonist/HMG superovulation for *in-vitro* fertilization. *Hum Reprod* 1991; **6**:933–937.

31. Dor J, Shulman A, Levran D, Ben-Rafael Z, Rudak E, Mashiach S. The treatment of patients with polycystic ovary syndrome by *in-vitro* fertilization: a comparison of results with those patients with tubal infertility. *Hum Reprod* 1990; **5**:816–818.

32. Homburg R, Berkowitz D, Levy T, Feldberg D, Ashkenazi J, Ben-Rafael Z. *In-vitro* fertilization and embryo transfer for the treatment of infertility associated with polycystic ovary syndrome. *Fertil Steril* 1993; **60**:858–863.

33. Mulders-Annemarie-G-M-G-J, Laven-Joop-S-E, Eijkemans-Marinus-J-C, de-Jong-Frank-H, Themmen-Axel-P-N, Fauser-Bart-C-J-M. Changes in anti-Müllerian hormone serum cocentrations over time suggest delayed ovarian ageing in normogonadotrophic anovulatory infertility. *Hum Reprod* Sep 2004; **19**(9):2036–2042.

34. Nikolaou-D, Gilling-Smith-C. Early ovarian ageing: are women with polycystic ovaries protected? *Hum Reprod* Oct 2004; **19**(10):2175–2179.

35. Dunaif A. Insulin resistance and the polycystic ovary syndrome: mechanisms and implication for pathogenesis. *Endocr Rev* 1997; **18**:774–800.

36. Bergh C, Carlsson B, Olsson JH, Selleskog U, Hillensjo T. Regulstion of androgen production in cultured human thecal cells by insulin-like growth factor I and insulin. *Fertil Steril* 1993; **59**:323–331.

5 Genetic Analyses of Polycystic Ovary Syndrome

Margrit Urbanek, PhD

Summary

Polycystic ovary syndrome (PCOS) is a very common endocrine disorder with a strong genetic component that is characterized by hyperandrogenemia and menstrual irregularity. Over the last decade, the roles of more than 70 candidate genes in the etiology of PCOS have been evaluated. However, because of genetic and phenotypic heterogeneity and underpowered studies as a consequence of analyzing insufficiently large cohorts, the results of many of these studies remain inconclusive. This chapter will discuss the factors contributing to the complexity of genetic studies of PCOS including (1) the heritability of PCOS, (2) phenotyping heterogeneity, (3) power and study design of past and future genetic studies of PCOS, and (4) the results of a select group of candidate genes. Owing to the large number of PCOS candidate genes that have been studied, we have limited our discussion of candidate genes to six candidate gene regions that are specifically promising or have been studied intensively. The six genes are CYP11A, insulin gene variable number of tandem repeats (VNTR), calpain-10, sex hormone-binding globulin (SHBG), androgen receptor (AR) and X-chromosome inactivation, and the chromosome 19p13.2 susceptibility locus, D19S844. While past genetic studies of PCOS have yielded only modest results, the resources and techniques to remedy the major deficits of these early studies have now been assembled, promising that the next few years will be a very exciting and rewarding era for the genetic analysis of PCOS.

Key Words: PCOS; genetic association; linkage; CYP11A; insulin gene VNTR; androgen receptor; calpain-10; SHBG; D19S884.

From: *Contemporary Endocrinology: Polycystic Ovary Syndrome*
Edited by: A. Dunaif, R. J. Chang, S. Franks, and R. S. Legro © Humana Press, Totowa, NJ

1. POLYCYSTIC OVARY SYNDROME

Polycystic ovary syndrome (PCOS) is a genetically complex disorder that is characterized by hyperandrogenemia and amenhorrea/oligomenhorrea, resulting in the most
frequent cause of infertility among reproductive age women. It is also the most common
endocrinopathy among reproductive age women (1,2) affecting approximately 105
million reproductive age women worldwide (3). In addition to its reproductive features,
PCOS is associated with an increased risk of developing obesity (4,5), insulin resistance (6–11), and type 2 diabetes mellitus (T2DM) (12). Although PCOS can only be
diagnosed in reproductive age women, first-degree relatives of women with PCOS also
have an increased incidence of obesity, insulin resistance, and elevated triglycerides
(13–17). As a consequence, PCOS and its associated pathologies contribute approximately $4.36 billion annually to the health burden of the USA (3).

2. FAMILIAL BASIS OF PCOS

It has long been recognized that both environmental and genetic factors contribute to
the etiology of PCOS. For example, Kiddy et al. (18) have shown that weight loss
can reverse symptoms of PCOS, whereas Norman and colleagues have shown that
lifestyle modifications like moderate weight loss and exercise significantly improve
the hormonal profiles of both the reproductive and metabolic aspects of PCOS
(19–22). On the other hand, there is also a large familial component to the etiology
of PCOS (23–26), for which both dominant and multigenic modes of inheritance have
been proposed (23–32). However, until recently, it was unclear whether this familial
component is due to genetic factors or a shared environment. Vink et al. (32) used a
twin study paradigm to demonstrate that there is a strong heritable component to the
etiology of PCOS. They characterized 1332 monozygotic (share ~100% of genetic
material) and 1873 dizygotic or singleton sister pairs (share ~50% of genetic material)
from the Netherlands Twin Registry. Overall heritability for PCOS was 0.72 with a
correlation of 0.71 and 0.38 for monozygotic and dizygotic twin or non-twin sister
pairs. In addition to demonstrating the strong heritability of the disorder, the relatively
high correlation between dizygotic twins and between non-twin sister pairs found in
the study indicates that the genetic component of PCOS is likely to be due to a few
genes with a significant impact rather than many genes with minimal effect sizes. If this
is the case, it supports the feasibility of studies searching for PCOS susceptibility genes.

3. CURRENT STATUS OF PCOS GENETIC STUDIES

Over the last decade, many studies have investigated the genetic contribution to the
etiology of PCOS. All of these studies have been candidate gene analyses, an approach
that is very powerful when the biology of a disorder is understood well enough
to provide legitimate functional candidates. Several metabolic and/or biochemical
pathways are implicated in the etiology of PCOS, including those that regulate
gonadotropin secretion, affect androgen production and action, and influence insulin
signaling (33,34). As the connection between PCOS and the metabolic syndrome
becomes more clearly established, genes implicated in the development of diabetes
and obesity have also become ideal candidates.

Table 1
Studies of Candidate Genes for PCOS: all have been evaluated at the DNA level

Gene	Chromosome location	Polymorphism/ allele	Study design	Ethnicity	Sample size	Findings
ACTR1	12q13.12	D12S347	TDT[a]	>90% US Cauc.	150 families	Negative[b] (33)
			Linkage	>90% US Cauc.	39 ASPs[c]	Negative[b] (33)
ACTR2A	2q22.2	D2S2335	TDT[a]	>90% US Cauc.	150 families	Negative[b] (33)
			Linkage	>90% US Cauc.	39 ASPs[c]	Not significant[d] (33)
ACTR2B	3p22	D3S1298	TDT[a]	>90% US Cauc.	150 families	Negative[b] (33)
			Linkage	>90% US Cauc.	39 ASPs[c]	Negative[b] (33)
ADIPOQ	3q27.3		cc[e]	Finnish Cauc.	143 cases/245 controls	Negative[b] (127)
ADIPOQ	3q27.3	G45T	cc[e]	Spanish Cauc.	72 PCOS/42 controls	Negative[b] (128)
		T276G				
ADRB3	8p12	Y64R	cc[e]	Chilean	106 cases/82 controls	Negative[b] (129)
AGT	1q24.2	M235T	cc[e]	Italian Cauc.	95 cases/64 controls	Positive[b] (130)
		Epsilon2				
APOE	19q13.32	Epsilon3	cc[e]	Finnish Cauc.	58 PCOS/91controls	Negative[b] (131)
		Epsilon4				
AR	Xq11.2	(CAG)n	TDT[a]	>90% US Cauc.	150 families	Negative[b] (33)
			Linkage	>90% US Cauc.	39 ASPs[c]	Not significant[d] (33)

(Continued)

Table 1
(Continued)

Gene	Chromosome location	Polymorphism/ Allele	Study Design	Ethnicity	Sample size	Findings
AR	Xq11.2	(CAG)n	cc[e]	US Hispanic	110 infertility patients	No association with measures hyperandrogenism (88)
AR	Xq11.2	(CAG)n	cc[e]	Chinese, Asian Indian	91 PCOS/112 controls	Shorter repeats associated with lower androgen levels (89)
AR	Xq11.2	(CAG)n	cc[e]	Australian Cauc.	205 PCOS/831 controls	Longer repeats associated with PCOS (86)
AR	Xq11.2	(CAG)n	cc[e]	Finnish Cauc.	106 cases/112 controls	Negative[b] (87)
CAPN10	2q37.3	SNP-43 SNP-19 SNP-63 SNP-44	cc[e]	African American US Cauc.	57 African American PCOS 124 Caucasian PCOS	Positive Association elevated insulin levels in OGTT in African American women (73)
CAPN10	2q37.3	SNP-43 SNP-19 SNP-63 SNP-44	TDT[a] cc[e]	Cauc.	146 trios 331 PCOS/525 controls	Negative[b] (74)

Gene	Location	Marker	Method	Population	Sample	Result
CAPN10	2q37.3	SNP-43 SNP-19 SNP-63	cc[e]	Spanish Cauc.	148 PCOS/93 controls	Positive SNP44 only (75, 76)
CYP1A	15q24.1	T6235C	cc[e]	South Indian	180 PCO/72 controls	Positive (132)
CYP11A	15q23	D19S519	Linkagec cc[e]	European and Asian European	20 multiplex families 97 PCOS/51 PCO[f]/59 controls	Positive (44) Positive (44)
CYP11A	15q23	D19S519	cc[e]	Greek Cauc.	80 PCOS/90 controls	Positive(45)
CYP11A	15q23	D19S519	cc[e]	Spanish Cauc.	92 hirsute women/33 controls	Negative[b] (47)
CYP11A	15q23	D19S519 D15S520	TDT[a] Linkage	>90% US Cauc. >90% US Cauc.	150 families 39 ASPs[c]	Negative[b] (33) Not significant[d] (33)

(Continued)

Table 1
(Continued)

Gene	Chromosome location	Polymorphism/ Allele	Study Design	Ethnicity	Sample size	Findings
CYP11A	15q23	D15S520 P4 repeat	cc[e] TDT[a]	Finish Cauc. British Cauc. British Cauc.	1589 population cohort440 PCOS/1062 controls 255 trios	Not significant[d] (48)
CYP17	10q24.3	−34 promoter	cc[e]	British Cauc	69 PCOS/63 CAH[g]/124 controls	Negative[b] (133)
CYP17	10q24.3	−34 promoter	cc[e]	CaucAsian	55 PCOS/56 controls	Negative[b] (134)
CYP17	10q24.3	−34 promoter	cc[e]	Polish Cauc.		Negative[b] (135)
CYP17	10q24.3	−34 promoter	cc[e]	Greek Cauc.	50 PCOS/50 controls	Possible increased risk with C/C genotype (136)
CYP17	10q24.3	D10S192	cc[e]	US Cauc.	85 PCOS/87 controls	Negative[b] (137)
CYP17	10q24.3	D10S192	TDT[a] Linkage	>90% US Cauc. >90% US Cauc.	150 families 39 ASPs[c]	Not significant[d] (33) Negative[b] (33)
CYP17	10q24.3	−34 promoter	cc[e]	US Cauc.	259 PCOS/161 controls	Negative[b] (138)
CYP19	15q21	CYP19	cc[e]	US Cauc	85 PCOS/87 controls	Negative[b] (137)

Gene	Location	Variant	Method	Population	Sample	Result (ref)
CYP19	15q21	CYP19 rs12907866 rs2414096	TDT[a] Linkage	>90% US Cauc. >90% US Cauc.	150 families 39 ASPs[c]	Not significant[d] (33) Negative[b] (33)
				Spanish Cauc.	186 PP[h]/71 controls	Positive for rs241096 and haplotype (139)
CYP19	15q21	SNP60 rs4646 Haplotype	cc[e]	UK (97% Cauc.)	224 women cohort	Positive for rs241096 (139)
CYP19	15q21	–	Mutation screen	Mexican-Mestizo	25 PCOS/50 controls	Negative[b] (140)
CYP21	6p21.1	V281L P30L Intron 2 I172N	cc[e]		30 HA[i] girls/14 controls	Increased heterozygosity in symptomatic hyperandrogenism (141)
CYP21	6p21.1	V281L Q318X R354W P453S	cc[e]	US Cauc.	109 PCOS/95 controls	Negative[b] (142)
DRD3	3q13.31	MscI	cc[e]	US Cauc.	152 PCOS/96 controls	Negative[b] (143)
DRD3	3q13.31	MscI Y113H	cc[e]	US Hispanic	180 women	Positive association w/irregular menses (144)

(Continued)

Table 1
(Continued)

Gene	Chromosome location	Polymorphism/ Allele	Study Design	Ethnicity	Sample size	Findings
EPHX	1q42.12	H139R	cc[e]	Finnish Cauc.	112 PCOS/115 controls	Positive haplotype only (145)
FS	5p14	Haplotype D5S474 D5S623	TDT[a]	>90% US Cauc.	150 families	Negative[b] (33)
		D5S822	Linkage	>90% US Cauc.	39 ASPs[c]	Positive (33)
FS	5p14	–	Mutation screen	Chinese	64 PCOS	no mutations (146)
FS	5p14	D5S474 D5S623	Mutation Screen	>90% US Cauc.	19 multiplex families	Negative[b] (147)
		D5S822	TDT[a]	>90% US Cauc.	324 trios	
		Exon 6 SNP	Linkage	>90% US Cauc.	75 ASPs	
FS	5p14	D5S474 D5S623	cc[e]	US Cauc	85 PCOS/87 controls	Negative[b] (137)
		D5S822				
FSHR	2p21	–	Mutation Screen	Japanese	15 POF/38 PCOS/3 controls	Negative[b] (148)

Gene	Locus	Variant	Method	Population	Sample	Result
FSHR	2p21	2p21	Mutation screen / cc^e	Singapore Chinese / Singapore Chinese	16 POF^i/124 PCOS124 PCOS/236 controls	Negative^b (149) / Negative^b (149)
FSHR	2p21	D2S1352	TDT^a / Linkage	>90% US Cauc. / >90% US Cauc.	150 families / 39 ASPs^c	Negative^b (33) / Negative^b (33)
FSHR	2p21	T307A N680S	cc^e	Japanese	522 cohort	Positive (150)
FSH-β	11p14.1	Exon 3 T/C	Mutation screen / cc^e	Singapore Chinese	135 PCOS/105 Controls	Possibly associated with PCOS (151)
GATA6	18q11.2	hCV7490431 hCV1892216 rs1941084	Mutation screen / TDT^a	>90% US Cauc. / >90% US Cauc.	15 PCOS/5 controls469 families	Negative^b (152)
GDF9	5q23.3	–	Mutation screen	Japanese	15 POF^i/38 PCOS/3 controls	No polymorphisms (153)
BMP15 (GDF9B)	Xq11.2	–	Mutation screen	Japanese	15 POF^i/38 PCOS/3 controls	No polymorphisms (153)
GnRH	8p21.2	–	Mutation screen	US Cauc.	80 PCOS	No mutations in exons (154)
GRL	5q32	Asn363Ser	cc^e		114 PCOS/92 controls	Negative^b (155)
GSTM1	1p13.3		cc^e	South Indian	180 PCO^f/72 controls	Negative^b (132)
GST1	22q11.23		cc^e	South Indian	180 PCO^f/72 controls	Negative^b (132)

(Continued)

Table 1
(Continued)

Gene	Chromosome location	Polymorphism/ Allele	Study Design	Ethnicity	Sample size	Findings
H6PD	1p36.22	R453Q	cc[e]	Spanish Cauc.	116 PCOS/76 controls	Positive (156)
HSD11B1	1q32.2	T1971G	cc[e]	Racially mixed	3551 population cohort	Negative[b] (157)
HSD11B1	1q32.2	83557insA	cc[e]	Spanish Cauc	116 PCOS/76 controls	Negative[b] (156)
HSD17B1	17q21.2	D17S934	TDT[a] Linkage	>90% US Cauc. >90% US Cauc.	150 families 39 ASPs[c]	Negative[b] (33) Negative[b] (33)
HSD17B2	16q24.1	HSD17B2	TDT[a] Linkage	>90% US Cauc. >90% US Cauc.	150 families 39 ASPs[c]	Not significant[d] (33) Negative[b] (33)
HSD1B3	9q22	D9S1809	TDT[a] Linkage	>90% US Cauc. >90% US Cauc.	150 families 39 ASPs[c]	Negative[b] (33) Negative[b] (33)
HSD17B3	9q22	Ser289Gly	cc[e]	US racially mixed	46 PCOS/32 controls	Negative[b] (158)
HSD17B5	10p15.1	G-71A	cc[e]	US racially mixed	121 PCOS/128 controls	Positive (159)
HSD3B1	1p31.1	D1S514	TDT[a] Linkage	>90% US Cauc. >90% US Cauc.	150 families 39 ASPs[c]	Negative[b] (33) Negative[b] (33)
HSD3B2	1p31.1	D1S514	TDT[a] Linkage	>90% US Cauc. >90% US Cauc.	150 families 39 ASPs[c]	Negative[b] (33) Negative[b] (33)

Gene	Locus	Marker	Method	Population	Sample	Result
IGF1	12q23.2	IGF1 STRP	TDT[a]	>90% US Cauc.	150 families	Negative[b] (33)
			Linkage	>90% US Cauc.	39 ASPs[c]	Negative[b] (33)
IGF1	12q23.2	IGF1 STRP	cc[e]	Spanish Cauc.	72 PCOS/42 controls	Negative[b] (127)
IGF1R	15q26.3	IGF1R	TDT[a]	>90% US Cauc.	150 families	Negative[b] (33)
			Linkage	>90% US Cauc.	39 ASPs[c]	Negative[b] (33)
IGF1R	15q26.3	IGF1R	cc[e]	Spanish Cauc.	72 PCOS/42 controls	Negative[b] (127)
IGF2	11p15.5	ApaI GA 3′ UTR	cc[e]	Spanish Cauc.	72 PCOS/42 controls	Positive (127)
IGF2R	6q25.3	ACAA in/del 3′ UTR	cc[e]	Spanish Cauc.	72 PCOS/42 controls	Negative[b] (127)
IGFBP1	7p13	D7S519	TDT[a]	>90% US Cauc.	150 families	Not significant[d] (33)
			Linkage	>90% US Cauc.	39 ASPs[c]	Negative[b] (33)
IGFBP3	7p13	D7S519	TDT[a]	>90% US Cauc.	150 families	Not significant[d] (33)
			Linkage	>90% US Cauc.	39 ASPs[c]	Negative[b] (33)
IL-6	G-174C		cc[e]	Austrian Cauc.	62 PCOS/94 controls	Negative[b][161]
INHA	2q35	D2S163	TDT[a]	>90% US Cauc.	150 families	Negative[b] (33)
			Linkage	>90% US Cauc.	39 ASPs[c]	Negative[b] (33)
INHBA	7p14.1	INHBA STRP	TDT[a]	>90% US Cauc.	150 families	Negative[b] (33)
			Linkage	>90% US Cauc.	39 ASPs[c]	Not significant[d] (33)

(Continued)

Table 1
(Continued)

Gene	Chromosome location	Polymorphism/Allele	Study Design	Ethnicity	Sample size	Findings
INHBB	2q14.2	D2S293	TDT[a] Linkage	>90% US Cauc. >90% US Cauc.	150 families 39 ASPs[c]	Not significant[d] (33) Not significant[d] (33)
INHC	12q13	D12S1691	TDT[a] Linkage	>90% US Cauc. >90% US Cauc.	150 families 39 ASPs[c]	Not significant[d] (33) Negative[b] (33)
INS	11p15.5	INS VNTR	TDT[a] cc[e]	>95% Cauc.	224 population cohort	Positive paternal transmission of class III allele (61)
INS	11p15.5	INS VNTR	cc[e] TDT Linkage	British Cauc. Racial Mixed Racial Mixed	59 PCOS/52 controls 17 multiplex families 17 multiplex families	Positive linkage & association with paternal transmission of class III allele (60)
INS	11p15.5	INS VNTR	TDT[a] Linkage	>90% US Cauc. >90% US Cauc.	150 families 39 ASPs[c]	Negative[b] (33) Negative[b] (33)
INS	11p15.5	INS VNTR	cc[e]	Spanish Cauc	96 HA[h]/38 controls	Negative[b] (62)
INS	11p15.5	INS VNTR	cc[e]	Czech Cauc.	38 PCOS/22 controls	Negative[b] (63)
INS	11p15.5	INS VNTR	cc[e] TDT[a]	Finish Cauc. British Cauc. British Cauc.	1589 pop. Cohort440 PCOS/1062 controls255 trios	Negative[b] (64)

Gene	Location	Marker	Method	Population	Sample	Result
INSR	19p13.3	INSR STRP	TDT[a] Linkage	>90% US Cauc. >90% US Cauc.	150 families 39 ASPs[c]	Negative[b] (33) Not significant[d] (33)
INSR	19p13.3	H1058H C/T	cc[e]	US Cauc.	99 PCOS/136 controls	Positive (161)
Chr19p3.13	19p13.3	D19S884	TDT[a] Linkage	>90% US Cauc. >90% US Cauc.	367 families 107 ASPs[c]	Positive (33, 94) Positive (94)
Chr19p3.13	19p13.3	D19S884	cc[e]	US Cauc.	85 PCOS/87 controls	Positive (137)
Chr19p3.13	19p13.3	D19S884	cc[e]	Spanish Cauc. Italian Cauc.	50 PCOS/37 controls 58 PCOS/29 controls	Negative[b] (96) Negative[b] (96)
INSL3 D19S410	19p13.2	D19S212	TDT[a] Linkage	>90% US Cauc. >90% US Cauc.	150 families 39 ASPs[c]	Negative[b] (33) Not significant[d] (33)
IRS1	2q36.3	IRS1 STRP	TDT[a] Linkage	>90% US Cauc. >90% US Cauc.	150 families 39 ASPs[c]	Negative[b] (33) Not significant[d] (33)
IRS1	2q36.3	Gly972Arg	Mutation screen cc[e]	Cauc. Cauc.	28 PCOS 53 PCOS/224 controls	Positive association with fasting insulin levels (162)
IRS1	2q36.3	Gly972Arg	cc[e]	Turkish Cauc.	60 PCOS/60 controls	Positive (163)
IRS1	2q36.3	Gly972Arg	cc[e]	Spanish Cauc.	103 cases/48 controls	Negative[b] (164)

(Continued)

Table 1
(Continued)

Gene	Chromosome location	Polymorphism/Allele	Study Design	Ethnicity	Sample size	Findings
IRS1	2q36.3	Gly972Arg	cc[e]	US Cauc.	109 cases/95 controls	Negative[b] (142)
IRS1	2q36.3	Gly972Arg	cc[e]	Chilean	146 PCOS/97controls	Positive (165)
IRS2	13q34	Gly1057Asp	cc[e]	Spanish Cauc.	103 cases/48 controls	Negative[b] (164)
IRS2	13q34	Gly1057Asp	Mutation screen cc[e]	Cauc. Cauc.	28 PCOS53 PCOS/224 controls	Negative[b] (162) Negative[b] (164)
LEP	7q32.1	D7S1875	TDT[a] Linkage	US Cauc.US Cauc.	150 families 39 ASPs[c]	Not significant[d] (33) Negative[b] (33)
LEP	7q32.1	–	Mutation screen cc[e]	Finnish Cauc. Finnish Cauc.	38 PCOS38 PCOS/122 controls	Negative[b] (166) Negative[b] (166)
LEPR	1p31	D1S198	TDT Linkage	US Cauc. US Cauc.	150 families 39 ASPs[c]	Negative[b] (33)
LEPR	1p31	K109R Q223R K656N 3' UTR	Mutation screen cc[e]	Finnish Cauc.Finnish Cauc	38 PCOS38 PCOS/122 controls	Negative[b] (33) Negative[b] (166) Negative[b] (166)
LEPR	1p31	Q223R	cc[e]	Turkish	56 PCOS/58 controls	Negative[b] (167)
LH-β	19q13.33	Trp8ArgIle 15Thr	cc[e]	Finnish, Dutch, UK, and US Cauc.	363 PCOS/944 controls	Positive for UK only (168)

Gene	Locus	Variant/Marker	Method	Population	Sample	Result (Ref.)
LH-β	19q13.33	Exon 3 (Gly102Ser)	cc[e]	Korean	68 PCOS/59 controls	Negative[b] (169)
LHCGR	2p21	D2S1352	TDT[a] Linkage	US Cauc. US Cauc.	150 families 39 ASPs[c]	Negative[b] (33) Negative[b] (33)
MADH4	18q21.1	D18S474	TDT[a] Linkage	US Cauc. US Cauc.	150 families 39 ASPs[c]	Not significant[d] (33) Negative[b] (33)
MIS	19p13.3	–	Mutation screen	Japanese	43 PCOS/20 controls	Negative[b] (170)
MC4R	18q21.32	D18S64	TDT[a] Linkage	US Cauc. US Cauc.	150 families 39 ASPs[c]	Negative[b] (33) Negative[b] (33)
MMP1	11q22.2	–1607 GG/G	cc[e]	Austrian Cauc.	62 cases/94 controls	Positive (171)
MTHFR	1p36.22	C677T	cc[e]	Italian Cauc	70 PCOS/70 controls	Negative[b] (172)
PAI1	7q22.1	4G/5G promoter	cc[e]	Austrian Cauc.	106 PCOS/102 controls	Negative[b] (173)
PAI1	7q22.1	4G/5G promoter	cc[e]	Greek Cauc	98 PCOS/ 64 controls	Positive (174)
PAI1	7q22.1	4G/5G promoter	cc[e]	Spanish Cauc.	72 PCOS/42 controls	Negative[b] (128)
PC-1	6q23.2	K121Q	cc[e]	Finnish Cauc.	143 PCOS/115 controls	Positive (175)
PC-1	6q23.2	K121Q	cc[e]	Spanish Cauc.	72 PCOS/42 controls	Negative[b] (128)
POMC	2p23	D2S131 C-108T	TDT Linkage	US Cauc. US Cauc.	150 families 39 ASPs[c]	Not significant[d] (33) Negative[b] (33)
PON1	7q21.3	L55M N192R	cc[e]	Spanish Cauc.	72 PCOS/42 controls	Positive C-108T only (128)

(Continued)

Table 1
(Continued)

Gene	Chromosome location	Polymorphism/ Allele	Study Design	Ethnicity	Sample size	Findings
PPARG	3p25.2	D3S1263	TDT[a]	US Cauc.	150 families	Negative[b] (33)
PPARG	3p25.2	Pro12Ala	Linkage	US Cauc.	39 ASPs[c]	Negative[b] (33)
PPARG	3p25.2	Pro12Ala	cc[e]	Cauc.	102 cases/104 controls	Negative[b] (176)
PPARG	3p25.2	Pro12AlaExon 6 C →T	cc[e]	Italian Cauc. Italian Cauc.	120 PCOS/120 controls100 PCOS/100 controls	Negative[b] (177, 178) Positive (178)
PPARG	3p25.2	Pro12Ala	cc[e]	Spanish Cauc.	72 PCOS/42 controls	Negative[b] (128)
PPARG	3p25.2	Pro12Ala	cc[e]	Finnish Cauc.	135 PCOS/115 controls	Negative[b] (179)
PTP1B	20q13.13	Ins/del 1484GC981T	cc[e]	Spanish Cauc.	72 PCOS/42 controls	Negative[b] (128)
RSTN	19p13.3	−420 C/G	TDT[a]	US Cauc.	258 families	Negative[b] (180)
SHBG	17p13.2	D17S1353	TDT[a]	US Cauc.	150 families	Negative[b] (33)
SHBG	17p13.2		Linkage	US Cauc.	39 ASPs[c]	Negative[b] (33)
SHBG	17p13.2	Promoter (TAAAA)$_n$	cc[e]	Greek Cauc.	185 PCOS/324 controls	Positive (83)
SORBS1	10q24.1	T228A	cc[e]	Spanish Cauc.	72 PCOS/42 controls	Negative[b] (128)
STAR	8p11.2	D8S1821	TDT[a]	US Cauc.	150 families	Negative[b] (33)
STAR	8p11.2		Linkage	US Cauc.	39 ASPs[c]	Negative[b] (33)
TNFα	6p21.1	−C-850T promoter	cc[e]	Finnish Cauc	87 PCOS/155 controls	Negative[b] (181)

Gene	Locus	Variant	Method	Population	Sample	Result
TNFα	6p21.1	−308 promoter M196R	cc[e]	Australian Cauc.	84 PCOS + 38 PCO/136 controls	Negative[b] (182)
TNFRSF1B	1p36.22	G1663A 3′UTR T1668G 3′UTR T1690C 3′UTR	cc[e]	Spanish Cauc. Italian Cauc.	42 PCOS/36 controls64 PCOS/29 controls	Positive M196R only (183)
UCP-2	11q13	D11S911	TDT[a] Linkage	US Cauc. US Cauc.	150 families 39 ASPs[c]	Negative[b] (33) Negative (33)
UCP-3	11q13	D11S911	TDT[a] Linkage	US Cauc. US Cauc.	150 families 39 ASPs[c]	Negative[b] (33) Negative[b] (33)

[a]TDT Transmission Disequilibrium Test, family based test for association in the presence of linkage.

[b]Negative absence of evidence for association.

[c]ASPs Affected sib pairs.

[d]Not significant nominal significant finding but not significant after correcting for multiple testing.

[e]cc case control population based association study.

[f]PCO polycystic ovarian morphology.

[g]CAH congenital adrenal hyperplasia

[h]PP premature pubarche.

[i]HA hyperandrogenemia.

[j]POF premature ovarian failure.

To date, the roles of more than 70 genes in the etiology of PCOS have been evaluated (see Table 1 for a summary of relevant PCOS genetic studies). However, with a few notable exceptions which an discussed below (i.e. the insulin gene VNTR, CYPIIA, and D195884), the findings of these studies have been ambiguous or lacked replication. This lack of reproducibility is endemic to association studies of common traits *(35–38)* and can be attributed to multiple factors that plague both the genetic analysis of complex diseases in general and specifically PCOS. These factors include (1) an absence of consistent phenotype criteria being used across studies, (2) limited sample sizes, and (3) incomplete characterization of candidate genes.

One obvious drawback of the candidate gene approach is that genes that are not a priori reasoned to play a role in the disorder will not be evaluated. In order to be able to fully assess the impact of genetic variation on the etiology of PCOS, a non-biased approach is required such as a whole genome linkage scan or a genome-wide association (WGA) study, neither one of which has been applied to PCOS. Linkage analysis with a few exceptions has not been a very successful approach for the identification of complex genetic disorders such as PCOS. Additionally, linkage analysis is dependent on co-segregation of the disease trait and a genetic marker(s) in *multiple* members of a family. Sufficient numbers of such families (>200 families) to carry out genome-wide linkage study have been very difficult to collect (1) because of the inability to assign a phenotype to male relatives and non-reproductive female relatives, (2) because of the inability to assign a phenotype to reproductive age women who are taking confounding medications such as oral contraceptives and insulin-sensitizing drugs both of which are very common occurrences in this group of women due to their age and the high incidence of insulin resistance in PCOS families, and (3) finally, because PCOS results in reduced fertility, families that segregate PCOS are more likely to be smaller than the norm making multiplex families relatively rare and/or the selection of multiplex (i.e., large) families results in a selection bias toward a subtype of PCOS with only a modest impact on fertility and which may not be representative of PCOS in the general population. The molecular and analytical techniques for WGA studies are just becoming available and are a promising approach for the genetic analysis of PCOS (see Heading 5).

3.1. Phenotyping

PCOS is a complex syndrome with multiple features (hyperandrogenism, menstrual irregularity, ovarian morphology, and gonadotropin dysregulation) contributing to the overall phenotype. Therefore, different aspects of the disease may be under the control of unique genes, and the specific characteristics that are emphasized in the assignment of the phenotype may affect the outcome of the genetic analysis. A useful approach for genetic analyses in this situation would be to restrict the phenotype to a limited number of phenotypic characteristics with the expectation that this phenotypically more homogeneous subset of patients is also genetically more homogeneous. For instance, we have limited our analyses to patients with biochemical hyperandrogenemia and fewer than six menses per year. We realize that these criteria do not include all possible PCOS patients but may instead identify a subset of families with the same underlying defect. In fact, this approach has allowed us to identify a PCOS susceptibility locus mapping to chr19p13.2.

In an attempt to standardize the definition of PCOS, guidelines for the designation of PCOS were established in 1990, and more recently in 2003. The 1990 NIH Criteria requires that two criteria be filled for the diagnosis of PCOS *(39)*: clinical (acne or hirsutism) or/and biochemical hyperandrogenemia (measured elevated androgen levels) and menstrual irregularity. The 2003 Rotterdam Criteria requires that two of the following three criteria need to be filled for the diagnosis of PCOS *(40)*. The Rotterdam criteria are as follows: (1) clinical (acne or hirsutism) or/and biochemical hyperandrogenemia (measured elevated androgen levels, (2) menstrual irregularity, and (3) polycystic ovarian morphology on ultrasound. However, although there is a large degree of overlap between these guidelines, they still allow for multiple designations of the phenotype and the actual definition of hyperandrogenism (clinical or biochemical), and irregular menses varies from investigator to investigator. Therefore, although a given set of criteria for the phenotype of PCOS is not necessarily better or more appropriate than another set of criteria, it is critical that investigators and readers of the literature are aware of the potential differences in phenotypic characterizations and the impact of such variability on the outcome of studies.

3.2. Sample Sizes

A major limitation of most of the PCOS studies conducted to date is that they are based on very small sample sizes (Table 1). From successful studies of other genetically complex diseases, it is now clear that most susceptibility alleles have relatively small effect sizes [reviewed in *(36,38)*] and as such require sample sizes of several hundred, if not thousand, patients. For instance, in the case of the peroxisome proliferator-activated receptor gamma (PPAR-γ) Pro12Ala polymorphism, one of the few unambiguous type 2 diabetes susceptibility alleles identified to date, the more common proline residue is associated with approximately 1.25 increased risk of developing T2DM and a population attributable risk for diabetes of 25% *(41)*. However, owing to the small relative risk associated with this variant, it required a meta-analysis of approximately 3000 individuals to definitively establish its role in the pathology of T2DM. Similarly, Grant et al. were able to identify transcription factor 7-like 2 (*TCF7L2*), a very promising susceptibility gene for T2DM associated with a relative risk of 1.5, in an association study of 1185 cases and 931 controls *(42)*. Given the large sample sizes required to detect these loci, the majority of PCOS genetic studies have been vastly underpowered. To date, studies from only a few groups have used samples sizes with greater than 300 probands (Table 1).

One reason for the small sample sizes used in the genetic studies of PCOS is that although PCOS is a very common disorder, it has been difficult to collect sufficiently large cohorts of patients due to multiple characteristics inherent to the disorder. One major limitation is that PCOS, as mentioned above, can only be accurately assessed in reproductive age women who are not taking several common medications (oral contraceptives, insulin-sensitizing medication, etc.). This also automatically excludes men, severely limits the pool from which women with PCOS can be recruited, and is even more detrimental to the recruitment of the affected family members critical for linkage studies. Although it is clear that male relatives of women with PCOS are at an increased risk of developing features of the metabolic syndrome *(16,17)*, it is currently impossible to unambiguously assign a phenotype to them. Finally, as PCOS is a disorder with reduced fertility, large families are uncommon and families with multiple eligible sisters are rare.

3.3. Variant Choice

For Mendelian traits, a single mutation within one gene often accounts for most, if not all, of the genetic variation contributing to the phenotype of the disease. By definition, genetically complex diseases like PCOS have multiple variants that contribute to the etiology of a disease due to genetic heterogeneity (variants in multiple genes) and/or allelic heterogeneity (multiple variants within one gene). In addition, susceptibility alleles for complex traits unlike of those of many Mendelian traits are not constrained to missense or nonsense mutations. As variants contributing to complex traits are expected to be common and therefore cannot be under strong selective pressure (36,37,43), they are expected to have more subtle consequences that are likely to affect transcript expression levels or processing. Such variants are much more difficult to recognize. It is therefore critical to characterize the genetic variation of an entire candidate gene, including the regulatory regions. For most genetic studies of PCOS, including most of our studies, only one or a few variants per gene have been tested, and very few studies have characterized the entire gene directly using SNPs or indirectly using haplotype analysis.

4. PCOS CANDIDATE GENES

To date greater than 70 PCOS candidate genes have been characterized using a variety of genetic approaches. Rather that discuss these genes individually, we have generated a table with the salient features of the study and appropriate references (Table 1), and we will focus our discussion on the several loci for which there is convincing evidence regarding their role in PCOS, for which a consensus may be reached in the near future, or which offer an interesting insight into their potential action in the etiology of PCOS. These loci include *CYP11A*, the insulin gene variable number of tandem repeats (VNTR), calpain-10, sex hormone-binding globulin (SHBG), the androgen receptor (AR) and X-inactivation, and D19S884, a dinucleotide repeat marker mapping to chr19p13.2.

4.1. CYP11A

CYP11A is an ideal functional candidate gene for PCOS because it encodes the gene for the cytochrome p450 side chain cleavage enzyme, the rate-limiting step in androgen biosynthesis. In 1997, Gharani et al. (44) showed evidence for linkage between *CYP11A* and PCOS. Subsequently, Urbanek et al. found modest evidence for linkage between PCOS and *CYP11A* [(33) and unpublished data]. Gharani et al. also found an association with allele 5 of D15S520, which is located in the promoter region of *CYP11A* although Urbanek et al. could not provide replication for association at D15S520 (33). Two additional studies by Diamanti-Kandarakis et al. (45) and Daneshmand et al. (46) did show evidence for association between CYP11A promoter alleles and PCOS. However, a study by San Millan et al. (47) in a Spanish cohort failed to show evidence for association between the D15S520 pentanucleotide repeat and PCOS.

More recently, Gaasenbeek et al. (48) assessed the role of CYP11A in the etiology of PCOS using a large scale family- and population-based association study including

371 PCOS patients and 331 population controls from the United Kingdom and 527 symptomatic women and 1062 cohort controls from the Northern Finland Birth Cohort of 1966. The UK cohort included 141 parent–offspring trios. Although the authors did detect a statistically significant difference in allele frequencies for both markers in the patients and controls from the United Kingdom, these results were in the opposite direction of that in previous findings (the alleles that are positively associated with PCOS in the current studies were not associated with PCOS in the initial studies) and the findings United Kingdom case-control cohort were not replicated in the trios or the Finnish cohort. There were no significant associations between the haplotypes of the two markers and PCOS in these samples.

Taken as a whole, the CYP11A genetic association studies indicate that there is no convincing evidence for association between genetic variants in the promoter of the gene and PCOS in the Caucasian population and inconclusive evidence for linkage. In addition, variants in the CYP11A gene that are not in linkage disequilibrium with the promoter variants have not been tested and could also play a role in the etiology of PCOS.

4.2. Insulin Gene VNTR

The insulin gene VNTR is a series of 14 or 15 base pair repeats that are located in the 5′ regulatory element of the insulin gene. Alleles of the insulin gene VNTR are divided into three classes dependent on the number of repeats: class I with an average length of 26–63 repeats, class II with an average of 64–140 repeats, and class III with an average of 141–209 repeats *(49)*. The VNTR regulates transcription of the insulin gene *(50–55)* and is associated with hyperinsulinemia *(55)*, susceptibility to T2DM *(51,56,57)*, birth weight *(57)*, fasting insulin levels *(58)*, and the development of childhood *(59)* and juvenile obesity *(58)*. In 1997, Waterworth et al. *(60)* showed evidence for modest linkage between PCOS and the insulin gene VNTR in 17 families and preferential transmission of the class III alleles of the insulin gene VNTR from the father to PCOS patients *(60)*. This positive association between paternally inherited class III alleles was subsequently confirmed by Michelmore et al. *(61)*. However, Urbanek et al. found no evidence for linkage between PCOS and the insulin VNTR in 28 multiplex families and no evidence of association between the insulin gene VNTR class III allele in general or specifically the paternally inherited allele in a much larger sample of 150 nuclear families *(33)* nor in an independent follow-up study of similar size by the same authors (unpublished data). In addition, Calvo et al. *(62)* failed to detect an association between the insulin gene VNTR and hyperandrogenemia in Spanish women, and Vankova et al. *(63)* failed to detect an association between the INS VNTR and PCOS in a Czech population *(63)*. Finally, in a large multicohort study including 255 parent–proband trios, 185 PCOS cases, and 1062 controls from the United Kingdom and 1599 women from the Northern Finland Birth Cohort of 1966, Powell et al. *(64)* failed to find evidence for association between the insulin gene VNTR Class III alleles and PCOS or testosterone levels. When data from all the studies are considered in their totality, it appears unlikely that the insulin gene VNTR plays an important role in the etiology of PCOS.

4.3. Calpain-10

The cysteine protease caplain-10 (CAPN10) maps to chromosome 2q37.3 and is expressed in all adult and fetal tissues examined to date. Calpain-10 was first identified as a susceptibility locus for T2DM in a genome-wide linkage scan for T2DM in Mexican Americans followed by positional cloning *(65,66)*, and it remains one of the few complex disease genes identified in this way. Association and linkage analysis identified two SNP haplotypes (designated 112 and 121) defined by three closely linked non-coding SNPs (UCSNP-43, -19, and -63) that conferred an increased risk for diabetes to individuals who were doubly heterozygous for the haplotypes (i.e., had the genotype 112/121) *(66)*. These findings were replicated in populations of Northern European descent *(66)* but not in a study of British diabetes patients *(67)* or Samoans with T2DM *(68)*. However, meta-analyses do support a modest role for *CAPN10* in susceptibility to T2DM in Europeans *(69–71)*, and *CAPN10* has been shown to be associated with insulin resistance *(72)*. Functional studies have shown that the G allele at UCSNP-43 is associated with reduced muscle mRNA levels of calpain-10 and insulin resistance in non-diabetic Pima Indians. Calpain-10 has also been found to play a role in insulin secretion and action. As T2DM and insulin resistance are often associated with PCOS, calpain-10, therefore, is also a plausible candidate gene for PCOS.

Multiple studies have examined the contribution of calpain-10 to the etiology of PCOS. Ehrmann et al. *(73)* tested 124 PCOS patients of European descent and 57 African American PCOS patients for association between the T2DM-associated DNA polymorphism and a series of phenotypic characteristics of PCOS and T2DM. They found no evidence for association between either the individual SNPs or the haplotype combinations and any of the phenotypic characteristics in PCOS patients of European descent. However, the 112/121 halpogenotype was found to be significantly associated with higher insulin levels in response to a glucose challenge in the African-American PCOS population. Haddad et al. *(74)* also found no evidence for association between the 112/121 genotype and PCOS or any intermediate traits in a sample 331 PCOS patients. We have tested for association between individual SNPs (UCSNPs 43, 44, 19, and 63) and haplotypes within the calpain-10 gene and PCOS in 390 PCOS trios of predominantly European ancestry. We did not detect any evidence for association between any *CAPN10* SNPs or haplotypes and PCOS (manuscript in preparation). Gonzalez et al. *(75,76)* found a modest association between UCSNP44 and the PCO phenotype (polycystic ovarian morphology) in a group of 148 PCOS patients *(75,76)*. Taken together, these studies indicate that calpain-10 is unlikely to play a major role in the etiology of PCOS in Europeans.

4.4. SHBG

Two central features of the PCOS phenotype are hyperandrogenemia and insulin resistance. One protein that functionally links these two apparently disparate phenotypes is SHBG. SHBG is a 373 amino acid glycoprotein that serves as the plasma transport protein for sex steroid hormones in humans. Sex steroids are rendered biologically inactive when bound by SHBG, thus levels of SHBGs directly impact the action of sex steroids. Insulin has been shown to inhibit SHBG secretion *(77,78)*; therefore, insulin resistance would lead to a decrease in SHBG levels and a subsequent increase in the availability of biologically active testosterone and hyperandrogenemia *(79)*. Variation in *SHBG* is therefore a promising contributor to the PCOS phenotype.

Two functional variants within *SHBG* have been tested for an association with PCOS and related phenotypes. The point mutation D327N in exon 8 of *SHBG* has previously been shown to result in an increase of the half-life of SHBG and higher SHBG levels in carriers of the arginine allele *(80,81)*. The second variant is a pentanucleotide repeat polymorphism $(TAAAA)_n$, which maps 800 bp upstream of the *SHBG* transcription start site. This site has been shown to bind a 46-kDa nuclear factor and affect transcriptional activity of the *SHBG* promoter *(82)*.

Xita et al. *(83)* have characterized the effect of variation at the pentanucleotide repeat on PCOS and SHBG levels in a study of 185 women with PCOS and 324 control women. They found that longer $(TAAAA)_n$ repeats were more common in women with PCOS than in unaffected women. In addition, affected women with longer $(TAAAA)_n$ repeats had significantly lower SHBG levels than women with shorter $(TAAAA)_n$ repeats *(83)*. Cousin et al. *(84)* genotyped the D327N and the $(TAAAA)_n$ *SHBG* polymorphisms in a cohort of 303 hirsute women of which 154 were women with PCOS. They found that D327N polymorphism contributed to SHBG concentrations independent of PCOS status and that shorter $(TAAAA)_n$ repeats were associated with higher SHBG levels *(84)*. As the relatively high degree of linkage disequilibrium between D327N and $(TAAAA)_n$ prevents these polymorphisms from being inherited independently, further experiments are needed to evaluate the significance of these findings.

In family-based studies of 150 PCOS families, we did not find statistically significant evidence for linkage or association between alleles of a dinucleotide repeat polymorphism (D17S1353) mapping approximately 85 kb centromeric to *SHBG* *(33)*. We did observe increased identity by descent (a measure of linkage), but this finding was not statistically significant and a larger, more informative data set is needed to test for statistically significant evidence for linkage. Additionally, because the marker that we tested, D17S1353, is located approximately 85 kb from the gene for *SHBG*, it is likely that degree of linkage disequilibrium between D17S1353 and variants within *SHBG* would be too low to detect an association between PCOS and variation within the *SHBG* gene using D17S1353 as a genetic marker. In summary, there is some very interesting evidence indicating that variation within the SHBG globulin gene predisposes to PCOS or modifies the PCOS phenotypes. However, it is critical to replicate these findings in some larger studies.

4.5. AR and X-inactivation

One very interesting area of research in PCOS is the investigation of the role of genetic variation in the *AR* gene and the role of X-inactivation in PCOS. As PCOS is a disorder of androgen excess, genes involved in androgen signaling are also believed to be important in the etiology of PCOS and related disorders. Several groups have tested for association between alleles of the polymorphic CAG repeat encoding the polyglutamine tract in the N-terminal transactivation domain of the androgen *AR* and PCOS and measures of hyperandrogenism in women *(85–90)*. In vitro studies demonstrating an inverse relationship between the length of the CAG repeat and receptor activity *(91,92)* suggest that the length of the CAG repeat could be expected to affect the degree of androgen sensitivity. Although Legro et al. *(88)* found no difference in CAG repeat number between normo-androgenic and hyperandrogenic Hispanic women, they did find an inverse relationship between repeat length and degree of hirsutism in normo-androgenic women with idiopathic hirsutism. These findings are consistent with increased androgen sensitivity with shorter repeat lengths. In contrast, Mifsud et al. *(89)* found significantly shorter CAG repeats for the shorter CAG allele in Chinese and Indian women with low androgen levels compared to those with high androgen level, while in a study of 106 non-diabetic women with PCOS and 112 non-hirsute fertile control women of northern European ethnicity, number Jaaskelainen et al. found no evidence for association between the *AR* CAG repeat and PCOS.

To date few studies have investigated the effect of the *AR* CAG repeat length on phenotypic variation in women with PCOS. However, Mohlig et al. have used multiple regression analysis to investigate the impact of the *AR* CAG repeat length polymorphism on insulin resistance in women with PCOS *(90)*. They found that 42.5% of the variation of the homeostatic model assessment of insulin resistance (HOMA-IR) in 63 women with PCOS with normal glucose tolerance is explained by testosterone levels and CAG repeat length. In the presence of shorter CAG repeat lengths (<21 repeats), elevated androgen levels reduce insulin sensitivity, whereas the opposite finding is seen with longer CAG repeat lengths (>23 repeats). Although this cohort is small, the findings are very intriguing and may explain some of the ambiguities observed in published studies of the effect of AR repeat length on the PCOS phenotype. It may, therefore, be the case that CAG repeat length may be important only in a subset of PCOS patients with particularly high androgen levels.

As the *AR* receptor gene is X-linked and one copy of the X-chromosome is inactivated in women, the pattern of X-inactivation could influence *AR* activity and PCOS. Hickey et al. *(86)* compared X-inactivation and CAG repeat length in 83 fertile and 122 infertile Australian Caucasian women with PCOS *(86)*. They observed a greater frequency of long CAG repeats (>22 CAG repeats) in infertile PCOS patients than in controls or the general population and saw preferential expression of the longer repeat in leukocytes from PCOS women *(86)*. The functional significance for other tissues is currently not known. More recently, Hickey and colleagues examined the *AR* polymorphism and X-inactivation pattern in sisters concordant and discordant for the PCOS phenotype *(93)*. In an analysis of X-inactivation of 88 sisters of women with PCOS, Hickey et al. found that sisters with the same *AR* CAG repeat genotype and the same clinical presentation (unaffected–unaffected or PCOS–PCOS) also more frequently showed the same pattern of X-inactivation than did sisters with different clinical presentations (85 vs. 16%) *(93)* but the same genotype. In other words, sister pairs in whom the same copy of the *AR* is transcriptionally active also have the same phenotype, whereas sister pairs with the same genotype but different transcriptionally active X-chromosomes do not have the same phenotype. These findings support the hypothesis that the *AR* CAG repeat number plays an important role in the etiology of PCOS. Furthermore, this study demonstrates that epigenetic factors like X-inactivation can have a significant effect on the expression of complex genetic diseases such as PCOS and may complicate the interpretation of genetic results. Owing to the relatively small sample of sisters analyzed in this study, it is critical that this study be replicated in an independent cohort.

In summary, variation in the *AR* CAG repeat length may be important in the etiology of PCOS, and gradually light is being shed on possible explanations for the contradictory results of previous studies. Further studies in larger cohorts are needed to confirm the importance of variation in the AR to the etiology of PCOS.

4.6. Chromosome 19p13.2 PCOS susceptibility locus (D19S884)

We have used family-based test for linkage and association to identify PCOS susceptibility genes. In an initial screen of 37 PCOS candidate genes in 150 families, the strongest evidence for association occurred with D19S884 *(33)*. D19S884 is a dinucleotide repeat polymorphism that maps 800 kb centromeric to the insulin receptor (*INSR*) on chromosome 19p13.2. This marker was originally selected to assess linkage between the PCOS candidate gene, *INSR*, and PCOS and is located too far from *INSR* to be considered a suitable marker for association with *INSR* as 800 kb exceeds the usual distance over which linkage disequilibrium (the biological basis for allelic association) is maintained. It is, therefore, unlikely that this variant is directly associated with genetic variation within the candidate gene *INSR* itself and that the association that we observe in our families with D19S884 is due to a variant outside of the *INSR* per se. Further characterization of this region with 18 additional markers and 217 additional families replicated the original findings and found that the strongest evidence for association is still with allele 8 (A8) of D19S884 *(94)*. Secondly, in the complete cohort of 367 families, the region of chr19p13.2 containing D19S884 also has the strongest evidence for linkage to PCOS of any of the 33 candidate gene regions tested in our families *(94)*. We, therefore, concluded that D19S884 or a very closely linked marker is the most likely PCOS susceptibility locus mapping to chromosome 19p13.2. In support of our conclusions are the findings in our data and the HAPMAP and Perlegen data that there is only limited linkage disequilibrium in the vicinity of D19S884 and that D19S884 itself maps directly within a recombination hotspot (http://genome.ucsc.edu).

Two relatively small case-control studies have tested for association between D19S884 and PCOS, one of which replicated our results *(95)* and one which did not *(96)*. Owing to the relatively small size of these studies, it is difficult to evaluate the significance of these findings.

D19S884 maps 105 bp 3′ to exon 55 of the fibrillin-3 gene (*FBN3*), the third member of the fibrillin extracellular matrix protein family, that shows strong sequence homology with fibrillin-1 and -2. Although very little is known about the function of *FBN3*, the strong sequence homology among members of the fibrillin gene family as well as molecular evidence for fibrillin-1 and -2 suggest that they function in a similar manner *(97–101)*. Because fibrillin-1 and -2 act through the transforming growth factor beta (TGF-β)-signaling pathway *(97,100,102–106)*, it follows that *FBN3* may do so as well. The TGF-β-signaling pathway has a wide range of biological actions including tissue differentiation, hormone regulation, cell proliferation, and the development of the immune system *(107–110)*. Multiple members of the TGF-β-signaling pathway play a role in the biology of the ovary and/or the pathology of PCOS including follistatin, activin, inhibin, and BMP proteins making *FBN3* a promising candidate gene for PCOS.

The functional role of D19S884 remains to be determined. However, variation in dinucleotide repeat polymorphisms like D19S884 have been shown to play a role in both transcriptional *(111–119)* and splicing enhancer *(120–123)* activity. Whether D19S884 acts as a distal enhancer element for the *INSR* (the candidate gene which directed our attention to this area of the genome) or whether it impacts the expression and/or splicing pattern of FBN3 are areas of active research in our laboratory and others. Preliminary evidence indicates that D19S884 and the sequences immediately flanking it have low levels of enhancer activity but that this activity is not correlated with allele status *(124)*. This makes it unlikely that D19S884 is affecting INSR gene expression and more likely that D19S884 has a more direct and localized activity (i.e., within the *FBN3*).

5. FUTURE DIRECTIONS

Although the above described summary of the current state of genetic studies of PCOS may seem rather discouraging, this is not so. We are currently at the brink of a very exciting and potentially extremely rewarding era for the identification of genetic determinants of PCOS due to the convergence of several critical factors. Within the last few years, new reagents and tools have been assembled to make successful analysis of genetically complex disorders eminently feasible. These tools include *(1)* a nearly complete catalog of common human genetic variation by the HAPMAP project *(125,126)*, *(2)* efficient and relatively inexpensive high volume genotyping technologies, *(3)* development of easily accessible analysis software, and *(4)* most importantly, the assembly of sufficiently large PCOS patient cohorts *(48,64,94)* to detect genetic variants with effect sizes observed in other complex diseases. When applied to candidate genes, these tools make it possible to fully explore the genetic relevance of these genes to the etiology of PCOS and may help to reconcile some of the discrepant results observed in studies of different variants within the same gene. Finally, it is now possible to carry out WGA studies of PCOS that will identify potentially novel and unexpected genes and variants contributing to the etiology of PCOS. The next 10 years, therefore, promise to be a very exciting and productive era in the genetic analysis of PCOS.

REFERENCES

1. Diamanti-Kandarakis E, Kouli CR, Bergiele AT, et al. A survey of the polycystic ovary syndrome in the Greek island of Lesbos: hormonal and metabolic profile. *J Clin Endocrinol Metab* 1999;84(11): 4006–11.
2. Knochenhauer ES, Key TJ, Kahsar-Miller M, Waggoner W, Boots LR, Azziz R. Prevalence of the polycystic ovary syndrome in unselected black and white women of the southeastern United States: a prospective study. *J Clin Endocrinol Metab* 1998;83(9):3078–82.
3. Azziz R, Marin C, Hoq L, Badamgarav E, Song P. Health care-related economic burden of the polycystic ovary syndrome during the reproductive life span. *J Clin Endocrinol Metab* 2005;90(8):4650–8.
4. Balen AH, Conway GS, Kaltsas G, et al. Polycystic ovary syndrome: the spectrum of the disorder in 1741 patients. *Hum Reprod* 1995;10:2107–11.
5. Conway GS, Honour JW, Jacobs HS. Heterogeneity of the polycystic ovary syndrome: clinical, endocrine and ultrasound features in 556 patients. *Clin Endocrinol (Oxf)* 1989;30:459–70.
6. Burghen GA, Givens JR, Kitabchi AE. Correlation of hyperandrogenism with hyperinsulinism in polycystic ovarian disease. *J Clin Endocrinol Metab* 1980;50:113–6.

7. Dunaif A, Segal KR, Futterweit W, Dobrjansky A. Profound peripheral insulin resistance, independent of obesity, in polycystic ovary syndrome. *Diabetes* 1989;38(9):1165–74.

8. Cotrozzi G, Matteini M, Relli P, Lazzari T. Hyperinsulinism and insulin resistance in polycystic ovarian syndrome: a verification using oral glucose, I.V. glucose and tolbutamide. *Acta Diabetologia Latina* 1983;20(2):135–42.

9. Ehrmann DA, Sturis J, Byrne MM, Karrison T, Rosenfield RL, Polonsky KS. Insulin secretory defects in polycystic ovary syndrome. Relationship to insulin sensitivity and family history of non-insulin-dependent diabetes mellitus. *J Clin Invest* 1995;96(1):520–7.

10. Dunaif A, Graf M, Mandeli J, Laumas V, Dobrjansky A. Characterization of groups of hyperandrogenic women with acanthosis nigricans, impaired glucose tolerance, and/or hyperinsulinemia. *J Clin Endocrinol Metab* 1987;65(3):499–507.

11. Dunaif A, Segal KR, Shelley DR, Green G, Dobrjansky A, Licholai T. Evidence for distinctive and intrinsic defects in insulin action in polycystic ovary syndrome. *Diabetes* 1992;41(10):1257–66.

12. Legro RS, Kunselman A, Dodson WC, Dunaif A. Prevalence and predictors of risk for type 2 diabetes mellitus and impaired glucose tolerance in polycystic ovary syndrome: a prospective, controlled study in 254 affected women. *J Clin Endocrinol Metab* 1999;84:165–9.

13. Yildiz BO, Yarali H, Oguz H, Bayraktar M. Glucose intolerance, insulin resistance, and hyperandrogenemia in first degree relatives of women with polycystic ovary syndrome. *J Clin Endocrinol Metab* 2003;88(5):2031–6.

14. Sam S, Legro RS, Bentley-Lewis R, Dunaif A. Dyslipidemia and metabolic syndrome in the sisters of women with polycystic ovary syndrome. *J Clin Endocrinol Metab* 2005;90(8):4797–802.

15. Sam S, Dunaif A. Polycystic ovary syndrome: syndrome XX? *Trends Endocrinol Metab* 2003;14(8):365–70.

16. Sir-Petermann T, Angel B, Maliqueo M, Carvajal F, Santos JL, Pâerez-Bravo F. Prevalence of type II diabetes mellitus and insulin resistance in parents of women with polycystic ovary syndrome. *Diabetologia* 2002;45(7):959–64.

17. Yilmaz M, Bukan N, Ersoy R, et al. Glucose intolerance, insulin resistance and cardiovascular risk factors in first degree relatives of women with polycystic ovary syndrome. *Hum Reprod (Oxf)* 2005;20(9):2414–20.

18. Kiddy DS, Hamilton-Fairley D, Bush A, et al. Improvement in endocrine and ovarian function during dietary treatment of obese women with polycystic ovary syndrome. *Clin Endocrinol* 1992;36(1):105–11.

19. Norman RJ, Noakes M, Wu R, Davies MJ, Moran L, Wang JX. Improving reproductive performance in overweight/obese women with effective weight management. *Hum Reprod Update* 2004;10(3):267–80.

20. Moran LJ, Noakes M, Clifton PM, Wittert G, Norman RJ. Short term energy restriction (using meal replacements) improves reproductive parameters in polycystic ovary syndrome. *Asia Pacific J Clin Nutr* 2004;13(Suppl):S88.

21. Moran L, Norman RJ. Understanding and managing disturbances in insulin metabolism and body weight in women with polycystic ovary syndrome. *Best practice Res Clin Obstet Gynaecol* 2004;18(5):719–36.

22. Norman RJ, Davies MJ, Lord J, Moran LJ. The role of lifestyle modification in polycystic ovary syndrome. *Trends Endocrinol Metab* 2002;13(6):251–7.

23. Cooper HE, Spellacy WN, Prem KA, Cohen WD. Hereditary factors in Stein-Leventhal syndrome. *Am J Obstet Gynecol* 1968;100:371–87.

24. Givens JR. Familial polycystic ovarian disease. *Endocrinol Metab Clin N Am* 1988;17(4):771–83.

25. Hague W, Adams J, Reeders S, Peto TA, Jacobs H. Familial polycystic ovaries: A genetic disease. *Clin Endocrinol* 1988;29:593–605.

26. Ferriman D, Purdie AW. The inheritance of polycystic ovarian disease and a possible relationship to premature balding. *Clin Endocrinol* 1979;11(3):291–300.

27. Carey AH, Chan KI, Short F, Williamson R, Franks S. Evidence for a single gene effect causing polycystic ovaries and male pattern baldness. *Clin Endocrinol* 1993;38:653–8.

28. Legro RS, Driscoll D, Strauss JF, Fox J, Dunaif A. Evidence for a genetic basis for hyperandrogenemia in polycystic ovary syndrome. *Proc Natl Acad Sci USA* 1998;95:14956–60.

29. Kahsar-Miller M, Azziz R. Heritability and the risk of developing androgen excess. *J Steroid Biochem Mol Biol* 1999;69(1–6):261–8.

30. Jahanfar S, Eden J, Nguyen T, Wang X, Wilcken D. A twin study of polycystic ovary syndrome and lipids. *Gynecol Endocrinol* 1997;11(2):111–7.

31. Kahsar-Miller MD, Nixon C, Boots LR, Go RC, Azziz R. Prevalence of polycystic ovary syndrome (PCOS) in first degree relatives of patients with PCOS. *Fertil Steril* 2001;75(1):53–8.

32. Vink J, Sadrzadeh SM, Lambalk CB, Boomsma DI. Heritability of polycystic ovary syndrome (PCOS) in a Dutch twin-family study. *J Clin Endocrinol Metab* 2005 [Epub ahead of print].

33. Urbanek M, Legro RS, Driscoll DA, et al. Thirty-seven candidate genes for polycystic ovary syndrome: strongest evidence for linkage is with follistatin. *Proc Natl Acad Sci USA* 1999;96(15):8573–8.

34. Escobar-Morreale HF, Luque-Ramâirez M, San Millâan JL. The molecular-genetic basis of functional hyperandrogenism and the polycystic ovary syndrome. *Endocr Rev* 2005;26(2):251–82.

35. Newton-Cheh C, Hirschhorn JN. Genetic association studies of complex traits: design and analysis issues. *Mutat Res* 2005;573(1–2):54–69.

36. Hirschhorn JN. Genetic approaches to studying common diseases and complex traits. *Pediatr Res* 2005;57(5):74R–7R.

37. Hirschhorn JN, Daly MJ. Genome-wide association studies for common diseases and complex traits. *Nat Rev Genet* 2005;6(2):95–108.

38. Hattersley AT, McCarthy MI. What makes a good genetic association study? *Lancet* 2005;366(9493):1315–23.

39. Zawadski JK, Dunaif A. Diagnostic criteria for polycystic ovary syndrome. In: Givens J, Haseltine F, Merriman G, eds. *The Polycystic Ovary Syndrome*. Cambridge, MA: Blackwell Scientific; 1992: 377–84.

40. The Rotterdam ESHRE/ASRM-sponsored PCOS consensus workshop group. Revised 2003 consensus on diagnostic criteria and long-term health risks related to polycystic ovary syndrome (PCOS). *Hum Reprod* 2004;19(1):41–7.

41. Altshuler D, Hirschhorn J, Klannemark M, et al. The common PPARγ Pro12Ala polymorphism is associated with decreased risk of type 2 diabetes. *Nat Genet* 2000;26(1):76–80.

42. Grant SF, Thorleifsson G, Reynisdottir I, et al. Variant of transcription factor 7-like 2 (TCF7L2) gene confers risk of type 2 diabetes. *Nat Genet* 2006;38(3):320–3.

43. Hirschhorn JN, Altshuler D. Once and again-issues surrounding replication in genetic association studies. *J Clin Endocrinol Metab* 2002;87(10):4438–41.

44. Gharani N, Waterworth DM, Batty S, et al. Association of the steroid synthesis gene CYP11a with polycystic ovary syndrome and hyperandrogenism. *Hum Mol Genet* 1997;6(3):397–402.

45. Diamanti-Kandarakis E, Bartzis MI, Bergiele AT, Tsianateli TC, Kouli CR. Microsatellite polymorphism (tttta)(n) at -528 base pairs of gene CYP11alpha influences hyperandrogenemia in patients with polycystic ovary syndrome. *Fertil Steril* 2000;73:735–41.

46. Daneshmand S, Weitsman SR, Navab A, Jakimiuk AJ, Magoffin DA. Overexpression of theca-cell messenger RNA in polycystic ovary syndrome does not correlate with polymorphisms in the cholesterol side-chain cleavage and 17alpha-hydroxylase/C(17–20) lyase promoters. *Fertil Steril* 2002;77(2):274–80.

47. San Millan JL, Sancho J, Calvo RM, Escobar-Morreale HF. Role of the pentanucleotide (tttta)(n) polymorphism in the promoter of the CYP11a gene in the pathogenesis of hirsutism. *Fertil Steril* 2001;75:797–802.

48. Gaasenbeek M, Powell BL, Sovio U, et al. Large-scale analysis of the relationship between CYP11A promoter variation, polycystic ovarian syndrome, and serum testosterone. *J Clin Endocrinol Metab* 2004;89(5):2408–13.

49. Bell GI, Selby MJ, Rutter WJ. The highly polymorphic region near the human insulin gene is composed of simple tandemly repeating sequences. *Nature* 1982;295(5844):31–5.

50. Bennett ST, Lucassen AM, Gough SC, et al. Susceptibility to human type 1 diabetes at IDDM2 is determined by tandem repeat variation at the insulin gene minisatellite locus. *Nat Genet* 1995;9(3): 284–92.

51. Bennett ST, Todd JA. Human type 1 diabetes and the insulin gene: principles of mapping polygenes. *Ann Rev Genet* 1996;30:343–70.

52. Vafiadis P, Bennett ST, Colle E, Grabs R, Goodyer CG, Polychronakos C. Imprinted and genotype-specific expression of genes at the IDDM2 locus in pancreas and leucocytes. *J Autoimmun* 1996;9(3):397–403.

53. Kennedy GC, German MS, Rutter WJ. The minisatellite in the diabetes susceptibility locus IDDM2 regulates insulin transcription. *Nat Genet* 1995;9(3):293–8.

54. Lucassen AM, Screaton GR, Julier C, Elliott TJ, Lathrop M, Bell JI. Regulation of insulin gene expression by the IDDM associated, insulin locus haplotype. *Hum Mol Genet* 1995;4(4):501–6.

55. Owerbach D, Gabbay KH. The search for IDDM susceptibility genes: the next generation. *Diabetes* 1996;45(5):544–51.

56. Huxtable SJ, Saker PJ, Haddad L, et al. Analysis of parent-offspring trios provides evidence for linkage and association between the insulin gene and type 2 diabetes mediated exclusively through paternally transmitted class III variable number tandem repeat alleles. *Diabetes* 2000;49(1):126–30.

57. Ong KK, Phillips DI, Fall C, et al. The insulin gene VNTR, type 2 diabetes and birth weight. *Nat Genet* 1999;21(3):262–3.

58. Le Stunff C, Fallin D, Schork NJ, Bougneres P. The insulin gene VNTR is associated with fasting insulin levels and development of juvenile obesity. *Nat Genet* 2000;26(4):444–6.

59. Le Stunff C, Fallin D, Bougneres P. Paternal transmission of the very common class I INS VNTR alleles predisposes to childhood obesity. *Nat Genet* 2001;29(1):96–9.

60. Waterworth DM, Bennett ST, Gharani N, et al. Linkage and association of insulin gene VNTR regulatory polymorphism with polycystic ovary syndrome. *Lancet* 1997;349(9057):986–90.

61. Michelmore K, Ong K, Mason S, et al. Clinical features in women with polycystic ovaries: relationships to insulin sensitivity, insulin gene VNTR and birth weight. *Clin Endocrinol (Oxf)* 2001;55(4):439–46.

62. Calvo RM, Telleráia D, Sancho J, San Millâan JL, Escobar-Morreale HF. Insulin gene variable number of tandem repeats regulatory polymorphism is not associated with hyperandrogenism in Spanish women. *Fertil Steril* 2002;77(4):666–8.

63. Vankova M, Vrbikova J, Hill M, Cinek O, Bendlova B. Association of insulin gene VNTR polymorphism with polycystic ovary syndrome. *Ann N Y Acad Sci* 2002;967:558–65.

64. Powell BL, Haddad L, Bennett A, et al. Analysis of multiple data sets reveals no association between the insulin gene variable number tandem repeat element and polycystic ovary syndrome or related traits. *J Clin Endocrinol Metab* 2005;90(5):2988–93.

65. Hanis CL, Boerwinkle E, Chakraborty R, et al. A genome-wide search for human non-insulin-dependent (type 2) diabetes genes reveals a major susceptibility locus on chromosome 2. *Nat Genet* 1996;13(2):161–6.

66. Horikawa Y, Oda N, Cox NJ, et al. Genetic variation in the gene encoding calpain-10 is associated with type 2 diabetes mellitus. *Nat Genet* 2000;26:163–75.

67. Evans JC, Frayling TM, Cassell PG, et al. Studies of association between the gene for calpain-10 and type 2 diabetes mellitus in the United Kingdom. *Am J Hum Genet* 2001;69(3):544–52.

68. Tsai HJ, Sun G, Weeks DE, et al. Type 2 diabetes and three calpain-10 gene polymorphisms in Samoans: no evidence of association. *Am J Hum Genet* 2001;69(6):1236–44.

69. Weedon MN, Schwarz PE, Horikawa Y, et al. Meta-analysis and a large association study confirm a role for calpain-10 variation in type 2 diabetes susceptibility. *Am J Hum Genet* 2003;73: 1208–12.

70. Song Y, Niu T, Manson JE, Kwiatkowski DJ, Liu S. Are variants in the CAPN10 gene related to risk of type 2 diabetes? A quantitative assessment of population and family-based association studies. *Am J Hum Genet* 2004;74(2):208–22.

71. Tsuchiya T, Schwarz P, Bosque-Plata L, et al. Association of the calpain-10 gene with type 2 diabetes in Europeans: results of pooled and meta-analyses. *Mol Genet Metab* 2006 [Epub ahead of print].

72. Baier LJ, Permana PA, Yang X, et al. A calpain-10 gene polymorphism is associated with reduced muscle mRNA levels and insulin resistance. *J Clin Invest* 2000;106(7):R69–73.

73. Ehrmann DA, Schwarz PE, Hara M, et al. Relationship of calpain-10 genotype to phenotypic features of polycystic ovary syndrome. *J Clin Endocrinol Metab* 2002;87(4):1669–73.

74. Haddad L, Evans JC, Gharani N, et al. Variation within the type 2 diabetes susceptibility gene calpain-10 and polycystic ovary syndrome. *J Clin Endocrinol Metab* 2002;87(6):2606–10.

75. Gonzalez A, Abril E, Roca A, et al. Specific CAPN10 gene haplotypes influence the clinical profile of polycystic ovary patients. *J Clin Endocrinol Metab* 2003;88(11):5529–36.

76. Gonzalez A, Abril E, Roca A, et al. CAPN10 alleles are associated with polycystic ovary syndrome. *J Clin Endocrinol Metab* 2002;87(8):3971–6.

77. Nestler JE. Sex hormone-binding globulin: a marker for hyperinsulinemia and/or insulin resistance? *J Clin Endocrinol Metab* 1993;76(2):273–4.

78. Plymate SR, Matej LA, Jones RE, Friedl KE. Inhibition of sex hormone-binding globulin production in the human hepatoma (Hep G2) cell line by insulin and prolactin. *J Clin Endocrinol Metab* 1988;67(3):460–4.

79. Pugeat M, Crave JC, Elmidani M, et al. Pathophysiology of sex hormone binding globulin (SHBG): relation to insulin. *J Steriod Biochem Mol Biol* 1991;40(4–6):841–9.

80. Cousin P, Dâechaud H, Grenot C, Lejeune H, Pugeat M. Human variant sex hormone-binding globulin (SHBG) with an additional carbohydrate chain has a reduced clearance rate in rabbit. *J Clin Endocrinol Metab* 1998;83(1):235–40.

81. Power SG, Bocchinfuso WP, Pallesen M, Warmels-Rodenhiser S, Van Baelen H, Hammond GL. Molecular analyses of a human sex hormone-binding globulin variant: evidence for an additional carbohydrate chain. *J Clin Endocrinol Metab* 1992;75(4):1066–70.

82. Hogeveen KN, Talikka M, Hammond GL. Human sex hormone-binding globulin promoter activity is influenced by a (TAAAA)n repeat element within an Alu sequence. *J Biol Chem* 2001;276(39): 36383–90.

83. Xita N, Tsatsoulis A, Chatzikyriakidou A, Georgiou I. Association of the (TAAAA)n repeat polymorphism in the sex hormone-binding globulin (SHBG) gene with polycystic ovary syndrome and relation to SHBG serum levels. *J Clin Endocrinol Metab* 2003;88(12):5976–80.

84. Cousin P, Calemard-Michel L, Lejeune H, et al. Influence of SHBG gene pentanucleotide TAAAA repeat and D327N polymorphism on serum sex hormone-binding globulin concentration in hirsute women. *J Clin Endocrinol Metab* 2004;89(2):917–24.

85. Jakubiczka S, Nedel S, Werder EA, et al. Mutations of the androgen receptor gene in patients with complete androgen insensitivity. *Hum Mutat* 1997;9(1):57–61.

86. Hickey T, Chandy A, Norman RJ. The androgen receptor CAG repeat polymorphism and X-chromosome inactivation in Australian Caucasian women with infertility related to polycystic ovary syndrome. *J Clin Endocrinol Metab* 2002;87(1):161–5.

87. Jèaèaskelèainen J, Korhonen S, Voutilainen R, Hippelèainen M, Heinonen S. Androgen receptor gene CAG length polymorphism in women with polycystic ovary syndrome. *Fertil Steril* 2005;83(6): 1724–8.

88. Legro R, Shahbahrami B, Lobo R, Kovacs B. Size polymorphisms of the androgen receptor among female Hispanics and correlation with androgenic characteristics. *Obstet Gynecol* 1994;83(5 Pt 1): 701–6.

89. Mifsud A, Ramirez S, Yong EL. Androgen receptor gene CAG trinucleotide repeats in annovulatory infertility and polycystic ovaries. *J Clin Endocrinol Metab* 2000;85:3484–8.

90. Mèohlig M, Jèurgens A, Spranger J, et al. Thc androgen receptor CAG repeat modifies the impact of testosterone on insulin resistance in women with polycystic ovary syndrome. *Eur J Endocrinol* 2006;155(1):127–30.

91. Mhatre AN, Trifiro MA, Kaufman M, et al. Reduced transcriptional regulatory competence of the androgen receptor in X-linked spinal and bulbar muscular atrophy. *Nat Genet* 1993;5(2):184–8.

92. Tut TG, Ghadessy FJ, Trifiro MA, Pinsky L, Yong EL. Long polyglutamine tracts in the androgen receptor are associated with reduced trans-activation, impaired sperm production, and male infertility. *J Clin Endocrinol Metab* 1997;82(11):3777–82.

93. Hickey TE, Legro RS, Norman RJ. Epigenetic modification of the X chromosome influences susceptibility to polycystic ovary syndrome. *J Clin Endocrinol Metab* 2006;91(7):2789–91.

94. Urbanek M, Woodroffe A, Ewens KG, et al. Candidate gene region for polycystic ovary syndrome on chromosome 19p13.2. *J Clin Endocrinol Metab* 2005;90(12):6623–9.

95. Tucci S, Futterweit W, Concepcion ES, et al. Evidence for association of polycystic ovary syndrome in caucasian women with a marker at the insulin receptor locus. *J Clin Endocrinol Metab* 2001;86(1): 446–9.

96. Villuendas G, Escobar-Morreale HF, Tosi F, Sancho J, Moghetti P, San Millan JL. Association between the D19S884 marker at the insulin receptor gene locus and polycystic ovary syndrome. *Fertil Steril* 2003;79(1):219–20.

97. Charbonneau NL, Ono RN, Corson GM, Keene DR, Sakai LY. Fine tuning of growth factor signals depends on fibrillin microfibril networks. *Birth Defects Res C Embryo Today* 2004;72(1):37–50.

98. Corson GM, Charbonneau NL, Keene DR, Sakai LY. Differential expression of fibrillin-3 adds to microfibril variety in human and avian, but not rodent, connective tissues. *Genomics* 2004;83(3): 461–72.

99. Pereira L, Andrikopoulos K, Tian J, et al. Targetting of the gene encoding fibrillin-1 recapitulates the vascular aspect of Marfan syndrome. *Nat Genet* 1997;17(2):218–22.

100. Arteaga-Solis E, Gayraud B, Lee SY, Shum L, Sakai L, Ramirez F. Regulation of limb patterning by extracellular microfibrils. *J Cell Biol* 2001;154(2):275–81.

101. Carta L, Pereira L, Arteaga-Solis E, et al. Fibrillins 1 and 2 perform partially overlapping functions during aortic development. *J Biol Chem* 2006;281(12):8016–23.

102. Neptune ER, Frischmeyer PA, Arking DE, et al. Dysregulation of TGF-beta activation contributes to pathogenesis in Marfan syndrome. *Nat Genet* 2003;33(3):407–11.

103. Kaartinen V, Warburton D. Fibrillin controls TGF-beta activation. *Nat Genet* 2003;33(3):331–2.

104. Kissin EY, Lemaire R, Korn JH, Lafyatis R. Transforming growth factor beta induces fibroblast fibrillin-1 matrix formation. *Arthritis Rheum* 2002;46(11):3000–9.

105. Isogai Z, Gregory KE, Ono RN, et al. Microfibrils and morphogenesis. In: Tamburro AM, Pepe A, eds. *Elastin*. Potenza, Italy; 2003:213–23.

106. Habashi JP, Judge DP, Holm TM, et al. Losartan, an AT1 antagonist, prevents aortic aneurysm in a mouse model of Marfan syndrome. *Science* 2006;312(5770):117–21.

107. Mehra A, Wrana JL. TGF-beta and the Smad signal transduction pathway. *Biochem Cell Biol* 2002;80(5):605–22.

108. Chang H, Brown CW, Matzuk MM. Genetic analysis of the mammalian transforming growth factor-beta superfamily. *Endocr Rev* 2002;23(6):787–823.

109. Findlay JK, Drummond AE, Dyson ML, Baillie AJ, Robertson DM, Ethier JF. Recruitment and development of the follicle; the roles of the transforming growth factor-beta superfamily. *Mol Cell Endocrinol* 2002;191(1):35–43.

110. Moustakas A, Souchelnytskyi S, Heldin CH. Smad regulation in TGF-beta signal transduction. *J Cell Sci* 2001;114(Pt):4359–69.

111. Gebhardt F, Zèanker KS, Brandt B. Modulation of epidermal growth factor receptor gene transcription by a polymorphic dinucleotide repeat in intron 1. *J Biol Chem* 1999;274:13176–80.

112. Dolan-O'Keefe M, Chow V, Monnier J, Visner GA, Nick HS. Transcriptional regulation and structural organization of the human cytosolic phospholipase A(2) gene. *Am J Physiol Lung Cell Mol Physiol* 2000;278:L649–57.

113. Hata R, Akai J, Kimura A, Ishikawa O, Kuwana M, Shinkai H. Association of functional microsatellites in the human type I collagen alpha2 chain (COL1A2) gene with systemic sclerosis. *Biochem Biophys Res Commun* 2000;272:36–40.

114. Rothenburg S, Koch-Nolte F, Rich A, Haag F. A polymorphic dinucleotide repeat in the rat nucleolin gene forms Z-DNA and inhibits promoter activity. *Proc Natl Acad Sci USA* 2001;98:8985–90.

115. Ferrand PE, Parry S, Sammel M, et al. A polymorphism in the matrix metalloproteinase-9 promoter is associated with increased risk of preterm premature rupture of membranes in African Americans. *Mol Hum Reprod* 2002;8:494–501.

116. Fornoni A, Lenz O, Striker LJ, Striker GE. Glucose induces clonal selection and reversible dinucleotide repeat expansion in mesangial cells isolated from glomerulosclerosis-prone mice. *Diabetes* 2003;52:2594–602.

117. Fenech AG, Billington CK, Swan C, et al. Novel polymorphisms influencing transcription of the human CHRM2 gene in airway smooth muscle. *Am J Respir Cell Mol Biol* 2004;30:678–86.

118. Huang TS, Lee CC, Chang AC, et al. Shortening of microsatellite deoxy(CA) repeats involved in GL331-induced down-regulation of matrix metalloproteinase-9 gene expression. *Biochem Biophys Res Commun* 2003;300:901–7.

119. Gao PS, Heller NM, Walker W, et al. Variation in dinucleotide (GT) repeat sequence in the first exon of the STAT6 gene is associated with atopic asthma and differentially regulates the promoter activity in vitro. *J Med Genet* 2004;41(7):535–9.

120. Gabellini N. A polymorphic GT repeat from the human cardiac Na+Ca2+ exchanger intron 2 activates splicing. *Eur J Biochem* 2001;268:1076–83.

121. Hui J, Stangl K, Lane WS, Bindereif A. HnRNP L stimulates splicing of the eNOS gene by binding to variable-length CA repeats. *Nat Struct Biol* 2003;10:33–7.

122. Hui J, Reither G, Bindereif A. Novel functional role of CA repeats and hnRNP L in RNA stability. *RNA* 2003;9:931–6.

123. Stangl K, Cascorbi I, Laule M, et al. High CA repeat numbers in intron 13 of the endothelial nitric oxide synthase gene and increased risk of coronary artery disease. *Pharmacogenetics* 2000;10:133–40.

124. Stewart DR, Dombroski BA, Urbanek M, et al. Fine mapping of genetic susceptibility to polycystic ovary syndrome on chromosome 19p13.2 and tests of regulatory activity. *J Clin Endocrinol Metab* 2006 [Epub ahead of print].

125. The International HapMap Consortium. The International HapMap Project. *Nature* 2003;426(6968):789–96.

126. Altshuler D, Brooks LD, Chakravarti A, Collins FS, Daly MJ, Donnelly P. A haplotype map of the human genome. *Nature* 2005;437(7063):1299–320.

127. Heinonen S, Korhonen S, Helisalmi S, et al. Associations between two single nucleotide polymorphisms in the adiponectin gene and polycystic ovary syndrome. *Gynecol Endocrinol* 2005;21(3):165–9.

128. San Millan JL, Cortâon M, Villuendas G, Sancho J, Peral B, Escobar-Morreale HF. Association of the polycystic ovary syndrome with genomic variants related to insulin resistance, type 2 diabetes mellitus, and obesity. *J Clin Endocrinol Metab* 2004;89(6):2640–6.

129. Perez-Bravo F, Echiburâu B, Maliqueo M, Santos JL, Sir-Petermann T. Tryptophan 64 –> arginine polymorphism of beta-3-adrenergic receptor in Chilean women with polycystic ovary syndrome. *Clin Endocrinol* 2005;62(2):126–31.

130. Zulian E, Sartorato P, Schiavi F, et al. The M235T polymorphism of the angiotensinogen gene in women with polycystic ovary syndrome. *Fertil Steril* 2005;84(5):1520–1.

131. Heinonen S, Korhonen S, Hippelainen M, Hiltunen M, Mannermaa A, Saarikoski S. Apolipoprotein E alleles in women with polycystic ovary syndrome. *Fertil Steril* 2001;75(5):878–80.

132. Babu KA, Rao KL, Kanakavalli MK, Suryanarayana VV, Deenadayal M, Singh L. CYP1A1, GSTM1 and GSTT1 genetic polymorphism is associated with susceptibility to polycystic ovaries in South Indian women. *Reprod Biomed online* 2004;9(2):194–200.

133. Techatraisak K, Conway GS, Rumsby G. Frequency of a polymorphism in the regulatory region of the 17 alpha-hydroxylase-17,20-lyase (CYP17) gene in hyperandrogenic states. *Clin Endocrinol* 1997;46(2):131–4.

134. Gharani N, Waterworth DM, Williamson R, Franks S. 5´ Polymorphism of the CYP17 gene is not associated with serum testosterone levels in women with polycystic ovaries. *J Clin Endocrinol Metab* 1996;81(11):4174.

135. Marszalek B, Laciânski M, Babych N, et al. Investigations on the genetic polymorphism in the region of CYP17 gene encoding 5'-UTR in patients with polycystic ovarian syndrome. *Gynecol Endocrinol* 2001;15(2):123–8.

136. Diamanti-Kandarakis E, Bartzis MI, Zapanti ED, et al. Polymorphism T–>C (-34 bp) of gene CYP17 promoter in Greek patients with polycystic ovary syndrome. *Fertil Steril* 1999;71(3):431–5.

137. Tucci S, Futterweit W, Concepcion FS, et al. Evidence for association of polycystic ovary syndrome in caucasian women with a marker at the insulin receptor gene locus. *J Clin Endocrinol Metabol* 2001;86(1):446–9.

138. Kahsar-Miller M, Boots LR, Bartolucci A, Azziz R. Role of a CYP17 polymorphism in the regulation of circulating dehydroepiandrosterone sulfate levels in women with polycystic ovary syndrome. *Fertil Steril* 2004;82(4):973–5.

139. Petry CJ, Ong KK, Michelmore KF, et al. Association of aromatase (CYP 19) gene variation with features of hyperandrogenism in two populations of young women. *Hum Reprod* 2005;20(7):1837–43.

140. Sèoderlund D, Canto P, Carranza-Lira S, Mâendez JP. No evidence of mutations in the P450 aromatase gene in patients with polycystic ovary syndrome. *Hum Reprod (Oxf)* 2005;20(4):965–9.

141. Witchel SF, Aston CE. The role of heterozygosity for CYP21 in the polycystic ovary syndrome. *J Pediatr Endocrinol Metab* 2000;13:1315–7.

142. Witchel SF, Kahsar-Miller M, Aston CE, White C, Azziz R. Prevalence of CYP21 mutations and IRS1 variant among women with polycystic ovary syndrome and adrenal androgen excess. *Fertil Steril* 2005;83(2):371–5.

143. Kahsar-Miller M, Boots LR, Azziz R. Dopamine D3 receptor polymorphism is not associated with the polycystic ovary syndrome. *Fertil Steril* 1999;71(3):436–8.

144. Legro R, Muhleman D, Comings D, Lobo R, Kovacs B. A dopamine D3 receptor genotype is associated with hyperandrogenic chronic anovulation and resistant to ovulation induction with clomiphene citrate in female Hispanics. *Fertil Steril* 1995;63(4):779–84.

145. Korhonen S, Romppanen EL, Hiltunen M, et al. Two exonic single nucleotide polymorphisms in the microsomal epoxide hydrolase gene are associated with polycystic ovary syndrome. *Fertil Steril* 2003;79(6):1353–7.

146. Liao WX, Roy AC, Ng SC. Preliminary investigation of follistatin gene mutations in women with polycystic ovary syndrome. *Mol Hum Reprod* 1999;6:587–90.

147. Urbanek M, Wu X, Vickery KR, et al. Allelic variants of the follistatin gene in polycystic ovary syndrome. *J Clin Endocrinol Metab* 2000;85(12):4455–61.

148. Takakura K, Takebayashi K, Wang HQ, Kimura F, Kasahara K, Noda Y. Follicle-stimulating hormone receptor gene mutations are rare in Japanese women with premature ovarian failure and polycystic ovary syndrome. *Fertil Steril* 2001;75(1):207–9.

149. Tong Y, Liao WX, Roy AC, Ng SC. Absence of mutations in the coding regions of follicle-stimulating hormone receptor gene in Singapore Chinese women with premature ovarian failure and polycystic ovary syndrome. *Horm Metab Res* 2001;33(4):221–6.

150. Sudo S, Kudo M, Wada S, Sato O, Hsueh AJ, Fujimoto S. Genetic and functional analyses of polymorphisms in the human FSH receptor gene. *Mol Hum Reprod* 2002;8(10):893–9.

151. Tong Y, Liao WX, Roy AC, Ng SC. Association of AccI polymorphism in the follicle-stimulating hormone beta gene with polycystic ovary syndrome. *Fertil Steril* 2000;74:1233–6.

152. Ho CK, Wood JR, Stewart DR, et al. Increased transcription and increased messenger ribonucleic acid (mRNA) stability contribute to increased GATA6 mRNA abundance in polycystic ovary syndrome theca cells. *J Clin Endocrinol Metab* 2005;90(12):6596–602.

153. Takebayashi K, Takakura K, Wang H, Kimura F, Kasahara K, Noda Y. Mutation analysis of the growth differentiation factor-9 and -9B genes in patients with premature ovarian failure and polycystic ovary syndrome. *Fertil Steril* 2000;74:976–9.

154. Cohen DP, Stein EM, Li Z, Matulis CK, Ehrmann DA, Layman LC. Molecular analysis of the gonadotropin-releasing hormone receptor in patients with polycystic ovary syndrome. *Fertil Steril* 1999;72(2):360–3.

155. Kahsar-Miller M, Azziz R, Feingold E, Witchel SF. A variant of the glucocorticoid receptor gene is not associated with adrenal androgen excess in women with polycystic ovary syndrome. *Fertil Steril* 2000;74(6):1237–40.

156. San Millâan JL, Botella-Carretero JI, Alvarez-Blasco F, et al. A study of the hexose-6-phosphate dehydrogenase gene R453Q and 11beta-hydroxysteroid dehydrogenase type 1 gene 83557insA polymorphisms in the polycystic ovary syndrome. *J Clin Endocrinol Metab* 2005;90(7):4157–62.

157. White PC. Genotypes at 11beta-hydroxysteroid dehydrogenase type 11B1 and hexose-6-phosphate dehydrogenase loci are not risk factors for apparent cortisone reductase deficiency in a large population-based sample. *J Clin Endocrinol Metab* 2005;90(10):5880–3.

158. Moghrabi N, Hughes IA, Dunaif A, Andersson S. Deleterious missense mutations and silent polymorphism in the human 17beta-hydroxysteroid dehydrogenase 3 gene (HSD17B3). *J Clin Endocrinol Metab* 1998;83(8):2855–60.

159. Qin K, Ehrmann DA, Cox N, Refetoff S, Rosenfield RL. Identification of a functional polymorphism of the human type 5 17beta-hydroxysteroid dehydrogenase gene associated with polycystic ovary syndrome. *J Clin Endocrinol Metab* 2006;91(1):270–6.

160. Walch K, Grimm C, Zeillinger R, Huber JC, Nagele F, Hefler LA. A common interleukin-6 gene promoter polymorphism influences the clinical characteristics of women with polycystic ovary syndrome. *Fertil Steril* 2004;81(6):1638–41.

161. Siegel S, Futterweit W, Davies TF, et al. A C/T single nucleotide polymorphism at the tyrosine kinase domain of the insulin receptor gene is associated with polycystic ovary syndrome. *Fertil Steril* 2002;78(6):1240–3.

162. El Mkadem SA, Lautier C, Macari F, et al. Role of allelic variants Gly972Arg of IRS-1 and Gly1057Asp of IRS-2 in moderate-to-severe insulin resistance of women with polycystic ovary syndrome. *Diabetes* 2001;50(9):2164–8.

163. Dilek S, Ertunc D, Tok EC, Erdal EM, Aktas A. Association of Gly972Arg variant of insulin receptor substrate-1 with metabolic features in women with polycystic ovary syndrome. *Fertil Steril* 2005;84(2):407–12.

164. Villuendas G, Botella-Carretero JI, Roldan B, Sancho J, Escobar-Morreale HF, San Millan JL. Polymorphisms in the insulin receptor substrate-1 (IRS-1) gene and the insulin receptor substrate-2 (IRS-2) gene influence glucose homeostasis and body mass index in women with polycystic ovary syndrome and non-hyperandrogenic controls. *Hum Reprod (Oxf)* 2005;20(11):3184–91.

165. Sir-Petermann T, Pâerez-Bravo F, Angel B, Maliqueo M, Calvillan M, Palomino A. G972R polymorphism of IRS-1 in women with polycystic ovary syndrome. *Diabetologia* 2001;44(9):1200–1.

166. Oksanen L, Tiitinen A, Kaprio J, Koistinen HA, Karonen S, Kontula K. No evidence for mutations of the leptin or leptin receptor genes in women with polycystic ovary syndrome. *Mol Hum Reprod* 2000;6:873–6.

167. Erel CT, Cine N, Elter K, Kaleli S, Senturk LM, Baysal B. Leptin receptor variant in women with polycystic ovary syndrome. *Fertil Steril* 2002;78(6):1334–5.

168. Tapanainen JS, Koivunen R, Fauser BC, et al. A new contributing factor to polycystic ovary syndrome: the genetic variant of luteinizing hormone. *J Clin Endocrinol Metab* 1999;84(5):1711–5.

169. Kim NK, Nam YS, Ko JJ, Chung HM, Chung KW, Cha KY. The luteinizing hormone beta-subunit exon 3 (Gly102Ser) gene mutation is rare in Korean women with endometriosis and polycystic ovary syndrome. *Fertil Steril* 2001;75(6):1238–9.

170. Wang HQ, Takakura K, Takebayashi K, Noda Y. Mutational analysis of the mullerian-inhibiting substance gene and its receptor gene in Japanese women with polycystic ovary syndrome and premature ovarian failure. *Fertil Steril* 2002;78(6):1329–30.

171. Walch K, Nagele F, Zeillinger R, Vytiska-Binstorfer E, Huber JC, Hefler LA. A polymorphism in the matrix metalloproteinase-1 gene promoter is associated with the presence of polycystic ovary syndrome in Caucasian women. *Fertil Steril* 2005;83(5):1565–7.

172. Orio F, Jr., Palomba S, Di Biase S, et al. Homocysteine levels and C677T polymorphism of methylenetetrahydrofolate reductase in women with polycystic ovary syndrome. *J Clin Endocrinol Metab* 2003;88(2):673–9.

173. Walch K, Grimm C, Huber JC, Nagele F, Kolbus A, Hefler LA. A polymorphism of the plasminogen activator inhibitor-1 gene promoter and the polycystic ovary syndrome. *Eur J Obstet Gynecol Reprod Biol* 2005;123(1):77–81.

174. Diamanti-Kandarakis E, Palioniko G, Alexandraki K, Bergiele A, Koutsouba T, Bartzis M. The prevalence of 4G5G polymorphism of plasminogen activator inhibitor-1 (PAI-1) gene in polycystic ovarian syndrome and its association with plasma PAI-1 levels. *Eur J Endocrinol* 2004;150(6):793–8.

175. Heinonen S, Korhonen S, Helisalmi S, Koivunen R, Tapanainen JS, Laakso M. The 121Q allele of the plasma cell membrane glycoprotein 1 gene predisposes to polycystic ovary syndrome. *Fertil Steril* 2004;82(3):743–5.

176. Hahn S, Fingerhut A, Khomtsiv U, et al. The peroxisome proliferator activated receptor gamma Pro12Ala polymorphism is associated with a lower hirsutism score and increased insulin sensitivity in women with polycystic ovary syndrome. *Clin Endocrinol* 2005;62(5):573–9.

177. Orio F, Jr., Palomba S, Cascella T, et al. Lack of an association between peroxisome proliferator-activated receptor-gamma gene Pro12Ala polymorphism and adiponectin levels in the polycystic ovary syndrome. *J Clin Endocrinol Metab* 2004;89(10):5110–5.

178. Orio F, Jr., Matarese G, Di Biase S, et al. Exon 6 and 2 peroxisome proliferator-activated receptor-gamma polymorphisms in polycystic ovary syndrome. *J Clin Endocrinol Metab* 2003;88(12):5887–92.

179. Korhonen S, Heinonen S, Hiltunen M, et al. Polymorphism in the peroxisome proliferator-activated receptor-gamma gene in women with polycystic ovary syndrome. *Hum Reprod* 2003;18(3):540–3.

180. Urbanek M, Du Y, Silander K, et al. Variation in resistin gene promoter not associated with polycystic ovary syndrome. *Diabetes* 2003;52(1):214–7.

181. Korhonen S, Romppanen EL, Hiltunen M, et al. Lack of association between C-850T polymorphism of the gene encoding tumor necrosis factor-alpha and polycystic ovary syndrome. *Gynecol Endocrinol* 2002;16(4):271–4.

182. Milner CR, Craig JE, Hussey ND, Norman RJ. No association between the -308 polymorphism in the tumour necrosis factor alpha (TNFalpha) promoter region and polycystic ovaries. *Mol Hum Reprod* 1999;5:5–9.

183. Peral B, San Millan JL, Castello R, Moghetti P, Escobar-Morreale HF. Comment: the methionine 196 arginine polymorphism in exon 6 of the TNF receptor 2 gene (TNFRSF1B) is associated with the polycystic ovary syndrome and hyperandrogenism. *J Clin Endocrinol Metab* 2002;87(8):3977–83.

6

Fetal Origins of Polycystic Ovary Syndrome

David H. Abbott, PhD,
Cristin M. Bruns, MD,
Deborah K. Barnett, PhD,
Alice F. Tarantal, PhD,
Sarah M. Hoffmann, MD,
Rao Zhou, MD, Jon E. Levine, MD,
and Daniel A. Dumesic, MD

CONTENTS

Summary

While the origins of polycystic ovary syndrome (PCOS) in humans are still debated, animal models reliably implicate a fetal origin. Androgen excess, one of the key diagnostic criteria for PCOS and one of its most reliably inherited traits, programs reproductive, adrenal and metabolic organs and tissues during fetal development, producing adult pathology that closely mimics PCOS. Differential gestational timing of androgen excess may also account for heterogeneity in the adult PCOS phenotype. Our fetal or developmental origins hypothesis predicts that development of therapeutic interventions designed to circumvent fetal programming by gestational androgen excess could well eliminate adult PCOS phenotypes.

From: *Contemporary Endocrinology: Polycystic Ovary Syndrome*
Edited by: A. Dunaif, R. J. Chang, S. Franks, and R. S. Legro © Humana Press, Totowa, NJ

Key Words: Animal model; fetal programming; androgen excess; anovulation; etiology of PCOS.

1. INTRODUCTION

Extant or latent ovarian androgen excess *(1)* is central to the diagnosis of polycystic ovary syndrome (PCOS) *(2,3)*. PCOS occurs in 6–7% of reproductive-aged women *(4)* and is highly familial *(5)* and heritable *(6)*, with hyperandrogenism being one of its most reliably inherited traits *(7)*. Hyperandrogenism is pronounced in adult PCOS women, is readily identifiable in adolescent PCOS girls *(8–10)*, and occurs in a subset of juvenile (5–8 year old) girls who are born small for gestational age *(11)* but develop PCOS in later adolescence *(12)*.

Such evidence for developmental progression of hyperandrogenic signs suggests fetal or early postnatal origins for the onset of PCOS *(13,14)*. Potentially in PCOS fetuses, embryonic differentiation of hyperandrogenic ovaries may result in fetal androgen excess during mid- to late gestation *(13)*, when ovarian androgen biosynthesis becomes established *(15)*, when ovarian androgen receptors are expressed *(16)*, and when the female urogenital tract is unresponsive to androgen re-programming *(17,18)*. Moreover, maternal circulating androgen levels are elevated in PCOS women during mid- to late pregnancy *(19)* and may further contribute to the circulating pool of fetal androgens *(20)*.

Molecular components of the hyperandrogenic PCOS phenotype include enhanced functional activity of P450 steroidogenic enzymes, 3-β-hydroxysteroid dehydrogenase II, and specific kinase signaling pathways that exaggerate theca cell androgen biosynthesis *(21–24)*. Up-regulation of genes encoding aldehyde dehydrogenase-6 and retinol dehydrogenase-2, involved in all-trans-retinoic acid synthesis and expression of the transcription factor GATA6, also increases expression of the androgen biosynthetic enzyme, P450c17 (17-α-hydroxylase/17,20-lyase) *(24)*. Dysregulation of the androgen receptor gene in PCOS women may further amplify androgen action cellularly *(25,26)*, whereas genetically determined variants of the gene regulating sex hormone-binding globulin (SHBG) expression may expose PCOS women to elevated circulating bio-available androgens levels *(27)*.

Although a genetic basis for PCOS remains undefined *(28)*, a gene locus centromeric to the insulin receptor gene on chromosome 19 (allele 8 of D19S884) has been the only gene to be repeatedly associated with a PCOS phenotype in several studies *(29–32)*. Studies on the involvement of allele 8 at gene locus D19S884 speculate that this gene locus affects signal transduction mechanisms in PCOS in a manner that (1) enhances theca cell androgen production, (2) regulates metabolism of skeletal muscle and adipose tissue, (3) stabilizes mRNA from degradation, and (4) alters the expression of fibrillin-3, a member of the fibrillin family of extracellular matrix proteins *(21,30,33)*.

Taken together, phenotypic and genotypic evidence strongly implicate a genetic origin for PCOS determined in early life. In this regard, fetal, rather than postnatal, programming of PCOS from androgen excess has one salient feature: it simultaneously exposes multiple organ systems to a specific developmental insult during cellular differentiation and maturation (Fig. 1). In support of fetal programming from hyperandrogenism, elevated human fetal testosterone levels are associated with increased numbers of fetal stem cells from umbilical cord blood and their ability to proliferate *(34)*, and exposure of female fetuses to androgen excess early in gestation produces

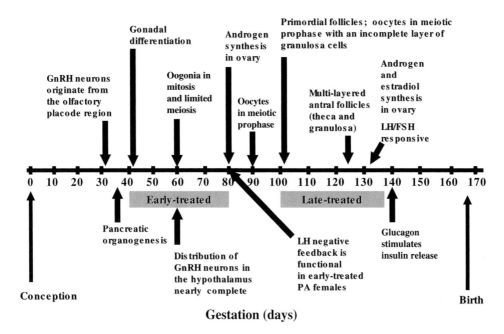

Fig. 1. Gestational progression of aspects of differentiation and maturation of hypothalamic–pituitary–ovarian function and pancreas and β-cell function in rhesus monkeys, modified from *(35)*. The timing of exposure of females to androgen excess (early or late in gestation) is indicated in relation to fetal developmental progress.

permanent alterations in structure and function, including permanent virilization of the female urogenital tract in many mammals, including humans *(35)*. The best example of fetal programming is described by Barker and colleagues *(36)*, in which human fetal undernutrition and low birth weight are associated with cardiovascular disease, hypertension, insulin resistance, type 2 diabetes in adulthood, and all metabolic components of the PCOS phenotype, apart from the reproductive elements required for the PCOS diagnosis.

As illustrated in Fig. 2 and in Table 1, early or late gestation exposure of the female rhesus monkey fetus to fetal male levels of testosterone *(37)* results in adult females with PCOS phenotypic traits that exceed those required for the PCOS diagnosis in women. The ability of this single endocrine disruption to produce a phenotypic mimic of PCOS implicates fetal androgen excess as the common denominator in the etiology of a syndrome that might otherwise appear to have multiple origins *(13)*. In other words, fetal androgen excess might be crucial for expression of the adult phenotype, regardless of whether single or multiple (albeit unidentified) PCOS-related genes exist, environmental factors modify PCOS phenotype *(38)* or epigenetic fetal programming also occurs *(35,39)*. Such a fetal origin for PCOS, with androgen excess at different gestational ages inducing different PCOS phenotypes *(35)* (Fig. 2 and Table 1), also provides a rationale for the heterogeneous reproductive and metabolic phenotypes variously present in PCOS women *(1,35,40)*.

This chapter examines the fetal origins of PCOS in prenatally androgenized female rhesus monkeys and the contribution of the fetal or developmental origins hypothesis

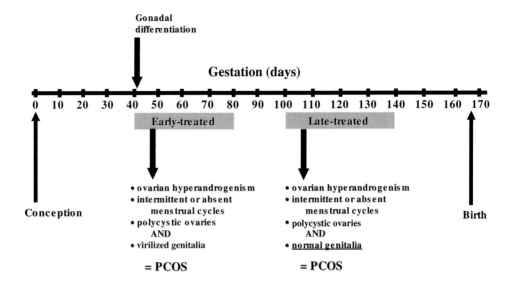

Fig. 2. Key polycystic ovary syndrome (PCOS) diagnostic traits shown by adult female rhesus monkeys exposed to androgen excess during early or late gestation.

(13,35) to our understanding of the pathophysiological mechanisms underlying this highly complex and multi-faceted syndrome.

2. PCOS IN PRENATALLY ANDROGENIZED FEMALE RHESUS MONKEYS

2.1. Fetus and Neonate

Circulating testosterone levels in female rhesus fetuses are elevated into the fetal male range (up to 5–6 ng/ml) when their mothers receive daily injections of testosterone propionate for discrete periods during gestation *(37)* (Abbott et al., unpublished results). Once fetal androgen excess treatment is concluded, prenatally androgenized fetal and newborn female monkeys exhibit hypersecretion of luteinizing hormone (LH) *(41,42)*, an antecedent of PCOS reproductive pathology that appears in adult, prenatally androgenized female monkeys exposed to androgen excess during early gestation *(35)*. The external genitalia are virilized only in prenatally androgenized females exposed to androgen excess during early gestation *(43)*. Following late gestation androgen excess, alterations of the external genitalia are limited to clitoromegaly *(43)*, a characteristic commonly found in women with androgen excess *(44,45)*.

Newborn weight is normal in prenatally androgenized female monkeys exposed to androgen excess during either early or late gestation (*n* = 31) *(35)*. This is in marked contrast to low birthweights and intra-uterine growth restriction (IUGR) in female rats *(46)* and ewes *(47)* exposed to fetal androgen excess. Experimentally induced maternal androgen excess appears to impair placental function in non-primate *(47)* but not primate mammals, possibly due to relatively diminished aromatase activity in non-primate compared to primate placentae *(48)*, thereby exposing the placenta and fetus to relatively greater, and potentially damaging, hyperandrogenic effects *(49,50)*.

Table 1
Dysfunctional Reproductive, Fertility, Adrenal, and Metabolic Defects Common to Both
PCOS Women and Prenatally Androgenized Female Rhesus Monkeys

Sign or symptom	PCOS women	Prenatally androgenized female monkeys	
		Early gestation exposure	Late gestation exposure
Reproductive/fertility defects			
Ovarian hyperandrogenism	+	+ [a]	+ [b]
Anovulation	+	+ [b]	+ [b]
Enlarged polyfollicular ovaries	+	+ [c]	+ [c]
LH hypersecretion	+	+ [d]	− [d]
Reduced steroid hormone negative feedback on LH	+	+ [b,e]	+ [b]
Abnormal ovarian endocrine response to hyperstimulation for IVF	+ (increased response)	+ [d,f]	+ [d,f]
Impaired embryo development after IVF	? (increased miscarriages)	+ [d]	+ [d]
Adrenal defects			
Adrenal hyperandrogenism	+	+ [g]	?
Metabolic defects			
Insulin resistance	+	+ [h]	− [i]
Impaired insulin secretion	+	+ [i]	− [i]
Impaired glucose tolerance	+	+ [h]	+ [h]
Increased type 2 diabetes	+	+ [h]	− [h]
Increased abdominal fat	+	+ [j]	+ [k]
Hyperlipidemia	+	+ [l]	− [l]

[a]Ref. 51
[b]Ref. 35
[c]Ref. 52
[d]Ref. 72
[e]Ref. 53
[f]Ref. 87
[g]Ref. 99
[h]Ref. 54
[i]Ref. 103
[j]Ref. 105
[k]Ref. 55
[l]Refs. 85, 104

There are conflicting reports about whether low birthweight is associated with pregnancy in PCOS women. In northern Spain *(9,11,12)*, IUGR and low birthweight, in association with later development of PCOS, are restricted to those individuals who also experience precocious puberty *(56)*. In a Spanish-speaking population in Chile, PCOS mothers deliver a greater proportion of low birthweight babies when compared to non-PCOS mothers *(57)*, whereas associations between low birthweight and PCOS in larger studies of northern European women have not revealed similar outcomes [Finland *(58)*, Netherlands *(59)*, and United Kingdom *(60)*]. Therefore, in certain human populations, maternal hyperandrogenism in pregnancy might impair placental function to such a degree that fetal development is compromised and birthweight is reduced. Such speculation is consistent with findings that impaired placental aromatization in human pregnancies is accompanied by low birthweight infants *(49,61)* and may be associated with reduced uteroplacental blood flow *(49)*. Furthermore, in non-primate mammals, such as rats, experimentally induced maternal hyperandrogenism increases the risk of low birthweight offspring in pregnancies exposed to a variety of stressors *(50)*, suggesting that hyperandrogensim during pregnancy may increase the risk of placental insufficiency.

2.2. Adolescence

Juvenile, prenatally androgenized female rhesus monkeys display enhanced frequencies of behaviors typically associated with juvenile males, regardless of whether they are exposed to androgen excess during early or late gestation *(62)* or whether they received exogenous testosterone or the non-aromatizable androgen, dihydrotestosterone (DHT) *(43)*. There is a tendency toward "tomboy" behavior in pre-adolescent PCOS girls *(63)*, whereas fetal androgen excess induced by classical congenital adrenal hyperplasia also produces "tomboy" behavior in affected girls *(64,65)*. Menarche is delayed in prenatally androgenized female monkeys exposed early in gestation to either testosterone or DHT, and luteal phase defects are unusually frequent following menarche *(66)*. Such adolescent menstrual cycle disorders precede oligomenorrhea and amenorrhea in adult prenatally androgenized female monkeys (Fig. 3), regardless of gestational timing of androgen excess.

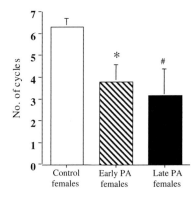

Fig. 3. Mean ± SEM menstrual cycles in six early- and five late-treated prenatally androgenized (PA) and six control female rhesus monkeys during a 6-month period between the months of September–May. Menstrual cycles were determined from at least two serum progesterone values =1 ng/ml obtained 15 days or less before menses *(66,67)*. Data from the months of June–August are omitted to avoid the seasonal time of increased incidence of amenorrhea, typical of this species *(68)*. *, $p < 0.04$ and #, $p < 0.02$, early- and late-treated PA females, respectively, versus controls. Control females: open bar; early-treated PA females: hatched bar; late-treated PA females: solid bar. Reprinted with permission *(35)*.

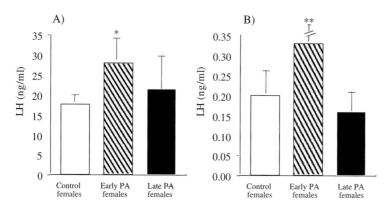

Fig. 4. Elevated circulating luteinizing hormone (LH) levels in early-treated prenatally androgenized (PA) and control rhesus monkeys after (**A**) immuno-determination from control (n = 24), early-treated PA (n = 10), and late-treated PA (n = 3) females; *, $p < 0.001$ versus controls, data modified from (67) and (**B**) bio-active determination from five control, early-treated and five late-treated PA females; **, $p < 0.03$ versus controls, data modified from (72). Control females: open bars; early-treated PA females: hatched bars; late-treated PA females: solid bars. Reprinted with permission (35).

Adolescent and young adult female prenatally androgenized monkeys, exposed to androgen excess during early gestation, exhibit a transient increase in body weight compared to non-exposed females at approximately 3–4 years of age (35,69). At this age, male rhesus monkeys also increase their body weights above those of non-exposed, control females (70), representing a sexually dimorphic trait maintained through adulthood in males but not in prenatally androgenized females. Whether the transient adolescent weight gain in prenatally androgenized females represents increased adiposity or another aspect of fetal programming or masculinization remains to be determined.

2.3. Adult—Reproductive Defects

Whether exposed to androgen excess during early or late gestation, adult, prenatally androgenized female rhesus monkeys exhibit oligomenorrhea or amenorrhea (Fig. 3), hyperandrogenism (35,39), and polycystic ovaries (13,71). The combination of these traits in monkeys also defines the diagnosis of PCOS in women, using either the "NIH" (2) or "Rotterdam" (3) criteria, or currently proposed amendments (1,40).

In addition to menstrual irregularity, hyperandrogenism, and polycystic ovaries, prenatally androgenized female monkeys exposed to androgen excess during early gestation show elevated circulating LH levels (Fig. 4) (35,39,71,72) and increased pituitary LH responsiveness to exogenous gonadotropin-releasing hormone (GnRH) stimulation (35). This LH excess may indicate enhanced endogenous GnRH release from the hypothalamus of such prenatally androgenized monkeys. The frequency of episodic release of hypothalamic GnRH is accelerated (Levine JE et al., 2006, unpublished results), a trait resembling that of PCOS women (73–75).

Recent studies of reproductive dysfunction in prenatally androgenized female sheep (76,77), mice (78), and rats (79) confirm and extend those of prenatally androgenized female monkeys. Regardless of species, all prenatally androgenized females express at least one PCOS diagnostic trait, with additional traits commonly associated with PCOS, including LH hypersecretion. Anovulation in prenatally androgenized female mice *(78)* and rats *(79)* is induced by fetal exposure to the non-aromatizable androgen, DHT, suggesting an androgen receptor-mediated neuroendocrine defect. In prenatally androgenized monkeys, although prenatal DHT exposure induces behavioral outcomes similar to those achieved by testosterone *(35)*, prenatally DHT-exposed animals are not currently available for PCOS studies. In prenatally androgenized adult female mice, however, administration of the anti-androgen, flutamide, restores ovulatory cycles, suggesting that androgen excess in adulthood can disrupt neuroendocrine control of ovulation through an androgen receptor-mediated mechanism *(78)*. In PCOS women, such anti-androgen treatment also reverses an attenuation in progesterone negative feedback on LH secretion but does not correct accelerated LH pulse frequency *(80)*. Prenatally androgenized female monkeys also show reduced progesterone-mediated LH negative feedback *(81)*. Whether accelerated GnRH release in prenatally androgenized monkeys is a primary hypothalamic defect programmed by fetal androgen excess, as suggested by studies in PCOS women *(74)*, or whether it is a consequence of reduced GnRH neuron sensitivity to progesterone-mediated negative feedback remains to be determined.

As in women with PCOS *(82–84)*, compensatory hyperinsulinemia from insulin resistance appears involved in the mechanism of anovulation in prenatally androgenized female rhesus monkeys *(39,85)*, with highly similar metabolic defects in both species *(35)* providing a crucial confluence in anovulatory mechanisms between the monkey model and PCOS women. Improving insulin sensitivity restores ovulatory function in many, but not all, PCOS women *(86)*, whereas chronic treatment of androgenized monkeys with an insulin sensitizer, pioglitazone, also normalizes menstrual cycles in most females, with a similar success rate to that achieved by insulin sensitizer treatment in PCOS women *(85)*. The presumed abnormal insulin signaling in association with ovulatory dysfunction in both prenatally androgenized female monkeys and PCOS women suggests remarkable parallels in reproductive pathologies, ranging from organ system defects to molecular dysfunction, and provides compelling evidence for fetal programming of PCOS and its relevant systemic and molecular defects.

2.4. Adult—Fertility Defects

In addition to hypothalamic–pituitary–ovarian dysfunction, prenatally androgenized female rhesus monkeys exhibit obvious fertility defects. Early gestation androgen excess results in a greater degree of oocyte developmental impairment in vitro, after controlled ovarian stimulation for in vitro fertilization (IVF), while both early and late gestation androgen excess result in reduced blastocyst development and abnormal follicular fluid steroid hormone levels *(71,87,88)*. These infertility findings are analogous to those found in women with PCOS, in whom reduced oocyte quality contributes to increased rates of implantation failure and pregnancy loss after IVF *(89–93)*.

Consistent with the ability of estradiol to enhance cleavage rates of in vitro matured rhesus monkey and human oocytes *(94–95)*, diminished follicular fluid concentrations of estradiol following controlled ovarian hyperstimulation for IVF using either recombinant human (rh) follicle-stimulating hormone (FSH), alone *(87,88)*, or combined rhFSH/rh chorionic gonadotropin *(72,88)* were associated with impaired oocyte developmental competence in prenatally androgenized females regardless of gestational age at the time of androgen excess exposure. Such diminished intra-follicular ovarian estrogenic responses to controlled ovarian hyperstimulation for IVF in prenatally androgenized female monkeys resemble those found in normal women who have reduced ovarian responses to controlled ovarian hyperstimulation for IVF *(96)* but are not found in women with PCOS undergoing similar treatment for IVF *(97)*. In PCOS women, intra-follicular androgen levels are elevated following controlled ovarian hyperstimulation for IVF *(97)*. Consequently, enhancing ovarian estrogenic responses to gonadotropin in prenatally androgenized monkeys may improve oocyte developmental deficiencies, whereas diminishing ovarian androgenic responses to gonadotropin may prove more successful in PCOS women.

Such functionally different responses between prenatally androgenized monkeys and women with PCOS with regard to controlled ovarian hyperstimulation for IVF may reveal a fundamental difference between the two PCOS phenotypes. PCOS women possess constitutively hyperandrogenic ovarian theca cells *(98)*, whereas ovarian hyperandrogenism in prenatally androgenized female monkeys is observed under basal or rhCG-stimulated conditions only *(35,39)*. The relatively greater ovarian hyperandrogenism in PCOS women may reflect a genetically determined ovarian trait that develops during fetal life, exposing female fetuses to androgen excess fetal programming *(13)* and persists into adulthood.

2.5. Adult—Adrenal Defects

Prenatally androgenized female monkeys, exposed to androgen excess during early gestation, display endogenous adrenal androgen excess in adulthood *(99)*. The most likely causes of the excessive adrenal androgen secretion appear to be increased activity of *(1)* P450c17, the rate-limiting step in androgen biosynthesis, in both the zona reticularis (ZR) and the zona fasciculata (ZF), and *(2)* 3-β-hydroxysteroid dehydrogenase II activity in at least the ZR and ZF *(99)*. These findings of adrenal hyperandrogenism in prenatally androgenized female monkeys closely resemble those observed in 25–60% of women with PCOS *(100–102)*. Although it is not yet known whether prenatally androgenized females exposed to androgen excess during late gestation also display adrenal androgen excess in adulthood, our findings suggest that differentiation of the adrenal cortex in a hyperandrogenic environment permanently up-regulates its androgenic capacity that is then retained in the development of mature, postnatal adrenal ZR and ZF. Taken together with our findings of ovarian hyperandrogenism in the same prenatally androgenized female monkeys, these results indicate a systemic enhancement of androgen biosynthesis from fetal programming.

2.6. Adult—Metabolic Defects

Adult female prenatally androgenized female monkeys display a variety of metabolic defects commonly found in PCOS women (Table 1) *(35)*. Fetal programming of metabolic dysfunction occurs when female monkeys are exposed to androgen excess during either early or late gestation. Early gestation-exposed females, however, manifest a more severe metabolic phenotype, exhibiting insulin resistance *(35)*, impaired insulin secretion *(103)*, hyperglycemia *(85)*, hyperlipidemia *(85,104)*, increased visceral adiposity *(105)*, and increased incidence of type 2 diabetes *(88)*. Three of these attributes—abdominal adiposity, hyperlipidemia, and hyperglycemia (Fig. 5)—closely mimic the diagnostic criteria for metabolic syndrome in humans *(106)*, a condition that is also prevalent among adolescent *(108)* and adult *(109,110)* women with PCOS. Late gestation-exposed female monkeys, on the other hand, show decrements in insulin sensitivity with increasing body mass index (BMI) *(103)*, hyperglycemia (Abbott DH et al., unpublished results), and total body adiposity *(55)* while preserving insulin secretory capacity *(103)*, lipid levels (Abbott DH et al., unpublished results), and glycemic control *(88)*.

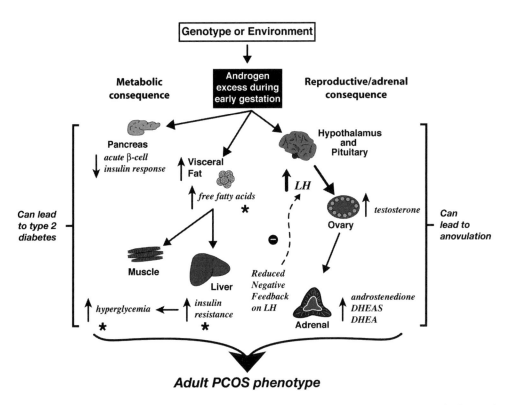

Fig. 5. Diagrammatic representation of our fetal or developmental origins hypothesis for early gestation, fetal androgen excess programming of adult polycystic ovary syndrome (PCOS) traits. Genetic or environmental mechanisms induce fetal hyperandrogenism (see text) that results in permanent changes in reproductive, adrenal, and metabolic function. Reproductive consequences include *(1)* altered hypothalamic–pituitary function leading to luteinizing hormone (LH) hypersecretion, *(2)* ovarian hyperandrogenism that may or may not be the result of LH hypersecretion, *(3)* reduced steroid hormone negative feedback regulation of LH, which may be a component of the initial permanent alteration in hypothalamic–pituitary function, and *(4)* increased anovulation. Adrenal consequences include adrenal hyperandrogenism. Metabolic consequences include *(1)* increased abdominal adiposity that may be responsible for increased circulation of total free fatty acid levels, *(2)* impaired pancreatic insulin secretory response to glucose, *(3)* impaired insulin action and compensatory hyperinsulinemia, *(4)* hyperglycemia, and *(5)* increased incidence of type 2 diabetes. Insulin resistance and compensatory hyperinsulinemia may be functionally implicated in the anovulatory mechanism. *, indicates three traits that closely mimic diagnostic criteria for metabolic syndrome in humans *(106)*: abdominal obesity, hyperlipidemia, and hyperglycemia. Modified from *(107)*.

Amelioration of impaired insulin action has beneficial glucoregulatory effects in both early and late gestation-exposed, prenatally androgenized female monkeys. Chronic pioglitazone therapy improves insulin sensitivity, normalizes fasting plasma glucose levels *(85)*, and reduces abdominal adiposity (Bruns CM, unpublished results). Overall, these metabolic findings in prenatally androgenized female monkeys suggest that *(1)* insulin secretion and insulin action are perturbed similarly in androgenized monkeys and in women with PCOS, *(2)* such insulin impairments in both primate species may develop from preferential accumulation of abdominal fat *(111,112)*, and *(3)* insulin impairments can be ameliorated by an insulin sensitizing agent. These parallels in metabolic defects between prenatally androgenized female monkeys and women with PCOS, together with heterogeneity of metabolic phenotypes, provide further evidence in support of fetal androgen excess programming of this syndrome in humans.

3. PCOS METABOLIC DEFECTS IN PRENATALLY ANDROGENIZED MALE RHESUS MONKEYS

"Prenatally androgenized" may be an oxymoron in terminology when referring to a male rhesus monkey, but it perhaps best describes those fetal males exposed to the same fetal androgen excess treatment as prenatally androgenized females. Prenatally androgenized monkeys generated 15–20 years ago were not selected based on gender *(113)*. Such prenatally androgenized males show no apparent reproductive endocrine defects analogous to those found in prenatally androgenized females, but they do display two key metabolic defects found in the females: insulin resistance and impaired insulin secretion *(113)*. Insulin resistance intensifies with increasing BMI in prenatally androgenized, but not control, male monkeys, raising the possibility of preferential accumulation of abdominal fat in prenatally androgenized males. The group of prenatally androgenized male monkeys comprises individuals exposed to androgen excess during early, mid-, and late gestation *(113)*.

Close male relatives of women with PCOS demonstrate metabolic abnormalities that parallel those found in their PCOS kin, including impaired glucose tolerance, type 2 diabetes, and hyperinsulinemia *(114–118)*. PCOS male kin also can exhibit adrenal hyperandrogenism *(119)* and can show an exaggerated androgenic response to leuprolide *(120)*. The similar metabolic phenotypes in prenatally androgenized male and female monkeys, and in women with PCOS and their male close relatives, suggest the intriguing possibility that metabolic programming from maternal or fetal androgen excess is central to adult metabolic dysfunction, regardless of the fetal sex.

4. FETAL OR DEVELOPMENTAL ORIGINS HYPOTHESIS FOR PCOS

In this chapter, we have provided overwhelming evidence in support of the fetal or developmental origins hypothesis for PCOS (Figs 2 and 5). Prenatally androgenized female rhesus monkeys recapitulate many of the traits found in PCOS women, regardless of the timing of gestational exposure to androgen excess. PCOS-like metabolic defects are also found in prenatally androgenized male monkeys and in close male relatives of women with PCOS. Female monkeys exposed to androgen excess during early gestation demonstrate a greater preponderance of reproductive and metabolic PCOS traits when compared to females exposed during late gestation (Table 1). This more pervasive expression of PCOS traits in female monkeys exposed to androgen excess during early gestation may reflect androgen exposure when many fetal organ systems are undergoing differentiation (Fig. 1). Late gestation-exposed females, on the other hand, experience androgen excess when most organ systems have completed differentiation but are still undergoing functional maturation. It is not surprising, therefore, that these two different gestational exposures to androgen excess yield different programming outcomes, with early gestational exposure altering structure and multiple aspects of function and late gestational exposure being more limited to modifying function and maturation *(35)* (Table 1). Such defined heterogeneity of PCOS phenotype in female monkeys may provide additional insight into the developmental origins of heterogeneity in PCOS women.

Our fetal or developmental hypothesis for PCOS, focusing on early gestation androgen excess, is illustrated in Fig. 5. We propose that early gestation androgen excess inflicts at least two, and possibly three, distinctive programming consequences on female reproductive, adrenal, and metabolic physiology. Whether significant components of reproductive and adrenal programming are secondary to hypothalamic dysregulation of pituitary LH and adrenocorticotropin (ACTH), respectively, or involve additional abnormalities of ovarian and adrenal origin remains to be determined. An analogous situation may also pertain to metabolic programming: are defects in insulin action and secretion secondary to abdominal adiposity and hyperlipidemia or do they represent abnormalities that are pancreatic in origin or involve insulin signaling mechanisms? Regardless, our proposed fetal androgen excess in PCOS women may still be induced by genetic, maternal, or in utero environmental mechanisms, or by a combination of all three (Fig. 5). The findings of PCOS-like metabolic defects in prenatally androgenized male monkeys, similar to those found in male close relatives of women with PCOS *(113)*, raise the possibility that such metabolic abnormalities have a common fetal origin in both sexes.

Our fetal or developmental origins hypothesis also predicts the increased prevalence of PCOS found in women with androgen excess disorders related to the fetal adrenal cortex, including 21-hydroxylase deficiency and congenital adrenal virilizing tumors *(121–124)*. The hypothesis further agrees with the increased prevalence of insulin resistance in men with 21-hydroxylase deficiency *(125)*. Supporting our hypothesis, umbilical cord sampling of 10 human female fetuses during early gestation demonstrates a 40% incidence of elevated serum testosterone levels into the fetal male range *(126)*, suggesting that human fetal androgen excess may frequently occur in humans.

As models for PCOS women and their close male relatives, prenatally androgenized female and male rhesus monkeys, respectively, implicate androgen excess (or its consequences) during critical periods of gestation in the pathogenesis of adult PCOS phenotypes in women and metabolic dysfunction in their male close relatives. Our fetal or developmental origins hypothesis (Fig. 5) opens new directions for clinical management of PCOS through increased understanding of hormonal disruption during intra-uterine life and the programming of target organ differentiation in developing fetuses of both sexes.

ACKNOWLEDGMENTS

We thank the many staff members of our respective laboratories and institutions for their multiple contributions to the work reported here. This work was supported by NIH grants P50 HD044405, U01 HD044650, R01 RR013635, R21 RR014093, T32 AG000268, P51 RR000167, and P51 RR000169 and was partly conducted at a facility constructed with support from Research Facilities Improvement Program grant numbers RR15459-01 and RR020141-01.

REFERENCES

1. Azziz R, Carmina E, Dewailly D, Diamanti-Kandarakis E, Escobar-Morreale HF, Futterweit W, Janssen OE, Legro RS, Norman RJ, Taylor AE, Witchel SF. Position statement: Criteria for defining polycystic ovary syndrome as a predominantly hyperandrogenic syndrome: An Androgen Excess Society guideline. *J Clin Endocrinol Metab*. 2006, 91:4237–4245.

2. Zawadzki JA, Dunaif A. Diagnostic criteria for polycystic ovary syndrome: towards a rational approach. In: Dunaif A, Givens JR, Haseltine FP, Merriam GR, eds. *Polycystic Ovary Syndrome*. Boston, MA: Blackwell Scientific. 1992, 377–384.

3. Rotterdam ESHRE/ASRM-Sponsored PCOS consensus workshop group. Revised 2003 consensus on diagnostic criteria and long-term health risks related to polycystic ovary syndrome (PCOS). *Hum Reprod* 2004, 19:41–47.

4. Azziz R, Woods KS, Reyna R, Key TJ, Knochenhauer ES, Yildiz BO. The prevalence and features of the polycystic ovary syndrome in an unselected population. *J Clin Endocrinol Metab* 2004, 89:2745–2749.

5. Diamanti-Kandarakis E, Piperi C. Genetics of polycystic ovary syndrome: searching for the way out of the labyrinth. *Hum Reprod Update* 2005, 11:631–643.

6. Vink JM, Sadrzadeh S, Lambalk CB, Boomsma DI. Heritability of polycystic ovary syndrome (PCOS) in a Dutch twin-family study. *J Clin Endocrinol Metab* 2006, 91: 2100–2104.

7. Legro RS, Driscoll D, Strauss JF 3rd, Fox J, Dunaif A. Evidence for a genetic basis for hyperandrogenemia in polycystic ovary syndrome. *Proc Natl Acad Sci USA* 1998, 95:14956–14960.

8. Chhabra S, McCartney CR, Yoo RY, Eagleson CA, Chang RJ, Marshall JC. Progesterone inhibition of the hypothalamic gonadotropin-releasing hormone pulse generator: evidence for varied effects in hyperandrogenemic adolescent girls. *J Clin Endocrinol Metab* 2005, 90:2810–2815.

9. Ibanez L, de Zegher FD. Low-dose flutamide-metformin therapy for hyperinsulinemic hyperandrogenism in non-obese adolescents and women. *Hum Reprod Update* 2006, 12:243–252.

10. Leibel NI, Baumann EE, Kocherginsky M, Rosenfield RL. Relationship of adolescent polycystic ovary syndrome to parental metabolic syndrome. *J Clin Endocrinol Metab* 2006, 91: 1275–1283.

11. Ibanez L, Potau N, Zampolli M, Prat N, Virdis R, Vicens-Calvet E, Carrascosa A. Hyperinsulinemia in postpubertal girls with a history of premature pubarche and functional ovarian hyperandrogenism. *J Clin Endocrinol Metab* 1996, 81:1237–1243.

12. Ibanez L, Potau N, Francois I, de Zegher F. Precocious pubarche, hyperinsulinism, and ovarian hyperandrogenism in girls: relation to reduced fetal growth. *J Clin Endocrinol Metab* 1998, 83: 3558–3562.

13. Abbott DH, Dumesic DA, Franks S. Developmental origin of polycystic ovary syndrome - a hypothesis. *J Endocrinol* 2002, 174:1–5.

14. Xita N, Tsatsoulis A. Fetal programming of polycystic ovary syndrome by androgen excess: evidence from experimental, clinical and genetic association studies. *J Clin Endocrinol Metab* 2006, 91: 1660–16666.

15. Ellinwood WE, McClellan MC, Brenner RM, Resko JA. Estradiol synthesis by fetal monkey ovaries correlates with antral follicle formation. *Biol Reprod* 1983, 28:505–516.

16. Wilson CM, McPhaul MJ. A and B forms of the androgen receptor are expressed in a variety of human tissues. *Mol Cell Endocrinol* 1996, 18:51–57.

17. Goy RW, Bercovitch FB, McBrair MC. Behavioral masculinization is independent of genital masculinization in prenatally androgenized female rhesus macaques. *Horm Behav* 1988, 22:552–571.

18. Quigley CA, De Bellis A, Marschke KB, el-Awady MK, Wilson EM, French FS. Androgen receptor defects: historical, clinical, and molecular perspectives. *Endocr Rev* 1995, 16:271–321.

19. Sir-Petermann T, Maliqueo M, Angel B, Lara HE, Perez-Bravo F, Recabarren SE. Maternal serum androgens in pregnant women with polycystic ovarian syndrome: possible implications in prenatal androgenization. *Hum Reprod* 2002, 17:2573–2579.

20. Gitau R, Adams D, Fisk NM, Glover V. Fetal plasma testosterone correlates positively with cortisol. *Arch Dis Child Fetal Neonatal Ed* 2005, 90:F166–F169.

21. Wood JR, Nelson VL, Ho C, Jansen E, Wang CY, Urbanek M, McAllister JM, Mosselman S, Strauss JF III. The molecular phenotype of polycystic ovary syndrome (PCOS) theca cells and new candidate PCOS genes defined by microarray analysis. *J Biol Chem* 2003, 278:26380–26390.

22. Wood JR, Ho CK, Nelson-Degrave VL, McAllister JM, Strauss JF III. The molecular signature of polycystic ovary syndrome (PCOS) theca cells defined by gene expression profiling. *J Reprod Immunol* 2004, 63:51–60.

23. Nelson-Degrave VL, Wickenheisser JK, Hendricks KL, Asano T, Fujishiro M, Legro RS, Kimball SR, Strauss JF III, McAllister JM. Alterations in mitogen-activated protein kinase and extracellular regulated kinase signaling in theca cells contribute to excessive androgen production in polycystic ovary syndrome. *Mol Endocrinol* 2005, 19:379–390.

24. Escobar-Morreale HF, Luque-Ramirez M, San Millan JL. The molecular-genetic basis of functional hyperandrogenism and the polycystic ovary syndrome. *Endocr Rev* 2005, 26:251–282.

25. Hickey T, Chandy A, Norman RJ. The androgen receptor CAG repeat polymorphism and X-chromosome inactivation in Australian Caucasian women with infertility related to polycystic ovary syndrome. *J Clin Endocrinol Metab* 2002, 87:161–165.

26. Ibanez L, Ong KK, Mongan N, Jaaskelainen J, Marcos MV, Hughes IA, de Zegher F, Dunger DB. Androgen receptor gene CAG repeat polymorphism in the development of ovarian hyperandrogenism. *J Clin Endocrinol Metab* 2003, 88:3333–3338.

27. Xita N, Tsatsoulis A, Chatzikyriakidou A, Georgiou I. Association of the (TAAAA)n repeat polymorphism in the sex hormone-binding globulin (SHBG) gene with polycystic ovary syndrome and relation to SHBG serum levels. *J Clin Endocrinol Metab* 2003, 88:5976–5980.

28. Legro RS and Strauss JF. Molecular progress in infertility: polycystic ovary syndrome. *Fertil Steril* 2003, 78:569–576.

29. Urbanek M, Legro RS, Driscoll DA, Azziz R, Ehrmann DA, Norman RJ, Strauss JF III, Spielman RS, Dunaif A. Thirty-seven candidate genes for polycystic ovary syndrome: strongest evidence for linkage is with follistatin. *Proc Natl Acad Sci USA* 1999, 96:8573–8578.

30. Urbanek M, Woodroffe A, Ewens KG, Diamanti-Kandarakis E, Legro RS, Strauss JF III, Dunaif A, Spielman RS. Candidate gene region for polycystic ovary syndrome on chromosome 19p13.2. *J Clin Endocrinol Metab* 2005, 90:6623–6629.

31. Tucci S, Futterweit W, Concepcion ES, Greenberg DA, Villanueva R, Davies TF and Tomer Y. Evidence for association of polycystic ovary syndrome in Caucasian women with a marker at the insulin receptor gene locus. *J Clin Endocrinol Metab* 2001, 86:446–449.

32. Villuendas G, Escobar-Morreale HF, Tosi F, Sancho J, Moghetti P, San Millan JL. Association between the D19S884 marker at the insulin receptor gene locus and polycystic ovary syndrome. *Fertil Steril* 2003, 79:219–220.

33. Strauss JF III. Some new thoughts on the pathophysiology and genetics of polycystic ovary syndrome. *Ann N Y Acad Sci* 2003, 997:42–48.

34. Baik I, Devito WJ, Ballen K, Becker PS, Okulicz W, Liu Q, Delpapa E, Lagiou P, Sturgeon S, Trichopoulos D, Quesenberry PJ, Hsieh CC. Association of fetal hormone levels with stem cell potential: evidence for early life roots of human cancer. *Cancer Res* 2005, 65:358–363.

35. Abbott DH, Barnett DK, Bruns CM, Dumesic DA. Androgen excess fetal programming of female reproduction: a developmental aetiology for polycystic ovary syndrome? *Hum Reprod Update* 2005, 11:357–374.

36. Barker DJP. *Mothers, Babies and Health in Later Life*. Edinburgh: Churchill Livingstone. 1994.

37. Resko JA, Buhl AE, Phoenix CH. Treatment of pregnant rhesus macaques with testosterone propionate: observations on its fate in the fetus. *Biol Reprod* 1987, 37:1185–1191.

38. Jahanfar S, Eden JA, Warren P, Seppala M, Nguyen TV. A twin study of polycystic ovary syndrome. *Fertil Steril* 1995, 63:478–486.

39. Abbott DH, Dumesic DA, Eisner JR, Colman RJ, Kemnitz JW. Insights into the development of PCOS from studies of prenatally androgenized female rhesus monkeys. *Trends Endocrinol Metab* 1998, 9:62–67.

40. Azziz R. Controversy in clinical endocrinology: diagnosis of polycystic ovarian syndrome: the Rotterdam criteria are premature. *J Clin Endocrinol Metab* 2006, 91:781–785.

41. Abbott DH, Dobbert MJW, Levine JE, Dumesic DA, Tarantal AF. *Androgen Excess Induces Fetal Programming of LH Hypersecretion in a Female Rhesus Monkey Model for Polycystic Ovary Syndrome (PCOS)*. Abstract #OR28–2 presented at the 87th Annual Meeting of the Endocrine Society, San Diego, CA, June 4–7, 2005.

42. Herman RA, Jones B, Mann DR, Wallen K. Timing of prenatal androgen exposure: anatomical and endocrine effects on juvenile male and female rhesus monkeys. *Horm Behav* 2000, 38:52–66.

43. Goy RW, Uno H, Sholl SA. Psychological and anatomical consequences of prenatal exposure to androgens in female rhesus. In: *Toxicity of Hormones in Perinatal Life*. Mori T, Nagasawa H, eds. Boca Raton, FL: CRC Press, Inc. 1988, 127–142.

44. Emans SJ, Grace E, Goldstein DP. Oligomenorrhea in adolescent girls. *J Pediatr* 1980, 97:815–819.

45. Jabbour SA. Cutaneous manifestations of endocrine disorders: a guide for dermatologists. *Am J Clin Dermatol* 2003, 4:315–331.

46. Slob AK, den Hamer R, Woutersen PJ and van der Werff ten Bosch JJ. Prenatal testosterone propionate and postnatal ovarian activity in the rat. *Acta Endocrinol (Copenh)* 1983, 103:420–427.

47. Manikkam M, Crespi EJ, Doop DD, Herkimer C, Lee JS, Yu S, Brown MB, Foster DL, Padmanabhan V. Fetal programming: prenatal testosterone excess leads to fetal growth retardation and postnatal catch-up growth in sheep. *Endocrinology* 2004, 145:790–798.

48. France JT, Mason JI, Magness RR, Murry BA, Rosenfeld CR. Ovine placental aromatase: studies of activity levels, kinetic characteristics and effects of aromatase inhibitors. *J Steroid Biochem* 1987, 28:155–160.

49. Tanguy G, Thoumsin HJ, Zorn JR, Cedard L. DHEA-S-loading test in cases of intrauterine growth retardation: relationship between the pattern of the maternal plasma metabolites and the fetoplacental dysfunction. *Gy necol Obstet Invest* 1981, 12:305–316.

50. McGivern RF. Low birthweight in rats induced by prenatal exposure to testosterone combined with alcohol, pair-feeding, or stress. *Teratology* 1989, 40:335–338.

51. Eisner JR, Barnett MA, Dumesic DA, Abbott DH. Ovarian hyperandrogenism in adult female rhesus monkeys exposed to prenatal androgen excess. *Fertil Steril*. 2002, 77:167–172.

52. Abbott DH, Eisner JR, Colman RJ, Kemnitz JW and Dumesic DA. Prenatal androgen excess programs for PCOS in female rhesus monkeys. In: *Polycystic Ovary Syndrome*. R.J. Chang, A. Dunaif and J. Hiendel (eds), Marcel Dekker, Inc., New York. 2002, 119–133.

53. Steiner RA, Clifton DK, Spies HG and Resko JA. Sexual differentiation and feedback control of luteinizing hormone secretion in the rhesus monkey. *Biol Reprod* 1976, 15:206–212.

54. Abbott DH, Bruns CM, Barnett DK, Zhou R, Colman RJ, Kemnitz JW, Padmanabhan V, Goodfriend TL, Dumesic DA. *Metabolic and reproductive consequences of prenatal testosterone exposure.* Abstract #S34-1 presented at the 85th Annual Meeting of the Endocrine Society, Philadelphia, PA, June 19–22, 2003.

55. Bruns CM, Baum ST, Colman RJ, Dumesic DA, Eisner JR, Jensen MD, Whigham LD, Abbott DH. Prenatal androgen excess negatively impacts body fat distriburion in a nonhuman primate model of polycystic ovary syndrome. *Int J Obes (Lond). 2007, May 1; [Epub ahead of print].*

56. Hokken-Koelega AC. Timing of puberty and fetal growth. *Best Pract Res Clin Endocrinol Metab* 2002, 16:65–71.

57. Sir-Petermann T, Hitchsfeld C, Maliqueo M, Codner E, Echiburu B, Gazitua R, Recabarren S, Cassorla F. Birth weight in offspring of mothers with polycystic ovarian syndrome. *Hum Reprod* 2005, 20:2122–2126.

58. Laitinen J, Taponen S, Martikainen H, Pouta A, Millwood I, Hartikainen AL, Ruokonen A, Sovio U, McCarthy MI, Franks S, Jarvelin MR. Body size from birth to adulthood as a predictor of self-reported polycystic ovary syndrome symptoms. *Int J Obes Relat Metab Disord* 2003, 27:710–715.

59. Sadrzadeh S, Klip WA, Broekmans FJ, Schats R, Willemsen WN, Burger CW, Van Leeuwen FE, Lambalk CB; OMEGA Project group. Birth weight and age at menarche in patients with polycystic ovary syndrome or diminished ovarian reserve, in a retrospective cohort. *Hum Reprod* 2003, 18:2225–2230.

60. Cresswell JL, Barker DJ, Osmond C, Egger P, Phillips DI, Fraser RB (1997) Fetal growth, length of gestation, and polycystic ovaries in adult life. *Lancet* 350, 1131–1135.

61. Thoumsin HJ, Alsat E, Cedard L. In vitro aromatization of androgens into estrogens in placental insufficiency. *Gynecol Obstet Invest* 1982, 13:37–43.

62. Goy RW, Bercovitch FB, McBrair MC. Behavioral masculinization is independent of genital masculinization in prenatally androgenized female rhesus macaques. *Horm Behav* 1988, 22:552–571.

63. Gorzynski G and Katz JL. The polycystic ovary syndrome:psychosexual correlates. *Arch Sex Behav* 1977, 6:215–222.

64. Dittmann RW, Kappes ME and Kappes MH. Sexual behavior in adolescent and adult females with congenital adrenal hyperplasia. *Psychoneuroendocrinology* 1992, 17:153–170.

65. Hall CM, Jones JA, Meyer-Bahlburg HF, Dolezal C, Coleman M, Foster P, Price DA and Clayton PE. Behavioral and physical masculinization are related to genotype in girls with congenital adrenal hyperplasia. *J Clin Endocrinol Metab* 2004, 89:419–424.

66. Goy RW and Robinson JA. Prenatal exposure of rhesus monkeys to patent androgens: morphological, behavioral, and physiological consequences. In *Banbury Report II: Environmental Factors in Human Growth and Development*, Cold Spring Harbor, New York: Cold Spring Harbor Laboratory, 1982, 355–378.

67. Dumesic DA, Abbott DH, Eisner JR, Goy RW. Prenatal exposure of female rhesus monkeys to testosterone propionate increases serum luteinizing hormone levels in adulthood. *Fertil Steril* 1997, 67:155–163.

68. Resko JA, Goy RW, Robinson JA, Norman RL. The pubescent rhesus monkey: some characteristics of the menstrual cycle. Biol Reprod. 1982, 27:354–361.

69. Wilen R, Goy RW, Resko JA, Naftolin F. Pubertal body weight and growth in the female rhesus pseudohermaphrodite. Biol of Reprod 1977, 16:470–473.

70. Kemnitz JW, Sladky KK, Flitsch TJ, Pomerantz SM, Goy RW. Androgenic influences on body size and composition of adult rhesus monkeys. Am J Physiol 1988, 255:E857–864.

71. Abbott DH, Dumesic DA, Eisner, J.W. Kemnitz JW, Goy RW. The prenatally androgenized female rhesus monkey as a model for polycystic ovarian syndrome. In: Azziz R, Nestler JE and Dewailly D, eds. *Androgen Excess Disorders in Women*. Philadelphia, PA: Lippencott-Raven Press. 1997, 369–382.

72. Dumesic DA, Schramm RD, Peterson E, Paprocki AM, Zhou R, Abbott DH. Impaired developmental competence of oocytes in adult prenatally androgenized female rhesus monkeys undergoing gonadotropin stimulation for *in vitro* fertilization. *J Clin Endocrinol Metab* 2002, 87:1111–1119.

73. Burger CW, Korsen T, van Kessel H, van Dop PA, Caron FJ, Schoemaker J. Pulsatile luteinizing hormone patterns in the follicular phase of the menstrual cycle, polycystic ovarian disease (PCOD) and non-PCOD secondary amenorrhea. *J Clin Endocrinol Metab* 1985, 61:1126–1132.

74. Eagleson CA, Bellows AB, Hu K, Gingrich MB and Marshall JC. Obese patients with polycystic ovary syndrome: evidence that metformin does not restore sensitivity of the gonadotropin-releasing hormone pulse generator to inhibition by ovarian steroids. *J Clin Endocrinol Metab* 2003, 88: 5158–5162.

75. McCartney CR, Prendergast S, Chhabra C, Chopra C and Marshall JC. *Neuroendcorine Connection in PCOS.* In Marco Filicori, ed., *Updates in Infertility Treatment* 2004. Bologna, Italy: Medimond, International Proceedings. 2004, 427–436.

76. West C, Foster DL, Evans NP, Robinson J and Padmanabhan V. Intra-follicular activin availability is altered in prenatally-androgenized lambs. *Mol Cell Endocrinol* 2001, 185:51–59.

77. Sarma HN, Manikkam M, Herkimer C, Dell'Orco J, Foster DL, Padmanabhan V. Fetal programming: excess prenatal testosterone reduces postnatal luteinizing hormone, but not follicle-stimulating hormone responsiveness, to estradiol negative feedback in the female. *Endocrinology* 2005, 146:4281–4291.

78. Sullivan SD, Moenter SM. Prenatal androgens alter GABAergic drive to gonadotropin-releasing hormone nerurons: implications for a common fertility disorder. *Proc Natl Acad Sci USA* 2004, 101:7129–7134.

79. Foecking EM, Szabo M, Schwartz NB, Levine JF. Neuroendocrine consequences of prenatal androgen exposure in the female rat: absence of luteinizing hormone surges, suppression of progesterone receptor gene expression, and acceleration of the gonadotropin-releasing hormone pulse generator. *Biol Reprod* 2005, 72:1475–1483.

80. Eagleson CA, Gingrich MB, Pastro CL, Arora TK, Burt CM, Evans WS, Marshall JC. Polycystic ovarian syndrome: evidence that flutamide restores sensitivity of the gonadotropin-releasing hormone pulse generator to inhibition by estradiol and progesterone. *J Clin Endocrinol Metab* 2000, 85:4047–4052.

81. Levine JE, Terasawa E, Hoffmann SM, Dobbert MJW, Foecking E, Abbott DH. *Luteinizing Hormone (LH) Hypersecretion and Diminished LH Responses to RU486 in a Nonhuman Primate Model for Polycystic Ovary Syndrome (PCOS).* Abstract #P1–85 presented at the 87th Annual Meeting of the Endocrine Society, San Diego, CA, June 4–7, 2005.

82. Dunaif A, Scott D, Finegood D, Quintana B and Whitcomb R. The insulin-sensitizing agent troglitazone improves metabolic and reproductive abnormalities in the polycystic ovary syndrome. *J Clin Endocrinol Metab* 1996, 81, 3299–3306.

83. Ehrmann DA, Schneider DJ, Sobel BE, Cavaghan MK, Imperial J, Rosenfield RL, Polonsky KS. Troglitazone improves defects in insulin action, insulin secretion, ovarian steroidogenesis and fibrinolysis in women with polycystic ovary syndrome. *J Clin Endocrinol Metab* 1997, 82: 2108–2116.

84. Nestler JE, Jakubowicz DJ, Evans WS and Pasquali R. Effects of metformin on spontaneous and clomiphene-induced ovulation in the polycystic ovary syndrome. *N Engl J Med* 1998, 338: 1876–1880.

85. Zhou R, Bruns CM, Bird IM, Kemnitz JW, Goodfriend TL, Dumesic DA, Abbott DH. Pioglitazone improves insulin action and normalizes menstrual cycles in a majority of prenatally androgenized female rhesus monkeys. *Reprod Toxicol.* 2007, 23:438–448.

86. Lord JM, Flight IH, Norman RJ. Metformin in polycystic ovary syndrome: systematic review and meta-analysis. *BMJ* 2003, 327:951–953.

87. Dumesic DA, Schramm RD, Bird IM, Peterson E, Paprocki AM, Zhou R, Abbott DH. Reduced intrafollicular androstenedione and estradiol levels in early-treated prenatally androgenized female rhesus monkeys receiving FSH therapy for in vitro fertilization. *Biol Reprod* 2003, 69: 1213–1219.

88. Dumesic DA, Schramm RD, Abbott DH. Early origins of polycystic ovary syndrome (PCOS). *Reprod Fertil Dev* 2005, 17:349–360.

89. Homburg R, Armar NA, Eshel A, Adams J and Jacobs HS. Influence of serum luteinising hormone concentrations on ovulation, conception, and early pregnancy loss in polycystic ovary syndrome. *BMJ* 1988, 297:1024–1026.

90. Sagle M, Bishop K, Ridley N, Alexander FM, Michel M, Bonney RC, Beard RW and Franks S. Recurrent early miscarriage and polycystic ovaries. *BMJ* 1988, 297:1027–1028.

91. Dor J, Shulman A, Levran D, Ben-Rafael Z, Rudak E and Mashiach S. The treatment of patients with polycystic ovarian syndrome by in-vitro fertilization and embryo transfer: a comparison of results with those of patients with tubal infertility. *Hum Reprod* 1990, 5:816–818.

92. Tarlatzis BC, Grimbizis G, Pournaropoulos F, Bontis J, Lagos S, Spanos E and Mantalenakis S. The prognostic value of basal luteinizing hormone : follicle-stimulating hormone ratio in the treatment of patients with polycystic ovarian syndrome by assisted reproduction techniques. *Hum Reprod* 1995, 10:2545–2549.

93. Ludwig M, Finas DF, Al-Hasani S, Diedrich K, Ortmann O. Oocyte quality and treatment outcome in intracytoplasmic sperm injection cycles of polycystic ovarian syndrome patients. *Hum Reprod* 1999, 14:354–358.

94. Tesarik J, Mendoza C. Nongenomic effects of 17β-estradiol on maturing human oocytes: relationship to oocyte developmental potential. *J Clin Endocrinol Metab* 1995, 80:1438–1443.

95. Zheng P, Wei S, Bavister BD, Yang J, Ding C, Ji W. 17β-estradiol and progesterone improve in-vitro cytoplasmic maturation of oocytes from unstimulated prepubertal and adult rhesus monkeys. *Hum Reprod* 2003, 18:2137–2144.

96. Foong SC, Abbott DH, Lesnick TG, Session DR, Walker DL, Dumesic DA. Diminished intrafollicular estradiol levels in in vitro fertilization cycles from women with reduced ovarian response to recombinant human follicle-stimulating hormone. *Fertil Steril* 2005, 83:1377–1383.

97. Foong SC, Abbott DH, Zschunke MA, Lesnick TG, Phy JL, Dumesic DA. Follicle luteinization in hyperandrogenic follicles of polycystic ovary syndrome (PCOS) patients undergoing gonadotropin therapy for in vitro fertilization (IVF). *J Clin Endocrinol Metab* 2006, 91: 2327–2333.

98. Nelson VL, Qin Kn KN, Rosenfield RL, Wood JR, Penning TM, Legro RS, Strauss JF III, McAllister JM. The biochemical basis for increased testosterone production in theca cells propagated from patients with polycystic ovary syndrome. *J Clin Endocrinol Metab* 2001, 86:5925–5933.

99. Zhou R, Bird IM, Dumesic DA, Abbott DH. Adrenal hyperandrogenism is induced by fetal androgen excess in a rhesus monkey model of polycystic ovary syndrome. *J Clin Endocrinol Metab* 2005, 90:6630–6637.

100. Wild RA, Umstot ES, Andersen RN, Ranney G, Givens JR. Androgen parameters and their correlation with body weight in one hundred thirty-eight women thought to have hyperandrogenism. *Am J Obstet Gynecol* 1983, 146:602–606.

101. Moran C, Knochenhauer E, Boots LR, Azziz R. Adrenal androgen excess in hyperandrogenism: relation to age and body mass. *Fertil Steril* 1999, 71:671–674.

102. Carmina E, Koyama T, Chang L, Stanczyk FZ, Lobo RA. Does ethnicity influence the prevalence of adrenal hyperandrogenism and insulin resistance in polycystic ovary syndrome? *Am J Obstet Gynecol* 1992, 167:1807–1812.

103. Eisner JR, Dumesic DA, Kemnitz JW, Abbott DH. Timing of prenatal androgen excess determines differential impairment in insulin secretion and action in adult female rhesus monkeys. *J Clin Endocrinol Metab* 2000, 85:1206–1210.

104. Abbott DH, Eisner JR, Goodfriend TL, Medley RD, Peterson EJ, Colman Ricki J, Kemnitz JW and Dumesic DA. *Leptin and Total Free Fatty Acids are Elevated in the Circulation of Prenatally Androgenized Female Rhesus Monkeys.* Abstract #P2–329, 84th Annual Meeting of the Endocrine Society, San Francisco, CA, June 2002.

105. Eisner JR, Dumesic DA, Kemnitz JW, Colman RJ, Abbott DH. Increased adiposity in female rhesus monkeys exposed to androgen excess during early gestation. *Obes Res* 2003, 11:279–286.

106. Ford ES, Giles WH, Dietz WH. Prevalence of the metabolic syndrome among US adults: findings from the third National Health and Nutrition Examination Survey. *JAMA* 2002, 287:356–359.

107. Abbott DH, Padmanabhan V and Dumesic DA. Contributions of androgen and estrogen to fetal programming of ovarian dysfunction. *Reproductive Biology and Endocrinology* 2006, 4:17.

108. Coviello AD, Legro RS, Dunaif A. Adolescent girls with polycystic ovary syndrome have an increased risk of the metabolic syndrome associated with increasing androgen levels independent of obesity and insulin resistance. *J Clin Endocrinol Metab* 2006, 91:492–497.

109. Carmina E, Napoli N, Longo RA, Rini GB, Lobo RA. Metabolic syndrome in polycystic ovary syndrome (PCOS): lower prevalence in southern Italy than in the USA and the influence of criteria for the diagnosis of PCOS. *Eur J Endocrinol* 2006, 154:141–145.

110. Ehrmann DA, Liljenquist DR, Kasza K, Azziz R, Legro RS, Ghazzi MN; PCOS/Troglitazone Study Group. Prevalence and predictors of the metabolic syndrome in women with polycystic ovary syndrome. *J Clin Endocrinol Metab* 2006, 91:48–53.

111. Wagenknecht LE, Langefeld CD, Scherzinger AL, Norris JM, Haffner SM, Saad MF, Bergman RN. Insulin sensitivity, insulin secretion, and abdominal fat: the Insulin Resistance Atherosclerosis Study (IRAS) Family Study. *Diabetes* 2003, 52:2490–2496.

112. Puder JJ, Varga S, Kraenzlin M, De Geyter C, Keller U, Muller B. Central fat excess in polycystic ovary syndrome: relation to low-grade inflammation and insulin resistance. *J Clin Endocrinol Metab* 2005, 90:6014–6021.

113. Bruns CM, Baum ST, Colman RJ, Eisner JR, Kemnitz JW, Weindruch R, Abbott DH. Insulin resistance and impaired insulin secretion in prenatally androgenized male rhesus monkeys. *J Clin Endocrinol Metab* 2004, 89:6218–6223.

114. Yildiz BO, Yarali H, Oguz H, Bayraktar M. Glucose intolerance, insulin resistance, and hyperandrogenemia in first degree relatives of women with polycystic ovary syndrome. *J Clin Endocrinol Metab* 2003, 88:2031–2036.

115. Fox R. Prevalence of a positive family history of type 2 diabetes in women with polycystic ovarian disease. *Gynecol Endocrinol* 1999, 13:390–393.

116. Sir-Petermann T, Maliqueo M, Angel B, Lara HE, Perez-Bravo F, Recabarren SE. Maternal serum androgens in pregnant women with polycystic ovarian syndrome: possible implications in prenatal androgenization. *Hum Reprod* 2002, 17:2573–2579.

117. Colilla S, Cox NJ, Ehrmann DA. Heritability of insulin secretion and insulin action in women with polycystic ovary syndrome and their first degree relatives. *J Clin Endocrinol Metab* 2001, 86:2027–2031.

118. Yilmaz M, Bukan N, Ersoy R, Karakoc A, Yetkin I, Ayvaz G, Cakir N, Arslan M. Glucose intolerance, insulin resistance and cardiovascular risk factors in first degree relatives of women with polycystic ovary syndrome. *Hum Reprod* 2005, 20:2414–2420.

119. Legro RS, Kunselman AR, Demers L, Wang SC, Bentley-Lewis R, Dunaif A. Elevated dehydroepiandrosterone sulfate levels as the reproductive phenotype in the brothers of women with polycystic ovary syndrome. *J Clin Endocrinol Metab* 2002, 87:2134–2138.

120. Sir-Petermann TS, Cartes A, Maliqueo M, Vantman D, Gutierrez C, Toloza H, Echiburu B, Recabarren SE. Patterns of hormonal response to the GnRH agonist leuprolide in brothers of women with polycystic ovary syndrome: a pilot study. *Hum Reprod* 2004, 19:2742–2747.

121. Barnes RB, Rosenfield RL, Ehrmann DA, Cara JF, Cuttler L, Levitsky LL, Rosenthal IM. Ovarian hyperandrogynism as a result of congenital adrenal virilizing disorders: evidence for perinatal masculinization of neuroendocrine function in women. *J Clin Endocrinol Metab* 1994, 79: 1328–1333.

122. Merke DP and Cutler GB Jr. New ideas for medical treatment of congenital adrenal hyperplasia. *Endocrinol Metab Clin North Am* 2001, 30:121–135.

123. Phocas I, Chryssikopoulos A, Sarandakou A, Rizos D and Trakakis E. A contribution to the classification of cases of non-classic 21-hydroxylase-deficient congenital adrenal hyperplasia. *Gynecol Endocrinol* 1995, 9:229–238.

124. Stikkelbroeck NM, Hermus AR, Braat DD and Otten BJ. Fertility in women with congenital adrenal hyperplasia due to 21-hydroxylase deficiency. *Obstet Gynecol Surv* 2003, 58:275–284.

125. Hautanen A, Raikkonen K, Adlercreutz H. Associations between pituitary-adrenocortical function and abdominal obesity, hyperinsulinaemia and dyslipidaemia in normotensive males. *J Intern Med* 1997, 241:451–461.

126. Beck-Peccoz P, Padmanabhan V, Baggiani AM, Cortelazzi D, Buscaglia M, Medri G, Marconi AM, Pardi G, Beitins IZ. Maturation of hypothalamic-pituitary-gonadal function in normal human fetuses: circulating levels of gonadotropins, their common alpha-subunit and free testosterone, and discrepancy between immunological and biological activities of circulating follicle-stimulating hormone. *J Clin Endocrinol Metab* 1991, 73:525–532.

7 Pubertal Precursors of the Polycystic Ovarian Syndrome

John C. Marshall, MD, PhD,
Christopher R. McCartney, MD,
Susan K. Blank, MD,
and Quirine Lamberts Okonkwo, MD

Contents

Summary

Polycystic ovarian syndrome (PCOS) is a disorder characterized by ovulatory dysfunction and hyperandrogenemia. In the majority of women with PCOS, luteinizing hormone (LH) [gonadotropin-releasing hormone (GnRH)] pulse frequency is persistently rapid, which favors synthesis of LH and elevated plasma LH that in turn stimulates increased androgen production. Rapid GnRH frequencies are not optimal for FSH synthesis and secretion, contributing to impaired follicular maturation. In normal women, luteal phase concentrations of progesterone markedly slow GnRH pulse frequency (to one pulse every 3–4 h), but in anovulatory women with PCOS, this does not occur. In part, this reflects the low levels of circulating progesterone, but studies have also demonstrated reduced hypothalamic sensitivity to progesterone inhibition of GnRH secretion. The reduced sensitivity to progesterone appears to be the result of elevated androgens, as sensitivity is restored following treatment with the anti-androgen, flutamide. In the etiology of the disorder PCOS, ovulatory and hormonal abnormalities are commonly observed during puberty, with plasma measurements revealing hyperandrogenemia. In some girls, impaired hypothalamic progesterone sensitivity is present, similar to that in adult women, though not all hyperandrogenemic adolescents are affected. We propose that the pre- and early-pubertal hyperandrogenemia interferes with normal ovarian hypothalamic regulation of GnRH pulse frequency, leading to a persistently rapid frequency of GnRH pulse secretion. This in turn favors LH synthesis and secretion, further stimulating ovarian testosterone secretion and impairing normal regulation of ovulatory function.

From: *Contemporary Endocrinology: Polycystic Ovary Syndrome*
Edited by: A. Dunaif, R. J. Chang, S. Franks, and R. S. Legro © Humana Press, Totowa, NJ

Key Words: Polycystic ovaries; puberty; androgens; gonadotropins; progesterone.

1. INTRODUCTION

Polycystic ovarian syndrome (PCOS) is a common disorder in adult women, affecting some 6–8% during their reproductive years. The disorder is heterogeneous, with variable presentations, and is defined clinically by ovulatory dysfunction and hyper-androgenism, with or without polycystic ovarian morphology, in the absence of other disease *(1,2)*. Oligomenorrhea or amenorrhea is associated with hyperandrogenism, and clinical manifestations of hirsutism or acne may be present. Obesity, insulin resistance, and hyperinsulinemia are also commonly associated *(3,4)* with a recognized increased risk for the development of disorders such as the metabolic syndrome and diabetes mellitus.

The etiology of PCOS remains unclear, and abnormal ovarian steroidogenesis, hyperinsulinemia, and neuroendocrine abnormalities have been proposed as a primary underlying abnormality. Abnormal steroidogenesis is suggested by studies showing that ovarian theca cells produce excessive androgens and show abnormal ovarian steroid responses to gonadotropins *(5–7)*. Hyperinsulinemia, as a consequence of insulin resistance, acts synergistically with luteinizing hormone (LH) to increase ovarian androgen production *(8,9)*. This together with suppression of sex hormone-binding globulin (SHBG) production by insulin results in high levels of free (unbound) testos-terone. Further support for the role of insulin is seen in the results of treatment to decrease plasma insulin, with reduction in hyperandrogenism and enhanced ovulatory function. Neuroendocrine abnormalities are manifested as excess LH pulsatile secretion and relative follicle-stimulating hormone (FSH) deficiency. Excess LH enhances androgen synthesis by ovarian theca cells, and the relative lack of FSH impairs induction of the aromatase enzyme complex and follicular maturation. Evidence supporting the central role for LH is found in the results of long-term gonadotropin-releasing hormone (GnRH) agonist treatment, where down-regulation of LH secretion is accompanied by reduction of ovarian androgen production to post-menopausal levels *(10)*.

A careful history in most women indicates that the disorder began during pubertal maturation, with many never establishing regular menstrual cycles. In addition, hyperandrogenic adolescents demonstrate abnormalities of LH secretion similar to those found in adults. In this chapter, we focus on the evolution of the neuroen-docrine abnormalities of LH secretion and its evolution through pre- and pubertal maturation.

2. GONADOTROPIN SECRETION DURING OVULATORY CYCLES AND IN WOMEN WITH PCOS

2.1. Gonadotropin Secretion During Ovulatory Cycles

Both LH and FSH secretion are closely regulated during ovulatory cycles, as a result of modulation of both GnRH secretion from the hypothalamic GnRH pulse generator and pituitary responsiveness to GnRH. A major factor in the regulation of LH and FSH secretion is the frequency of the GnRH pulse stimulus, and changes in GnRH pulse frequency are one mechanism by which preferential synthesis and secretion of LH and FSH occurs during ovulatory cycles *(11)*. A pulsatile GnRH stimulus is essential for gonadotropin synthesis, and more rapid frequencies, one pulse every hour, favor LH synthesis and secretion, whereas slower pulses, one pulse every 3–4 h, favor FSH secretion. The effects of GnRH pulse frequency are modulated at the level of the LH-β and FSH-β gene, and frequency directly stimulates gene transcription *(12)*. In addition, GnRH frequency modulates the complex gonadotrope mechanism whereby follistatin production (increased by rapid pulses) can inactivate intragonadotrope activin, reducing FSH-β transcription and mRNA expression *(13)*.

In women, modulation of GnRH pulse frequency is effected predominantly by ovarian hormones, with major regulation occurring during the luteal phase *(14)*. Progesterone from the corpus luteum acts to enhance hypothalamic opioid activity, which in turn slows GnRH pulse secretion to one pulse every 3–4 h *(15)*. As noted above, this favors FSH synthesis and constitutes an important part of the mechanisms favoring preferential FSH secretion in the late luteal phase, which in turn stimulates the next wave of cyclic ovarian follicular maturation. In humans, the maximum GnRH pulse frequency is approximately one pulse per hour, a frequency that is initially achieved during pubertal maturation. In adult women during the follicular phase, inhibition of the slow luteal GnRH frequency is gradually released *(16)*, so that by the mid-cycle LH surge GnRH pulses occur approximately once per hour. Indeed one pulse per hour appears to be the intrinsic GnRH frequency in adult women, and reduction of this frequency is predominately effected by luteal progesterone. Estradiol plays a permissive role, in that it is required for expression of hypothalamic progesterone receptors *(17)*. In addition, estradiol, in concert with inhibin A from the corpus luteum, acts to directly suppress gonadotrope FSH synthesis and release during the mid-luteal phase. Estradiol in the concentrations seen in the late follicular phase can also elicit positive feedback, enabling marked enhancement of LH release in response to GnRH.

Thus, the ability to secrete GnRH at a frequency of one pulse per hour is achieved during pubertal maturation. Thereafter, the predominant regulation of GnRH secretion appears to be the combined effects of luteal progesterone and estradiol to inhibit GnRH frequency, thus favoring FSH production. As FSH release is restrained by both estradiol and inhibin A in the luteal phase, gonadotrope FSH stores are enhanced, providing a pool for release following the demise of the corpus luteum. The monotropic FSH stimulus facilitates recruitment of the next cohort of ovarian follicles, and GnRH pulse frequency gradually rises during the follicular phase, reflecting the gradual loss of the restraining influence of prior exposure to luteal progesterone *(11)*.

2.2. GnRH and Gonadotropin Secretion in Adult Women with PCOS

When recent spontaneous ovulation has been excluded, abnormal gonadotropin secretion is commonly observed in adult women with PCOS. Taylor et al. *(18)* demonstrated that 75% of women had elevated LH levels and over 90% had an elevated LH/FSH ratio. Spontaneous LH pulse amplitude is increased and LH responses to exogenous GnRH exaggerated while plasma FSH levels are relatively low *(19,20)*.

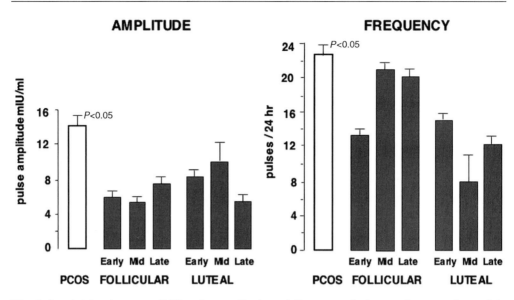

Fig. 1. Luteinizing hormone (LH) pulse amplitude and frequency during ovulatory cycles and in women with polycystic ovarian syndrome (PCOS). Spontaneous ovulation had not occurred within the week prior to study in women with PCOS.

These abnormalities appear to reflect a persistently, rapid GnRH pulse frequency *(21)* with LH (GnRH) pulses occurring approximately one per hour. The normal luteal slowing seen during ovulatory cycles does not occur (Fig. 1). This, in turn, favors LH secretion while FSH is restrained by the consistent presence of plasma estradiol. Measured against the background of the normal variations seen during ovulatory cycles, the persistent rapid frequency of GnRH pulse secretion appears to reflect failure to suppress the inherent post-pubertal GnRH pulse generator firing of one pulse per hour.

2.3. Etiology of Abnormal Gonadotropin Secretion

Convincing evidence of abnormalities of hypothalamic function in women is lacking, and the majority of studies have not shown consistent abnormalities of neurotransmitter function.

2.3.1. HYPOTHALAMIC NEUROTRANSMITTERS

Animal studies indicated that noradrenergic neurons were stimulatory, whereas dopamine and opioid neurons inhibited GnRH secretion. Studies in humans have attempted to define abnormalities of these central pathways. Investigations are by necessity indirect in women and reflect the use of medications that inhibit or stimulate these pathways. Initial studies suggested that diminished dopaminergic tone may be a factor, based on the moderate degree of hyperprolactinemia commonly present in women with PCOS. However, use of dopamine agonists did not improve clinical or biochemical function and results have been inconclusive *(22)*. Recognition that slowing of GnRH pulses during the luteal phase reflected the action of opioids suggested diminished hypothalamic opioid tone as a factor in the persistently rapid GnRH secretion

(23). In primates, hypophyseal-portal endorphin concentrations are increased during the luteal phase *(24)*. However, evidence showing that progesterone administration can slow GnRH pulses in women with PCOS suggested that progesterone induction of enhanced opioid tone was not significantly impaired in PCOS *(25)*. Other studies have assessed both noradrenergic and GABAergic pathways following administration of thymoxamine (α-1-adreno receptor antagonist) or valproate to increase GABA, but studies have not documented consequent changes in mean LH or LH pulse frequency *(26,27)*. Thus, evidence to date has failed to identify a primary hypothalamic abnormality and suggests that the observed abnormalities of GnRH secretion are secondary to the abnormal hormonal milieu in plasma.

2.3.2. ESTROGENS

The observation that estrogens could enhance LH secretion at mid-cycle suggested that excess androstenedione, peripherally aromatized to estrone, could enhance LH secretion *(28)*. Estrone levels are increased in PCOS, but administration of exogenous estrone or the use of a peripheral aromatase inhibitor did not augment GnRH-stimulated LH secretion or reduce LH pulse frequency *(29)*.

2.3.3. HYPERINSULINEMIA

A majority of obese and, to a lesser degree, lean women with PCOS exhibit insulin resistance with consequent compensatory increase of insulin secretion *(3,4,30)*. Type II diabetes is significantly more prevalent in women with PCOS compared to age- and weight-matched controls *(31)*. As noted, excess insulin acts synergistically with LH to stimulate ovarian androgen production and to suppress hepatic production of SHBG, resulting in elevated free testosterone. Reduction of insulin resistance following treatment with metformin, or thiazolidinediones, results in moderate reduction in hyperandrogenemia and improved ovulatory function *(32–34)*. Thus, in vivo evidence, together with in vitro data showing a direct effect on steroidogenesis, clearly indicates a role for hyperinsulinemia in the pathogenesis of PCOS. However, its potential role in the neuroendocrine abnormalities is unclear, and insulin does not augment gonadotrope responses to GnRH nor do insulin infusions alter LH secretion *(35,36)*. In a similar vein, insulin sensitization with metformin or pioglitazone did not result in reduced LH secretion *(37)* despite evidence of improved insulin sensitivity. In sum, the data do not provide evidence that hyperinsulinemia directly causes neuroendocrine abnormalities but may play a role through its action of increasing hyperandrogenemia.

2.3.4. PROGESTERONE

Chronic anovulation in PCOS results in reduced progesterone in plasma, which removes the predominant agent that slows GnRH pulse secretion during ovulatory cycles. Although low progesterone associated with anovulation clearly plays a role in the persistently rapid GnRH pulse secretion in PCOS, it does not appear to account for the neuroendocrine abnormalities. Anovulatory cycles can occur in otherwise normally cycling women, and spontaneous infrequent ovulation occurs in PCOS. In the latter circumstance, progesterone transiently reduces LH pulse frequency, but LH levels are again elevated with rapid frequency, some 10–14 days after progesterone falls *(18)*. In addition, adolescents with hyperandrogenemia exhibit abnormally rapid LH/GnRH

pulse secretion, even before menarche when ovulatory cycles have not yet been established *(38)*. However, as progesterone is the major physiologic inhibitor of GnRH
pulse frequency, the abnormalities of GnRH pulse secretion in PCOS suggest the possibility of reduced sensitivity to progesterone feedback. This concept is supported by
evidence following oral contraceptive therapy, which slowed LH pulses in hyperandrogenemic women but not to the same degree as normal controls *(39)*. Subsequent studies
have administered luteal concentrations of estradiol and progesterone to women with
PCOS and carefully monitored GnRH pulse frequency before and after exposure to
ovarian steroids. Women with PCOS require higher concentrations of progesterone to
suppress GnRH frequency to the same degree as ovulatory controls *(40)*. The reduced
sensitivity to progesterone reflects the actions of elevated androgens, as pretreatment
with the androgen receptor blocker, flutamide, can restore normal progesterone sensitivity, indicating that the impaired progesterone sensitivity is a reversible hypothalamic
abnormality *(41)*. Of interest, similar observations have recently been made in some
adolescents with hyperandrogenemia (*see* Subheading 3.1).

2.3.5. HYPERANDROGENEMIA

Elevated plasma androgens appear to be an important factor in modulating normal
neuroendocrine responses. While early in vitro evidence suggested that androgens
increased GnRH pulse frequency, data in women did not confirm this observation.
Basal LH pulsatility was not changed by androgen infusion or blockade of androgen
action *(41,42)*. However, as noted above, flutamide can restore normal hypothalamic
sensitivity to progesterone, and longer term administration has restored regular cyclical
regulation in some women with PCOS *(43)*. Exposure to excess androgens during fetal
life, however, appears to exert significant effects on hypothalamic function during
subsequent pubertal maturation. Exposure to high concentrations of androgens during
early fetal life in monkeys, sheep, and rats results in increased LH secretion and
GnRH pulse frequency during subsequent pubertal maturation *(44–47)*. In addition, in
sheep models of fetal hyperandrogenemia, sensitivity to progesterone was impaired as
seen in women. In rodent models, reduced basal and estradiol induction of hypothalamic progesterone receptors have been reported *(47)*. Similarly, in mice, prenatal
exposure to androgen enhances GABAergic drive to GnRH neurons that can be
reversed by flutamide *(48)*. These animal models provide compelling evidence that
prenatal androgen exposure can markedly modify neuroendocrine regulation during
subsequent puberty. However, few data are available in women though androgen
exposure may be increased during pregnancy in women with PCOS *(49)*, perhaps
reflecting genetic causes, the latter suggested by PCOS clustering in certain families
(50). Overall, androgens appear to exert significant modulation of normal endocrine
function, particularly impairment of hypothalamic progesterone sensitivity. The latter
may reflect reduced availability of hypothalamic progesterone receptors, resulting in
reduced responsiveness to lower concentrations of progesterone. It is of interest that
the consequences of prenatal androgenization are manifest during subsequent pubertal
maturation, suggesting that the earlier exposure to androgen excess may have permanently modified the normal set points for regulation of GnRH pulse secretion by
ovarian steroids.

3. GONADOTROPIN SECRETION IN NORMAL PUBERTY AND ADOLESCENTS WITH HYPERANDROGENEMIA

3.1. Regulation During Normal Pubertal Maturation

During the first 6 months of life, the GnRH pulse generator is active with plasma gonadotropins approximating adult values. Subsequently, LH and FSH levels fall, and GnRH pulses occur at low amplitude every 4–6 h, resulting in a relative predominance of FSH over LH during childhood (51). The resumption of GnRH activity occurs several years before clinical evidence of puberty is manifested (52–54). Initially, increased LH pulse amplitude and frequency occur during sleep, with associated overnight increases in sex steroids, testosterone, progesterone, and to a lesser degree, estradiol (55,56) (Fig. 2).

With the progression of maturation, daytime LH pulse secretion increases, and sleep-associated increases in LH pulsatility are less evident. The mechanisms governing the diurnal changes in GnRH secretion in early puberty are unclear. The close association of increased LH secretion with the onset of sleep (57) suggests higher central nervous system (CNS) center activation, but this may be modified by the overnight changes in sex steroids. The latter may facilitate modified higher CNS functions or may directly impair GnRH pulse generator activity during daytime (awake) hours. Evidence to support a role for the small increases in sex steroids in daytime inhibition of GnRH secretion is found in studies of diurnal changes in LH pulse frequency in girls with and without ovarian function. The increased frequency in association with sleep is not seen in girls with gonadal dysgenesis. LH pulse frequencies are similar before and during the onset of sleep, suggesting that GnRH frequency was not suppressed during the daytime hours (51) (Fig. 3).

These data suggest the influence of an ovarian factor(s) in modulating the day–night difference in early pubertal GnRH pulse secretion. In addition, estradiol infusion in early pubertal girls reduces the nocturnal increase in LH (58), and while data are not

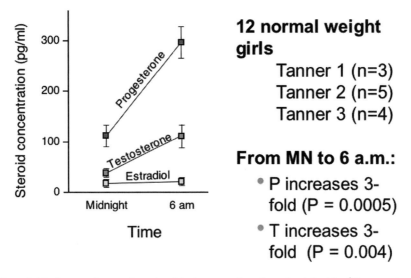

Fig. 2. Overnight changes in ovarian steroids in normal early pubertal girls (Tanner stages I–III). See insert for color figure.

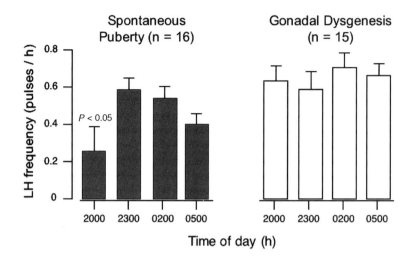

Fig. 3. Day/night luteinizing hormone (LH) (GnRH) pulse frequency in normal early pubertal girls and girls with gonadal dysgenesis. Reproduced with permission *(51)*.

available in girls, testosterone exerts similar actions in boys *(59)*. These studies suggest a role for gonadal steroids at the early stages of pubertal maturation, and they may be involved in the relative quiescence of GnRH pulse secretion during childhood. The hypothalamus is very sensitive to sex steroid feedback during childhood, but sensitivity appears to be lost during maturation *(60,61)*. The etiology of the decreasing sensitivity to feedback is uncertain, but analogy to studies in adults suggests that it may reflect an action of the gradual increase in androgen secretion. In pre- and early-pubertal girls, plasma testosterone concentrations exceed those of estradiol and remain so until later stages of puberty *(56)*. Thus, the progressive increase in testosterone during normal female puberty may modulate a reduced sensitivity of the GnRH pulse generator to inhibition by estradiol and progesterone.

While the above concept remains to be proven, hyperandrogenism during adolescence has been shown to modify progesterone inhibition of GnRH secretion in some girls during puberty. Chhabra et al. *(62)* showed that approximately 50% of hyperandrogenemic adolescents exhibit relative insensitivity of GnRH secretion to the feedback actions of progesterone and estradiol (Fig. 4). These studies mimic earlier observations in adults *(41)* and again suggest a role for androgens in the evolution of GnRH and gonadotropin secretion during puberty. This is supported by studies showing elevated LH, LH pulse frequency, and amplitude in hyperandrogenic adolescents *(63)*. In addition, hyperandrogenic girls have higher daytime GnRH pulse frequency, and the diurnal variation is less evident *(64)*. Detailed studies have suggested that the daytime increase of LH secretion is advanced by some 2 years in the presence of elevated plasma androgens *(38)*.

Taken together, the data suggest that ovarian steroids may play significant roles, either by direct action on the GnRH pulse generator or by modifying higher CNS centers, during both the period of childhood quiescence and the evolution of diurnal changes during subsequent puberty. The predominance of androgens in early pubertal blood in normal girls suggests that androgens may play a role in reducing hypothalamic

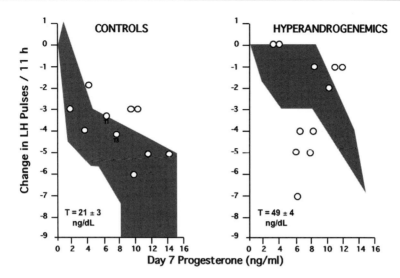

Fig. 4. The suppression of GnRH pulse frequency by progesterone in normal and hyperandrogenemic adolescent girls. Girls received estradiol (orally in a constant daily dosage) and variable amounts of oral progesterone suspension every 8 h for 7 days. The reduction in luteinizing hormone (LH) (GnRH) pulse frequency, during 11 h runs of q 10-min sampling in day 1 and day 7, is shown as a function of the mean plasma progesterone on day 7. T, mean total testosterone for the group; T_1 and T_3, indicate subjects at Tanner stages I and III, whereas the remaining subjects were at pubertal stage IV or V on the Tanner scale. Reproduced with permission *(62)*.

sensitivity to ovarian steroid feedback, resulting in the elevated LH and ovarian steroid concentrations seen later in puberty and adult women.

3.2. The Origin and Role of Excess Androgens and the Pubertal Evolution of PCOS

Data from animal studies, particularly those in monkeys *(46)*, clearly indicate that fetal exposure to excess androgens can modify neuroendocrine function during subsequent pubertal maturation. In several regards—elevated LH, rapid GnRH pulses, and impaired progesterone feedback *(45)*—the changes observed are similar to those seen in hyperandrogenic adolescents and women with PCOS. Although data in humans are lacking, the potential for excess exposure to androgens in fetal life may be a factor in the evolution of these disorders. Similarly, in prepubertal girls, excess androgens are associated with increased risk of PCOS in adulthood *(65)*. Some studies have suggested that this may reflect precocious adrenarche, which appears to be more common in some girls with low birth weight. The mechanisms are unclear, but a "catch-up" phenomenon is proposed in which hyperinsulinemia may be a factor. Studies in normal girls clearly indicate that androgen secretion exceeds that of estrogen during early puberty and thus may form part of the mechanism for reducing sensitivity to estradiol and progesterone regulation of GnRH pulse secretion during pubertal maturation. Few detailed studies are available in adolescent girls, but analogy to the effects of progesterone in adults suggests that this may be part of the mechanisms allowing increased GnRH, gonadotropin, and steroid secretion during maturation. In addition, the abnormalities of GnRH and LH secretion in hyperandrogenic adolescents resemble those seen in adult women with PCOS. Thus, it is feasible that excess androgens from any cause, during fetal life, associated with premature adrenache *(65)*, obesity *(66,67)*, hyperinsulinemia *(68)*, or reflecting inherent abnormalities of ovarian steroidogenesis *(6)*, may lead to feedback abnormalities in the diurnal control of pulsatile GnRH secretion by ovarian steroids. As the effect would be to impair inhibition of GnRH secretion, the persistently fast GnRH pulse secretion would favor increased LH, relatively decreased FSH, and further contribute to ovarian androgen production and ovulatory dysfunction.

In this regard, the increased prevalence of obesity in pre- and pubertal girls over the last quarter century may be a significant factor *(69,70)*. Studies *(66,67)* have emphasized the hyperandrogenemia associated with obesity (Fig. 5). Although the exact mechanisms remain to be elucidated, this may reflect the synergistic action of hyperinsulinemia augmenting early pubertal gonadotropin stimulation of the ovary.

Together, these data suggest a sequence that results in impaired regulation of diurnal changes in GnRH pulse frequency. Analogy to studies in adults and rodents suggests that the slow prepubertal GnRH pulse stimulation would favor FSH secretion during childhood. The augmentation of GnRH frequency and amplitude during sleep would gradually favor a change to LH synthesis, with the latter acting to enhance ovarian steroid secretion. In early pubertal girls, the overnight increase in ovarian steroids may in turn mediate the subsequent decline in GnRH secretion during the next day. We propose that exposure to excess androgens at a stage prior to or during the pubertal maturational process results in perturbation of these normal regulatory mechanisms. The net effect would be to diminish ovarian steroid inhibition of GnRH pulse frequency, resulting in increasing LH and decreasing FSH synthesis and secretion. This in turn

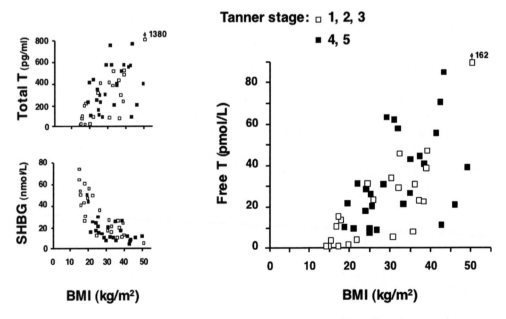

Fig. 5. Total plasma testosterone, sex hormone-binding globulin (SHBG), calculated free testosterone, as a function of BMI in early (Tanner I–III) and late (Tanner IV and V) stages of pubertal maturation. Open square, Tanner I–III subjects; closed square, Tanner IV and V.

will be reflected by enhanced ovarian production of androgen and impaired follicular maturation—circumstances that could be the forerunner of PCOS in adults.

In sum, present evidence is incomplete, but existing data suggest that hyperandrogenemia may play a central role in the evolution of altered hypothalamic sensitivity to ovarian steroid feedback during normal pubertal maturation. In turn, this would suggest that exposure to excess androgens might accelerate this process, resulting in earlier increase in daytime GnRH pulse secretion and a more rapid progression to the adult pattern. This concept is supported by available evidence to date, and further studies are required to elucidate the precise nature of this interaction. Establishing the role of androgens during pubertal maturation is of import, as it offers the potential for reversing or ameliorating the proposed sequence leading to PCOS in adults. Data using androgen blockade in adults have demonstrated that sensitivity to progesterone can be restored following administration of flutamide *(41)*. By analogy, it would suggest that early recognition and reduction in androgen production, or blockade of androgen action, during early puberty may lead to normalization of the pubertal transition, potentially preventing the evolution of the full neuroendocrine abnormalities seen in adult women with PCOS. In this regard, efforts to reduce the increased prevalence in childhood obesity may be particularly important, as recent data suggest that this is a potent cause of elevated androgens in a majority of girls. However, the degree of hyperandrogenemia associated with obesity varies, and not all girls with hyperandrogenemia exhibit impaired sensitivity to steroid feedback *(62)*. Thus, factors that determine the degree and the effects of hyperandrogenemia may well vary in individual adolescent girls, and further study to elucidate factors determining these changes will allow more complete understanding of the cause and effects of pubertal hyperandrogenemia.

ACKNOWLEDGMENTS

We recognize the important contributions of clinical fellows in these research studies and thank S. Chhabra, MD, C. A. Eagleson, MD, C. L. Pastor, MD, and K. A. Prendergast, MD for their contributions. In addition, the invaluable assistance of research coordinators A. Bellows, PhD and C. Chopra is recognized as are the contributions of the GCRC staff and nurses and the availability of the Ligand Core Lab of the Center for Research in Reproduction at the University of Virginia.

This work was supported by NIH grants: R01 HD34179 and R01 HD33039 (JCM), K23 HD044742 (CRM), and T32 HD-07382 (SKB). We also recognize the support of the Specialized Cooperative Centers Program in Research in Reproduction and Infertility through grant U54 HD28934 (JCM) and the GCRC grant M01 RR00847.

REFERENCES

1. Zawadski J, Dunaif A. Diagnostic criteria for polycystic ovary syndrome: towards a rational approach. In: Dunaif A, Givens J, Haseltine F, Merriam G, eds. *Polycystic Ovary Syndrome*. Oxford, England: Blackwell Scientific; 1992:377–84.

2. Rotterdam ESHRE/ASRM-Sponsored PCOS Consensus Workshop Group. Revised 2003 consensus on diagnostic criteria and long-term health risks related to polycystic ovary syndrome. *Fertil Steril* 2004;81(1):19–25.

3. Legro RS, Finegood D, Dunaif A. A fasting glucose to insulin ratio is a useful measure of insulin sensitivity in women with polycystic ovary syndrome. *J Clin Endocrinol Metab* 1998;83(8):2694–8.

4. DeUgarte CM, Bartolucci AA, Azziz R. Prevalence of insulin resistance in the polycystic ovary syndrome using the homeostasis model assessment. *Fertil Steril* 2005;83(5):1454–60.

5. Gilling-Smith C, Willis DS, Beard RW, Franks S. Hypersecretion of androstenedione by isolated thecal cells from polycystic ovaries. *J Clin Endocrinol Metab* 1994;79(4):1158–65.

6. Ehrmann DA, Barnes RB, Rosenfield RL. Polycystic ovary syndrome as a form of functional ovarian hyperandrogenism due to dysregulation of androgen secretion. *Endocr Rev* 1995;16(3):322–53.

7. Gilling-Smith C, Story H, Rogers V, Franks S. Evidence for a primary abnormality of thecal cell steroidogenesis in the polycystic ovary syndrome. *Clin Endocrinol (Oxf)* 1997;47(1):93–9.

8. Barbieri RL, Makris A, Randall RW, Daniels G, Kistner RW, Ryan KJ. Insulin stimulates androgen accumulation in incubations of ovarian stroma obtained from women with hyperandrogenism. *J Clin Endocrinol Metab* 1986;62(5):904–10.

9. Nestler JE, Jakubowicz DJ, de Vargas AF, Brik C, Quintero N, Medina F. Insulin stimulates testosterone biosynthesis by human thecal cells from women with polycystic ovary syndrome by activating its own receptor and using inositolglycan mediators as the signal transduction system. *J Clin Endocrinol Metab* 1998;83(6):2001–5.

10. Chang RJ, Laufer LR, Meldrum DR, et al. Steroid secretion in polycystic ovarian disease after ovarian suppression by a long-acting gonadotropin-releasing hormone agonist. *J Clin Endocrinol Metab* 1983;56(5):897–903.

11. Marshall JC, Kelch RP. Gonadotropin-releasing hormone: role of pulsatile secretion in the regulation of reproduction. *N Engl J Med* 1986;315(23):1459–68.

12. Burger LL, Dalkin AC, Aylor KW, Haisenleder DJ, Marshall JC. GnRH pulse frequency modulation of gonadotropin subunit gene transcription in normal gonadotropes-assessment by primary transcript assay provides evidence for roles of GnRH and follistatin. *Endocrinology* 2002;143(9):3243–9.

13. Kirk SE, Dalkin AC, Yasin M, Haisenleder DJ, Marshall JC. Gonadotropin-releasing hormone pulse frequency regulates expression of pituitary follistatin messenger ribonucleic acid: a mechanism for differential gonadotrope function. *Endocrinology* 1994;135(3):876–80.

14. Soules MR, Steiner RA, Clifton DK, Cohen NL, Aksel S, Bremner WJ. Progesterone modulation of pulsatile luteinizing hormone secretion in normal women. *J Clin Endocrinol Metab* 1984;58(2):378–83.

15. Filicori M, Santoro N, Merriam GR, Crowley WF, Jr. Characterization of the physiological pattern of episodic gonadotropin secretion throughout the human menstrual cycle. *J Clin Endocrinol Metab* 1986;62(6):1136–44.

16. McCartney CR, Gingrich MB, Hu Y, Evans WS, Marshall JC. Hypothalamic regulation of cyclic ovulation: evidence that the increase in gonadotropin-releasing hormone pulse frequency during the follicular phase reflects the gradual loss of the restraining effects of progesterone. *J Clin Endocrinol Metab* 2002;87(5):2194–200.

17. Romano GJ, Krust A, Pfaff DW. Expression and estrogen regulation of progesterone receptor mRNA in neurons of the mediobasal hypothalamus: an in situ hybridization study. *Mol Endocrinol* 1989;3(8):1295–300.

18. Taylor AE, McCourt B, Martin KA, et al. Determinants of abnormal gonadotropin secretion in clinically defined women with polycystic ovary syndrome. *J Clin Endocrinol Metab* 1997;82(7):2248–56.

19. Taylor AE. Polycystic ovary syndrome. *Endocrinol Metab Clin North Am* 1998;27(4):877–902, ix.

20. Marshall JC, Eagleson CA. Neuroendocrine aspects of polycystic ovary syndrome. *Endocrinol Metab Clin North Am* 1999;28(2):295–324.

21. Waldstreicher J, Santoro NF, Hall JE, Filicori M, Crowley WF, Jr. Hyperfunction of the hypothalamic-pituitary axis in women with polycystic ovarian disease: indirect evidence for partial gonadotroph desensitization. *J Clin Endocrinol Metab* 1988;66(1):165–72.

22. Buvat J, Buvat-Herbaut M, Marcolin G, et al. A double blind controlled study of the hormonal and clinical effects of bromocriptine in the polycystic ovary syndrome. *J Clin Endocrinol Metab* 1986;63(1):119–24.

23. Cumming DC, Reid RL, Quigley ME, Rebar RW, Yen SS. Evidence for decreased endogenous dopamine and opioid inhibitory influences on LH secretion in polycystic ovary syndrome. *Clin Endocrinol (Oxf)* 1984;20(6):643–8.

24. Wardlaw SL, Wehrenberg WB, Ferin M, Antunes JL, Frantz AG. Effect of sex steroids on beta-endorphin in hypophyseal portal blood. *J Clin Endocrinol Metab* 1982;55(5):877–81.

25. Berga SL, Yen SS. Opioidergic regulation of LH pulsatility in women with polycystic ovary syndrome. *Clin Endocrinol (Oxf)* 1989;30(2):177–84.

26. Paradisi R, Venturoli S, Capelli M, et al. Effects of alpha 1-adrenergic blockade on pulsatile luteinizing hormone, follicle-stimulating hormone, and prolactin secretion in polycystic ovary syndrome. *J Clin Endocrinol Metab* 1987;65(5):841–6.

27. Popovic V, Spremovic S. The effect of sodium valproate on luteinizing hormone secretion in women with polycystic ovary disease. *J Endocrinol Invest* 1995;18(2):104–8.

28. Yen S, Chaney C, Judd H. Functional aberrations of the hypothalamic-pituitary system in PCOS - a consideration for pathogenesis. In: *The Endocrine Function of the Human Ovary*. New York: Academic Press; 1976:273.

29. Chang RJ, Mandel FP, Lu JK, Judd HL. Enhanced disparity of gonadotropin secretion by estrone in women with polycystic ovarian disease. *J Clin Endocrinol Metab* 1982;54(3):490–4.

30. Dunaif A, Segal KR, Futterweit W, Dobrjansky A. Profound peripheral insulin resistance, independent of obesity, in polycystic ovary syndrome. *Diabetes* 1989;38(9):1165–74.

31. Ehrmann DA, Barnes RB, Rosenfield RL, Cavaghan MK, Imperial J. Prevalence of impaired glucose tolerance and diabetes in women with polycystic ovary syndrome. *Diabetes Care* 1999;22(1):141–6.

32. Nestler JE, Jakubowicz DJ. Decreases in ovarian cytochrome P450c17 alpha activity and serum free testosterone after reduction of insulin secretion in polycystic ovary syndrome. *N Engl J Med* 1996;335(9):617–23.

33. Dunaif A, Scott D, Finegood D, Quintana B, Whitcomb R. The insulin-sensitizing agent troglitazone improves metabolic and reproductive abnormalities in the polycystic ovary syndrome. *J Clin Endocrinol Metab* 1996;81(9):3299–306.

34. Lord JM, Flight IH, Norman RJ. Insulin-sensitising drugs (metformin, troglitazone, rosiglitazone, pioglitazone, D-chiro-inositol) for polycystic ovary syndrome. *Cochrane Database Syst Rev* 2003(3):CD003053.

35. Dunaif A, Graf M. Insulin administration alters gonadal steroid metabolism independent of changes in gonadotropin secretion in insulin-resistant women with the polycystic ovary syndrome. *J Clin Invest* 1989;83(1):23–9.

36. Mehta RV, Patel KS, Coffler MS, et al. Luteinizing hormone secretion is not influenced by insulin infusion in women with polycystic ovary syndrome despite improved insulin sensitivity during pioglitazone treatment. *J Clin Endocrinol Metab* 2005;90(4):2136–41.

37. Eagleson CA, Bellows AB, Hu K, Gingrich MB, Marshall JC. Obese patients with polycystic ovary syndrome: evidence that metformin does not restore sensitivity of the gonadotropin-releasing hormone pulse generator to inhibition by ovarian steroids. *J Clin Endocrinol Metab* 2003;88(11):5158–62.

38. Apter D, Butzow T, Laughlin GA, Yen SS. Accelerated 24-hour luteinizing hormone pulsatile activity in adolescent girls with ovarian hyperandrogenism: relevance to the developmental phase of polycystic ovarian syndrome. *J Clin Endocrinol Metab* 1994;79(1):119–25.

39. Daniels TL, Berga SL. Resistance of gonadotropin releasing hormone drive to sex steroid-induced suppression in hyperandrogenic anovulation. *J Clin Endocrinol Metab* 1997;82(12):4179–83.

40. Pastor CL, Griffin-Korf ML, Aloi JA, Evans WS, Marshall JC. Polycystic ovary syndrome: evidence for reduced sensitivity of the gonadotropin-releasing hormone pulse generator to inhibition by estradiol and progesterone. *J Clin Endocrinol Metab* 1998;83(2):582–90.

41. Eagleson CA, Gingrich MB, Pastor CL, et al. Polycystic ovarian syndrome: evidence that flutamide restores sensitivity of the gonadotropin-releasing hormone pulse generator to inhibition by estradiol and progesterone. *J Clin Endocrinol Metab* 2000;85(11):4047–52.

42. Dunaif A. Do androgens directly regulate gonadotropin secretion in the polycystic ovary syndrome? *J Clin Endocrinol Metab* 1986;63(1):215–21.

43. De Leo V, Lanzetta D, D'Antona D, la Marca A, Morgante G. Hormonal effects of flutamide in young women with polycystic ovary syndrome. *J Clin Endocrinol Metab* 1998;83(1):99–102.

44. Dumesic DA, Abbott DH, Eisner JR, Goy RW. Prenatal exposure of female rhesus monkeys to testosterone propionate increases serum luteinizing hormone levels in adulthood. *Fertil Steril* 1997;67(1):155–63.

45. Robinson JE, Forsdike RA, Taylor JA. In utero exposure of female lambs to testosterone reduces the sensitivity of the gonadotropin-releasing hormone neuronal network to inhibition by progesterone. *Endocrinology* 1999;140(12):5797–805.

46. Abbott DH, Barnett DK, Bruns CM, Dumesic DA. Androgen excess fetal programming of female reproduction: a developmental aetiology for polycystic ovary syndrome? *Hum Reprod Update* 2005;11(4):357–74.

47. Foecking EM, Szabo M, Schwartz NB, Levine JE. Neuroendocrine consequences of prenatal androgen exposure in the female rat: absence of luteinizing hormone surges, suppression of progesterone receptor gene expression, and acceleration of the gonadotropin-releasing hormone pulse generator. *Biol Reprod* 2005;72(6):1475–83.

48. Sullivan SD, Moenter SM. Prenatal androgens alter GABAergic drive to gonadotropin-releasing hormone neurons: implications for a common fertility disorder. *Proc Natl Acad Sci USA* 2004;101(18):7129–34.

49. Sir-Petermann T, Maliqueo M, Angel B, Lara HE, Perez-Bravo F, Recabarren SE. Maternal serum androgens in pregnant women with polycystic ovarian syndrome: possible implications in prenatal androgenization. *Hum Reprod* 2002;17(10):2573–9.

50. Kahsar-Miller MD, Nixon C, Boots LR, Go RC, Azziz R. Prevalence of polycystic ovary syndrome (PCOS) in first-degree relatives of patients with PCOS. *Fertil Steril* 2001;75(1):53–8.

51. Cemeroglu AP, Foster CM, Warner R, Kletter GB, Marshall JC, Kelch RP. Comparison of the neuroendocrine control of pubertal maturation in girls and boys with spontaneous puberty and in hypogonadal girls. *J Clin Endocrinol Metab* 1996;81(12):4352–7.

52. Wu FC, Borrow SM, Nicol K, Elton R, Hunter WM. Ontogeny of pulsatile gonadotrophin secretion and pituitary responsiveness in male puberty in man: a mixed longitudinal and cross-sectional study. *J Endocrinol* 1989;123(2):347–59.

53. Wennink JM, Delemarre-van de Waal HA, Schoemaker R, Schoemaker H, Schoemaker J. Luteinizing hormone and follicle stimulating hormone secretion patterns in girls throughout puberty measured using highly sensitive immunoradiometric assays. *Clin Endocrinol (Oxf)* 1990;33(3):333–44.

54. Jakacki RI, Kelch RP, Sauder SE, Lloyd JS, Hopwood NJ, Marshall JC. Pulsatile secretion of luteinizing hormone in children. *J Clin Endocrinol Metab* 1982;55(3):453–8.

55. Ankarberg C, Norjavaara E. Diurnal rhythm of testosterone secretion before and throughout puberty in healthy girls: correlation with 17-beta-estradiol and dehydroepiandrosterone sulfate. *J Clin Endocrinol Metab* 1999;84(3):975–84.

56. Mitamura R, Yano K, Suzuki N, Ito Y, Makita Y, Okuno A. Diurnal rhythms of luteinizing hormone, follicle-stimulating hormone, testosterone, and estradiol secretion before the onset of female puberty in short children. *J Clin Endocrinol Metab* 2000;85(3):1074–80.

57. Boyar R, Finkelstein J, Roffwarg H, Kapen S, Weitzman E, Hellman L. Synchronization of augmented luteinizing hormone secretion with sleep during puberty. *N Engl J Med* 1972;287(12):582–6.

58. Cemeroglu AP, Kletter GB, Guo W, et al. In pubertal girls, naloxone fails to reverse the suppression of luteinizing hormone secretion by estradiol. *J Clin Endocrinol Metab* 1998;83(10):3501–6.

59. Kletter GB, Foster CM, Brown MB, Beitins IZ, Marshall JC, Kelch RP. Nocturnal naloxone fails to reverse the suppressive effects of testosterone infusion on luteinizing hormone secretion in pubertal boys. *J Clin Endocrinol Metab* 1994;79(4):1147–51.

60. Kelch RP, Kaplan SL, Ghumbach MM. Suppression of urinary and plasma follicle-stimulating hormone by exogenous estrogens in prepubertal and pubertal children. *J Clin Invest* 1973;52(5): 1122–8.

61. Rapisarda JJ, Bergman KS, Steiner RA, Foster DL. Response to estradiol inhibition of tonic luteinizing hormone secretion decreases during the final stage of puberty in the rhesus monkey. *Endocrinology* 1983;112(4):1172–9.

62. Chhabra S, McCartney CR, Yoo RY, Eagleson CA, Chang RJ, Marshall JC. Progesterone inhibition of the hypothalamic gonadotropin-releasing hormone pulse generator: evidence for varied effects in hyperandrogenemic adolescent girls. *J Clin Endocrinol Metab* 2005;90(5):2810–5.

63. Venturoli S, Porcu E, Fabbri R, et al. Postmenarchal evolution of endocrine pattern and ovarian aspects in adolescents with menstrual irregularities. *Fertil Steril* 1987;48(1):78–85.

64. Zumoff B, Freeman R, Coupey S, Saenger P, Markowitz M, Kream J. A chronobiologic abnormality in luteinizing hormone secretion in teenage girls with the polycystic-ovary syndrome. *N Engl J Med* 1983;309(20):1206–9.

65. Ibanez L, Dimartino-Nardi J, Potau N, Saenger P. Premature adrenarche–normal variant or forerunner of adult disease? *Endocr Rev* 2000;21(6):671–96.

66. Wabitsch M, Hauner H, Heinze E, et al. Body fat distribution and steroid hormone concentrations in obese adolescent girls before and after weight reduction. *J Clin Endocrinol Metab* 1995;80(12): 3469–75.

67. Reinehr T, de Sousa G, Ludwig Roth C, Andler W. Androgens before and after weight loss in obese children. *J Clin Endocrinol Metab* 2005;90(10):5588–5595.

68. Dunaif A. Insulin resistance and the polycystic ovary syndrome: mechanism and implications for pathogenesis. *Endocr Rev* 1997;18(6):774–800.

69. Ogden CL, Flegal KM, Carroll MD, Johnson CL. Prevalence and trends in overweight among US children and adolescents, 1999–2000. *JAMA* 2002;288(14):1728–32.

70. Hedley AA, Ogden CL, Johnson CL, Carroll MD, Curtin LR, Flegal KM. Prevalence of overweight and obesity among US children, adolescents, and adults, 1999–2002. *JAMA* 2004;291(23):2847–50.

8 Variations in the Expression of the Polycystic Ovary Syndrome Phenotype

Enrico Carmina, MD

Contents

Summary

Three main polycystic ovary syndrome (PCOS) phenotypes may be distinguished. The most common, including at least two-thirds of the patients, is classic PCOS with an anovulatory hyperandrogenic phenotype. In 90% of the patients, polycystic ovaries are present. Obesity is common, but the prevalence varies largely among populations. Diabetes, altered glucose tolerance, metabolic syndrome, and increased circulating cardiovascular risk factors are also present, but their prevalence is largely influenced by body weight. The second phenotype, ovulatory PCOS, identifies patients presenting with hyperandrogenism and polycystic ovaries but ovulatory cycles. These patients seem to present a mild form of PCOS with insulin resistance and hyperinsulinemia being less severe and with a lower prevalence of metabolic and cardiovascular risk factors than in patients with classic PCOS. In these patients, body weight is often normal or only slightly increased, and changes in body weight may move the patients from one hyperandrogenic phenotype to another. The last main phenotype, normoandrogenic PCOS, is present in women with chronic anovulation and polycystic ovaries but normal androgen levels. Data on this group of patients are few and more studies are needed.

Key Words: PCOS; hyperandrogenism; androgen excess; insulin resistance; hyperinsulinemia; obesity.

From: *Contemporary Endocrinology: Polycystic Ovary Syndrome*
Edited by: A. Dunaif, R. J. Chang, S. Franks, and R. S. Legro © Humana Press, Totowa, NJ

1. INTRODUCTION

For many years, after the original description of Stein and Leventhal *(1)*, the association of menstrual irregularities, hirsutism, obesity, and polycystic ovaries was considered characteristic of patients with polycystic ovary syndrome (PCOS) *(2)*. Later, after an international NIH-sponsored meeting in 1990, most experts agreed that the key diagnostic features were chronic anovulation and hyperandrogenism, whereas obesity and polycystic ovaries were common but not specific *(3)*. Endocrine study was considered important to exclude some well-defined hyperandrogenic disorders (androgen secreting tumors, non-classic adrenal enzymatic deficiency, and Cushing's syndrome) *(3)*.

However, these criteria were also criticized. Several studies showed that anovulation is not an obligatory feature of PCOS *(4–7)*, and some researchers suggested that, because of the heterogeneity of the syndrome, it was better to base the diagnosis on ovarian morphology (polycystic ovaries) than on clinical features *(8)*.

Recently new guidelines, labeled The Rotterdam Criteria, have been suggested and widely adopted *(9,10)*. The new criteria are more extensive, because they permit the diagnosis of PCOS in patients with at least two of the following three criteria: chronic anovulation, hyperandrogenism (clinical or biologic), and polycystic ovaries. The same uncommon androgen excess disorders must first be excluded.

Using these new criteria, PCOS now includes patients with very different clinical appearances. In fact, the diagnosis of PCOS is assigned to patients who present with three main phenotypes. We have used the following names (in parentheses) to define these three phenotypes *(11,12)*:

1. Hyperandrogenism and chronic anovulation (or classic PCOS).
2. Hyperandrogenism and polycystic ovaries but ovulatory cycles (or ovulatory PCOS).
3. Chronic anovulation and polycystic ovaries but no clinical or biochemical hyperandrogenism (or normoandrogenic PCOS).

At the moment, it is unclear whether these different phenotypes are really part of the same syndrome or whether the Rotterdam's compromise has joined together disorders that have different characteristics and pathogenesis. Probably, only a better knowledge of the pathogenesis of PCOS will answer this question, but until that moment, it is important to determine the similarities and the differences between these three phenotypes. To date, only few studies have been dedicated to evaluate the characteristics of the different phenotypes. Therefore, in this chapter, I will use mostly personal data to describe the characteristics of the PCOS phenotypes. The factors that may influence the appearance of a single phenotype or permit the passage from one phenotype to another will also be discussed.

2. CLASSIC PCOS PHENOTYPE

This phenotype is well known and has been extensively studied. These patients present two main features: chronic anovulation and clinical or biologic hyperandrogenism *(3)*. Irregular menses (oligomenorrhea or amenorrhea) are generally found, but in some patients, chronic anovulation may be present despite a pattern of regular vaginal bleeding, suggestive of normal menses. Although this phenomenon is uncommon in the general population *(13)*, it may be relatively common in some disorders *(14,15)*, including PCOS *(6,16)*. In fact, normal menses with concurrent ovulatory dysfunction has been observed in about 15% of patients with classic PCOS *(16)*.

Increased androgen levels, generally high free and total testosterone, are observed in about 80% of women with classic PCOS *(17)*. It means that in 20% of patients with classic PCOS, only clinical hyperandrogenism (generally hirsutism, but sometimes acne or alopecia) is found. About 25–40% of patients with classic PCOS present an increase of adrenal androgen secretion *(18,19)*, but in most of them, ovarian androgens are also increased. An exclusive increase of DHEAS is uncommon, being observed only in about 5% of these patients *(19)*.

The third main feature of PCOS, polycystic ovaries, is present in the large majority of patients with the classic phenotype. I have recently observed that 90% of women with classic PCOS have polycystic ovaries and that about 50% also have increased ovarian size *(20)*.

Although obesity is not needed for diagnosis of classic PCOS (or for the diagnosis of PCOS in general), increased body weight is common and varies with the population studied. In different studies, we have observed that mean body weight is significantly higher in patients living in USA than in Mediterranean countries *(21,22)*. However, also in Italy, although only 30% of patients with classic PCOS have obesity (BMI > 30), many are overweight (BMI between 25 and 30), and therefore increased body weight is present in two-thirds of women with classic PCOS, a prevalence much higher than that found in general population *(12)*. In the USA, increased body weight is present in 90% of patients with the classic phenotype with more than 70% obese and another 15–20% overweight *(23,24)*. Figure 1 shows distribution of body weight in US and Italian women with classic phenotype of PCOS. All these data suggest that increased body weight, although influenced by genetic and environmental components, is an important component of the classic phenotype of PCOS *(25)*.

Another well-known feature of patients with classic PCOS is insulin resistance *(26)*, which may be present also in patients with normal body weight *(27)*. However, patients

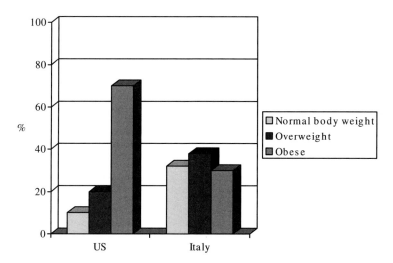

Fig. 1. Distribution of body weight in US and Italian women with the classic polycystic ovary syndrome (PCOS) phenotype. See insert for color figure.

with increased body weight have more severe insulin resistance with higher insulin and androgen levels *(26,28)*. In general, patients with classic PCOS, who are also obese, display most of the features of the syndrome *(17)*. Because of the combined effect of insulin resistance and increased body weight, PCOS patients with the classic phenotype have a high prevalence of metabolic disorders including diabetes mellitus *(29)*, altered glucose tolerance *(29)*, metabolic syndrome *(24,30)*, and abnormal levels of cardiovascular risk markers *(30–32)*. As with obesity, the prevalence of the metabolic disorders in classic PCOS is highly influenced by the studied population. In fact, altered glucose tolerance during reproductive age is found in 33% of US women *(29)* and in 15% of Italian women *(33)*. Similarly, diabetes mellitus is present in 5% of US classic PCOS *(29)* and in 2.5% of Italian classic PCOS *(33)*. The prevalence of metabolic syndrome is almost 50% in USA but less than 10% in Italy *(34)* and in other European countries *(35)*. However, similar to the USA, the prevalence of altered tolerance, diabetes, and metabolic syndrome is much higher in women with classic PCOS than in general population in Mediterranean countries *(34)*. We have found that metabolic syndrome is four times more common in Italian women with PCOS than in general female population of similar age *(34)*.

Owing to the major difference among the different populations with PCOS in regards to body weight, these data suggest that metabolic consequences are present in all ethnic groups of women with classic phenotype but that their prevalence is strongly influenced by an increase in body weight and therefore by a combination of genetic and environmental factors *(36)*. In conclusion, among patients with NIH-defined PCOS, about 90% present with three of the main features of the syndrome: chronic anovulation, hyperandrogenism, and polycystic ovaries. Increased body weight is more variable, being influenced by genetic and environmental factors, but it is present in 90% of US patients and in 70% of Italian patients with classic PCOS.

3. OVULATORY PCOS PHENOTYPE

The clinical features of patients with ovulatory PCOS are similar to those of the patients with Classic PCOS but with some important differences. The most obvious is the absence of ovulatory dysfunction. Not only are menstrual cycles normal but ovulation is regular and no impairment of fertility has been found. In fact, while it was initially suggested that these patients may have an alteration in the luteal phase *(37)*, successive studies have failed to observe any alteration of progesterone production *(38)*. On the contrary, there are no differences in androgen levels or in severity and prevalence of clinical signs of hyperandrogenism *(11)*. Most differences between the two phenotypes of hyperandrogenic PCOS regard metabolic abnormalities. In fact, while patients with ovulatory PCOS have high insulin levels and reduced insulin sensitivity in comparison to normal women *(7)*, serum insulin is lower and insulin resistance is less severe in patients with the ovulatory PCOS than in patients with classic PCOS *(11)*.

Although no data on the prevalence of diabetes or altered glucose tolerance in ovulatory PCOS are available, we have found that these patients present with an increased cardiovascular risk profile in comparison to normal women *(11,34)*. In fact, they have an altered lipid profile and increased circulating C-reactive protein *(11)*. In addition, the prevalence of metabolic syndrome is double in patients with ovulatory PCOS than in normal women (Fig. 2) *(34)*, and 38% of these patients present at least one

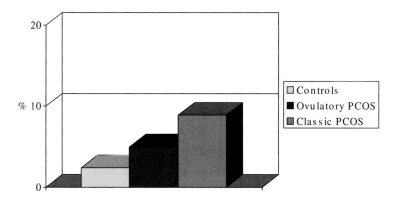

Fig. 2. Prevalence of the metabolic syndrome in Italian normal women aged 20–39 years and in Italian polycystic ovary syndrome (PCOS) patients with the classic or ovulatory hyperandrogenic phenotype. See insert for color figure.

altered cardiovascular risk marker (Fig. 3) *(11)*. All of these metabolic alterations are similar but less common and generally less severe than in classic PCOS (Figs 2 and 3) *(11,25)*.

Many of the differences in severity of metabolic alterations between ovulatory and classic PCOS are probably explained by differences in body weight. In fact, women with ovulatory PCOS are, on average, leaner than patients with classic PCOS, and their body weight is only slightly higher than normal women *(11)*. Obesity (BMI > 30) is present in only 8% of women with ovulatory PCOS although another 30–35% are overweight (Fig. 4). Therefore, in patients with ovulatory PCOS, only a mild increase of body weight is present, and it is associated with less severe insulin resistance and fewer metabolic and cardiovascular consequences than those observed in women with classic PCOS. In summary, patients with ovulatory PCOS are hyperandrogenic women

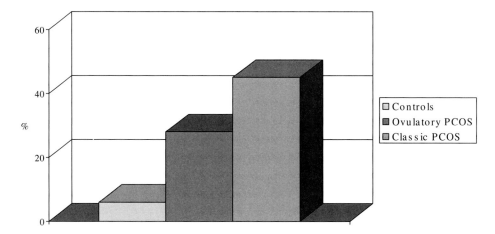

Fig. 3. Prevalence of the finding of at least one altered cardiovascular risk factor in Italian polycystic ovary syndrome (PCOS) patients with classic or ovulatory hyperandrogenic phenotype. See insert for color figure.

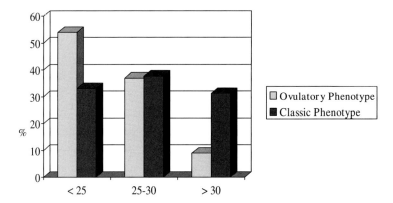

Fig. 4. Distribution of body weight in Italian polycystic ovary syndrome (PCOS) patients with classic or ovulatory hyperandrogenic phenotype. See insert for color figure.

who present many of the features of patients with classic PCOS but seem to have a less severe form of the syndrome.

4. NORMOANDROGENIC PCOS PHENOTYPE

The third main phenotype of PCOS regroups patients with chronic anovulation, polycystic ovaries but no clinical or biologic signs of hyperandrogenism. This phenotype has stimulated a large debate. In fact, very few data exist on clinical and endocrine characteristics of this subgroup of patients, and on the other hand, all actual animal models of PCOS have been obtained by inducing androgen excess during fetal life *(39)*. Because of it, some authors have suggested that, because of the main role of androgen excess in pathogenesis of PCOS, patients without signs of androgen excess should be part of a different syndrome and should not be included in the group of patients with PCOS *(40)*. However, others researchers believe that these patients should be included in PCOS not only because they present two main features of the syndrome, but also because the absence of clinical or biologic signs of hyperandrogenism does not exclude the existence of increased androgen production inside the ovary *(41)*. It is clear that only a better knowledge of the pathogenesis of PCOS will solve this question.

At this moment, we need to have more data on patients with this particular phenotype. Few studies to date have been specifically designed to study this group of patients. In the past, we have studied a small group (24 women) of anovulatory normoandrogenic patients *(42)*. Although this study was not designed to evaluate patients with normoandrogenic PCOS, most patients (80%) had polycystic ovaries and should be actually considered to be affected with PCOS. As a group, the patients had normal serum androgens but increased body weight and insulin levels and reduced insulin sensitivity. However, the severity of alterations was lower than in patients with classic PCOS with BMI, insulin levels, and insulin sensitivity being intermediate between normal controls and patients with classic PCOS (Fig. 5). Interestingly, metformin has been able to induce ovulation in 50% of these patients (Dewailly D, personal communication) with a prevalence of positive results that is not different from what we should expect in patients with classic PCOS *(42)*.

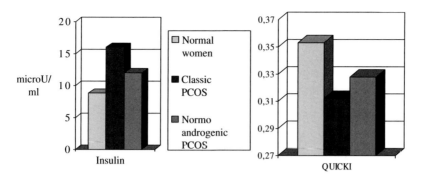

Fig. 5. Insulin serum levels and insulin sensitivity (by QUICKI) in Italian normal women and in Italian PCOS patients with classic hyperandrogenic or with normoandrogenic phenotype. See insert for color figure.

More recently Dewailly et al. *(41)* and Barber et al. *(43)* have reported that patients with a normoandrogenic PCOS phenotype present important similarities with the patients having the classic phenotype. However, the number of studied patients was relatively small and many more studies are needed. In fact, it is probable that this phenotype is heterogeneous and that may include patients with different disorders. Because of it, we have agreed for the time being to separate these patients from other PCOS patients, at least until more data are available *(44)*.

5. DIFFERENCES BETWEEN THE HYPERANDROGENIC PCOS PHENOTYPES AND FACTORS THAT PROMOTE PHENOTYPE SHIFT

As we have shown, the differences between the two hyperandrogenic PCOS phenotypes (classic and ovulatory) are mostly linked to changes in severity of the syndrome. In fact, patients with the ovulatory phenotype seem to represent a milder form of the syndrome. An important question is what are the factors that determine the expression of a mild or severe phenotype in the syndrome.

Of course, the ready response is that different genetic combinations may induce a different severity of phenotypes. PCOS is a heterogeneous genetic syndrome that is probably determined by the combination of multiple genetic factors *(36,45)*, and it should not be surprising that the syndrome presents with phenotypes of different severity. However, the possibility that, at least in hyperandrogenic forms of PCOS, environmental factors may determine the expressed phenotypes should not be underestimated *(36)*. One of the main features of PCOS, excessive body weight, is more common in patients with classic PCOS than in patients with ovulatory PCOS *(11,12)*, and it is well known that body weight is highly influenced by both genetic and environmental factors *(46,47)*.

We have hypothesized that changes in body weight, depending by sociocultural factors, may be one of the main factors that modifies the PCOS phenotype *(25)*. In fact, reduction of body weight constitutes one of the main strategies to induce ovulation *(48)* and therefore may be able to reverse the phenotype from the severe anovulatory to the mild anovulatory. The opposite possibility is also common *(49)*, and therefore patients may move from a mild ovulatory to a more severe anovulatory phenotype by increasing their body weight. In conclusion, while genetic factors clearly contribute to the severity of androgen excess and/or insulin resistance in the PCOS phenotype, environmental factors, affecting body weight, may be equally relevant.

REFERENCES

1. Stein I, Leventhal M. Amenorrhoea associated with bilateral polycystic ovaries. *Am J Obstet Gynecol* 1935; 29:181–185.
2. Goldzieher JW, Axelrod LR. Clinical and biochemical features of polycystic ovarian disease. *Fertil Steril* 1963; 14: 631–653.
3. Zawdaki JK, Dunaif A. Diagnostic criteria for polycystic ovary syndrome: towards a rationale approach. In: Dunaif A, Givens JR, Haseltine F, Merriam GR, eds. *Polycystic Ovary Syndrome.* Boston, MA: Blackwell Scientific Publications; 1992:377–384.
4. Gilling-Smith C, Willis DS, Beard RW, Franks S. Hypersecretion of androstenedione by isolated theca cells from polycystic ovaries. *J Clin Endocrinol Metab* 1994, 79:1158–1165.
5. Carmina E, Wong L, Chang L, Paulson RJ, Sauer MV, Stanczyk FZ, Lobo RA. Endocrine abnormalities in ovulatory women with polycystic ovaries on ultrasound. *Hum Reprod* 1997, 12: 905–909.
6. Carmina E, Lobo RA. Do hyperandrogenic women with normal menses have polycystic ovary syndrome? *Fertil Steril* 1999; 71:319–322.
7. Carmina E, Lobo RA. Polycystic ovaries in women with normal menses. *Am J Med* 2001; 111: 602–606.
8. Balen AH, Conway GS, Kaltsas G, Techatrasak K, Manning PJ, West C, Jacobs HS. Polycystic ovary syndrome: the spectrum of the disorder in 1741 patients. *Hum Reprod* 1995; 10: 1207–1211.
9. Rotterdam ESHRE/ASRM-Sponsored PCOS Consensus Workshop Group. Revised 2003 consensus on diagnostic criteria and long-term health risks related to polycystic ovary syndrome. *Fertil Steril* 2004; 81: 19–25.
10. Rotterdam ESHRE/ASRM-Sponsored PCOS Consensus Workshop Group. Revised 2003 consensus on diagnostic criteria and long-term health risks related to polycystic ovary syndrome. *Hum Reprod* 2004; 19: 41–47.
11. Carmina E, Longo RA, Rini GB, Lobo RA. Phenotypic variation in hyperandrogenic women influences the finding of abnormal metabolic and cardiovascular risk parameters. *J Clin Endocrinol Metab* 2005; 90: 2545–2549.
12. Carmina E, Rosato F, Jannì A, Rizzo M, Longo RA. Relative prevalence of different androgen excess disorders in 950 women referred because of clinical hyperandrogenism. *J Clin Endocrinol Metab* 2006; 91: 2–6.
13. Malcolm CE, Cumming DC. Does anovulation exist in eumenorrheic women? *Obstet Gynecol* 2003; 102:317–318.
14. Petsos P, Mamtora H, Ratcliffe WA, Anderson DC. Inadequate luteal phase usually indicates ovulatory dysfunction: observations from serial hormone and ultrasound monitoring of 115 cycles. *Gynecol Endocrinol* 1987; 1:37–45.
15. Page LA, Beauregard LJ, Bode HH, Beitins IZ. Hypothalamic-pituitary-ovarian function in menstruating women with Turner syndrome (45,X). *Pediatr Res* 1990; 28:514–517.
16. Azziz R, Woods KS, Reyna R, Key TJ, Knochenhauer ES, Yildiz BO. The prevalence and features of the polycystic ovary syndrome in an unselected population. *J Clin Endocrinol Metab* 2004; 89: 2745–2749.
17. Chang WY, Knochenhauer ES, Bartolucci AA, Azziz R. Phenotypic spectrum of polycystic ovary syndrome: clinical and biochemical characterization of the three major clinical subgroups. *Fertil Steril* 2005; 83:1717–1723.

18. Kumar A, Woods KS, Bartolucci AA, Azziz R. Prevalence of adrenal androgen excess in patients with the polycystic ovary syndrome (PCOS). *Clin Endocrinol (Oxf)* 2005; 62:644–649.

19. Carmina E, Lobo RA. Prevalence and metabolic characteristics of adrenal androgen excess in hyperandrogenic women. *J Endocrinol Invest* 2007; 30:111–116.

20. Carmina E, Koyama T, Chang L, Stanczyk FZ, Lobo RA. Does ethnicity influence the prevalence of adrenal hyperandrogenism and insulin resistance in polycystic ovary syndrome? *Am J Obstet Gynecol* 1992; 167: 1807–1812.

21. Carmina E, Orio F, Palomba S, Longo RA, Lombardi G, Lobo RA. Ovarian size and blood flow in women with polycystic ovary syndrome (PCOS) and their correlations with some endocrine parameters. *Fertil Steril* 2005; 84: 413–419.

22. Carmina E, Legro RS, Stamets K, Lowell J, Lobo RA. Difference in body weight between American and Italian women with polycystic ovary syndrome: influence of the diet. *Hum Reprod* 2003; 11: 2289–2293.

23. Apridonidze T, Essah PA, Iuorno MJ, Nestler JE. Prevalence and characteristics of the metabolic syndrome in women with polycystic ovary syndrome. *J Clin Endocrinol Metab* 2005; 90(4):1929–1935.

24. Essah PA, Nestler JE, Carmina E. Differences in dyslipidemia between American and Italian women with polycystic ovary syndrome. *J Endocrinol Invest* in press.

25. Carmina E. The spectrum of Androgen Excess Disorders. *Fertil Steril* 2006; 85: 1582–1585.

26. Dunaif A. Insulin resistance and the polycystic ovary syndrome: mechanisms and implications for pathogenesis. *Endocr Rev* 1997; 18: 774–800.

27. Dunaif A, Segal K, Futterweit W, Dobrjansky A. Profound peripheral insulin resistance, independent of obesity, in polycystic ovary syndrome. *Diabetes* 1989; 38: 1165–1174.

28. Pasquali R, Casimirri F. The impact of obesity on hyperandrogenism and polycystic ovary in premenopausal women. *Clin Endocrinol (Oxf)* 1993; 39:1–16.

29. Glueck CJ, Papanna R, Wang P, Goldenberg N, Sieve-Smith L. Incidence and treatment of metabolic syndrome in newly referred women with confirmed polycystic ovarian syndrome. *Metabolism* 2003; 52: 908–915.

30. Legro RS, Kunselman AR, Dunaif A. Prevalence and predictors of dyslipidemia in women with polycystic ovary syndrome. *Am J Med* 2001; 111: 607–613.

31. Kelly CJ, Speirs A, Gould GW, Petrie JR, Lyall H, Connell JM. Altered vascular function in young women with polycystic ovary syndrome. *J Clin Endocrinol Metab* 2002; 87: 742–746.

32. Ehrmann DA. Polycystic ovary syndrome. *N Engl J Med* 2005; 352: 1223–1236.

33. Gambineri A, Pelusi C, Manicardi E, Vicennati V, Cacciari M, Morselli-Labate AM, Fagotto U, Pasquali R. Glucose intolerance in a large cohort of Mediterranean women with polycystic ovary syndrome. Phenotype and associated factors. *Diabetes* 2004; 53:2353–2358.

34. Carmina E, Napoli N, Longo R A, Rini GB, Lobo RA. Metabolic syndrome in polycystic ovary syndrome (PCOS): lower prevalence in southern Italy than in the USA and the influence of criteria for the diagnosis of PCOS. *Eur J Endocrinol* 2006; 154: 141–145.

35. Vrbikova J, Vondra K, Cibula D, Dvorakova K, Stanicka S, Sramkova D, Sindelka G, Hill M, Bendlova B, Skrha J. Metabolic syndrome in young Czech women with polycystic ovary syndrome. *Hum Reprod* 2005; 20: 3328–3332.

36. Carmina E. Genetic and environmental aspects of polycystic ovary syndrome. *J Endocrinol Invest* 2003; 26: 1151–1159.

37. Joseph-Home R, Mason H, Batty S, White D, Hillier S, Urquhart M, Franks S. Luteal phase progesterone excretion in ovulatory women with polycystic ovaries. *Hum Reprod* 2002; 17: 1459–1463.

38. Hart R, Hickey M, Franks S. Definitions, prevalence and symptoms of polycystic ovaries and polycystic ovary syndrome. *Best Pract Res Clin Obstet Gynaecol* 2004; 18: 671–683.

39. Abbott DH, Barnett DK, Bruns CM, Dumesic DA. Androgen excess fetal programming of female reproduction: a developmental aetiology for polycystic ovary syndrome? *Hum Reprod Update* 2005; 11: 357–374.

40. Azziz RA. Androgen excess is the key element in polycystic ovary syndrome. *Fertil Steril* 2003; 80: 252–254.

41. Dewailly D, Catteau-Jonard S, Reyss AC, Leroy M, Pigney P. Oligoanovulation with polycystic ovaries but not overt hyperandrogenism. *J Clin Endocrinol Metab* 2006; 91: 3922–7.

42. Carmina E, Lobo RA. Does metformin induce ovulation in normoandrogenic anovulatory women? *Am J Obstet Gynecol* 2004; 191: 1580–1584.

43. Barber TM, Wass JA, McCarthy MI, Franks S. Metabolic characteristics of women with polycystic ovaries and oligo-amenorrhea but normal androgen levels: implications for the management of polycystic ovary syndrome. *Clin Endocrinol (Oxf)* 2007; 66: 513–7.

44. Nestler JE, Stovall D, Akhter N, Iuorno MJ, Jakubowicz DJ. Strategies for the use of insulin-sensitizing drugs to treat infertility in women with polycystic ovary syndrome. *Fertil Steril* 2002; 77:209–215.

45. Escobar-Morreale HF, Luque-Ramirez M, San Millan JL. The molecular-genetic basis of functional hyperandrogenism and the polycystic ovary syndrome. *Endocr Rev* 2005; 26: 251–282.

46. Clement K. Genetics of human obesity. *Proc Nutr Soc* 2005; 64: 133–142.

47. Marti A, Moreno-Aliaga MJ, Hebebrand J, Martinez JA. Genes, lifestyle and obesity. *Int J Obes Relat Metab Disord* 2004; 28 (Suppl 3): S29-S36.

48. Huber-Buckholz MM, Carey DG, Norman RJ. Restoration of reproductive potential by lifestyle modification in obese polycystic ovary syndrome: role of insulin sensitivity and luteinizing hormone. *J Clin Endocrinol Metab* 1999; 84:1470–1474.

49. Carmina E. Mild androgen phenotypes. *Best Pract Res Clin Endocrinol Metab* 2006; 20(2):207–220.

9

Acquired Polycystic Ovary Syndrome
Epilepsy, Bipolar Disorder, and the Role of Anti-Epileptic Drugs

Richard S. Legro, MD, and Elizabeth A. Winans, PHARMD, BCPP

CONTENTS

1 INTRODUCTION
2 EPILEPSY AND MENSTRUAL DISORDERS
3 PCOS AND BIPOLAR DISEASE
4 ARE ORAL CONTRACEPTIVE PILLS PROTECTIVE?
5 VALPROATE-ASSOCIATED PCOS: CURRENT THEORIES
6 CONCLUSION

Summary

Neurologic and psychiatric disorders offer a unique opportunity to study the polycystic ovary syndrome (PCOS) phenotype. Menstrual disorders are frequently associated with the presentation of epilepsy and bipolar disorder, and common factors and pathways may be involved. Some treatments of these conditions, for instance valproate, are thought to bring out stigmata of PCOS in susceptible individuals. The prevalence of PCOS appears higher in women with epilepsy and bipolar disorder. In addition, studies suggest that anti-epileptic drugs (AEDs), particularly valproate, may heighten a woman's risk for developing PCOS, especially with concomitant weight gain. Preliminary evidence suggests that oral contraceptives may be protective in certain instances. Further prospective studies are needed to better quantify the effects of treatment as well as the underlying disorder itself on development of the PCOS phenotype.

Key Words: hyperandrogenism, epilepsy, bipolar disease, anovulation, hirsutism.

1. INTRODUCTION

Polycystic ovary syndrome (PCOS) is a heterogeneous syndrome of androgen excess and chronic anovulation due to unknown cause. As with comparable psychiatric and neurologic syndromes, the clinical features of PCOS cluster in affected individuals, but only rarely (fortuitously) do all appear in a given individual. The putative causes of PCOS include a primary hypothalamic abnormality in gonadotropin secretion leading

From: *Contemporary Endocrinology: Polycystic Ovary Syndrome*
Edited by: A. Dunaif, R. J. Chang, S. Franks, and R. S. Legro © Humana Press, Totowa, NJ

to inappropriate ovarian sex steroid secretion and anovulation, a fundamental ovarian defect, for instance in steroidogenesis leading to androgen excess and secondary inappropriate feedback centrally at the hypothalamic–pituitary axis, and finally some extrinsic factor that affects both brain and ovary. Currently, the most likely candidate for this latter factor appears to be a disorder of insulin action leading to peripheral insulin resistance, compensatory hyperinsulinemia, and related gonadotropin and sex steroid abnormalities (1). Family studies have shown that these disorders cluster in families implying a genetic abnormality or predisposition that leads to the PCOS phenotype (2).

Neurologic and psychiatric disorders offer a unique opportunity to study the PCOS phenotype. One is because menstrual disorders appear intimately connected with the presentation of these conditions, especially given the putative central nervous system (CNS) link between neurologic, psychiatric, and reproductive disorders. Second is because some treatments, for instance valproate, are thought to bring out stigmata of PCOS in susceptible individuals. Thus, a closer study of these disorders might highlight the role of central hypothalamic–pituitary dysfunction in the etiology of PCOS as well as lend credence to the hypothesis that there are environmental modifiers—that is, anti-epileptic drugs or AEDs—that can initiate a PCOS phenotype.

In the absence of clear evidence-based guidelines, diagnosis often is settled by medical opinion. The most recent expert consensus conference, held in 2003, recommended diagnosing of PCOS (after exclusion of other disorders that mimic PCOS) when two of the three following criteria are present: (1) chronic anovulation, (2) hyperandrogenism, and (3) polycystic ovaries (3,4). This chapter will examine the prevalence of menstrual disorders and PCOS among women with epilepsy and bipolar disorder and explore the effects of AEDs on the PCOS phenotype.

2. EPILEPSY AND MENSTRUAL DISORDERS

Wallace et al. (5) also reported significantly reduced fertility among women with epilepsy, and although potential causes were not addressed, it is reasonable to assume that anovulatory infertility was a significant factor. Menstrual disorders have been reported to be more common among women with epilepsy. For instance, Herzog et al. (6,7) reported in a case-control study of a hospital-based population that menstrual disorders were 2.5 times more common among women with epilepsy. However, many of these studies are limited as they are reflective of an outpatient or inpatient neurology service and may not represent the true prevalence in the larger population with epilepsy. Svalheim et al. (8) conducted a community-based survey of females aged 18–45. Females with epilepsy (n = 265) were matched with a normal control for age and lifestyle (n = 142). Menstrual disorders were more common in patients and correlated somewhat with the severity of their epilepsy. Subjects on multiple medications were more likely to have a menstrual disorder compared to subjects on monotherapy. Similarly subjects with increased seizure frequency (five or more seizures/year) were more likely to have a menstrual disorder. The highest frequency of menstrual disorders was found among women on valproate.

The type of seizure disorder may also influence the risk for a menstrual disorder. For instance, Morrell et al. (9) found a trend toward more anovulatory cycles in subjects with idiopathic generalized epilepsy than among those with localization-related epilepsy. It is important to note that a menstrual disorder per se does not equate with a diagnosis of PCOS. Women with epilepsy experience the full range of menstrual abnormalities, including those due to hypothalamic amenorrhea, hyperprolactinemia, and premature ovarian failure *(10)*. However, PCOS is probably the most common cause of menstrual disorder that these women experience.

2.1. PCOS and Epilepsy

Prevalence rates of PCOS among women with epilepsy have been found to be much higher (10–26%) than in the general population (4–7%) *(10)*. Epileptic discharges may affect the secretion of GnRH from the hypothalamus. Herzog et al. *(11)* studied 50 women with partial temporal lobe epilepsy, 19 of whom had reproductive endocrine disorders. They reported that left-sided interictal epileptic activity appeared to be closely associated with PCOS with increased luteinizing hormone (LH) pulse frequencies characteristic of PCOS. The investigators theorized that left-sided epileptic discharges disrupt hypothalamic–pituitary–ovary regulation, leading to alterations in gonadotropin secretion. Right laterality has been associated with hypothalamic amenorrhea.

Further, these investigators have noted that some hormonal changes, for instance prolactin and gonadotropin levels, show a close temporal relationship to the occurrence of interictal discharges *(6,12)*. Anovulation may lower the limbic seizure threshold, as circulating progesterone produced during the luteal phase after an ovulation may stabilize seizure risk *(13)*. Similarly, unopposed circulating estrogen, characteristic of PCOS, may exacerbate seizure risk due to tempero-limbic effects *(11)*.

2.2. Epilepsy, AEDs, and PCOS

The link between AEDs and stigmata of PCOS was first made by the Isojarvi group *(14)*, and they have published a number of articles examining the effects of AEDs on the reproductive phenotype in women with epilepsy. These articles have had tremendous impact on the prescribing of AEDs in women with both epilepsy and bipolar disorders. However, it is important to note their limitations. Most of these reports took place in a Finnish or Scandinavian population, and these findings may not extrapolate to multi-cultural populations or those with varying racial background and lifestyles. Secondly, these were retrospective studies or at best observational studies, and their findings should not be confused with those from prospective randomized controlled trials. Nonetheless, their impact merits closer scrutiny.

In their first article, they retrospectively assessed the prevalence of PCOS and hyperandrogenism in 238 women with epilepsy *(14)*. Thirteen of 29 patients treated with valproate monotherapy reported menstrual abnormalities compared with 23 of 120 treated with carbamazepine monotherapy, 3 of 12 treated with carbamazepine and valproate in combination, and 8 of 62 who received other AEDs. Fifteen patients were untreated. Of those treated with valproate, 43% had polycystic ovaries and 17% had elevated serum testosterone levels in the absence of polycystic ovaries. Eighty percent of women who began taking valproate before age 20 demonstrated polycystic ovaries or hyperandrogenism. Although this study had limitations (small size and retrospective design), it suggests that valproate treatment may be associated with development of hyperandrogenism and polycystic ovaries, especially if treatment is initiated in early adulthood.

The same investigators also presented additional data assessing possible connections between AEDs and PCOS *(15)*. [None of these studies utilized the 1990 National Institutes of Health (NIH) diagnostic criteria for PCOS *(16)* or subsequent Rotterdam Criteria *(3,4)*.] In this small study of eight women with epilepsy, sex hormone levels and menstrual abnormalities were assessed before and after 1 and 5 years of carbamazepine therapy. Although none of the patients reported menstrual abnormalities prior to the study, two experienced menstrual abnormalities during the trial period and three patients demonstrated elevated sex hormone-binding globulin (SHBG) levels at year 5 of treatment.

In a separate cross-sectional study reported in the same article, Isojarvi et al. *(15)* assessed the influence of carbamazepine on endocrine function after 5 years of treatment for epilepsy. Of 56 women who participated, 14 (25%) experienced menstrual abnormalities and 5 had both menstrual abnormalities and elevated LH levels. However, no significant changes in androgen levels were associated with carbamazepine treatment. The investigators failed to note whether any of the menstrual abnormalities preceded treatment. Further, there was no untreated control group, making it difficult to determine whether the reported abnormalities were due to carbamazepine or to epilepsy.

In a further study of epileptic women who were switched from valproate to lamotrigine and then followed for a year, Isojarvi et al. *(17)* found an improvement in the PCOS phenotype. The body mass index and fasting serum insulin and testosterone concentrations (Fig. 1) decreased during the first year after replacing valproate with lamotrigine, whereas the high-density lipoprotein (HDL) cholesterol/total cholesterol ratios increased from 0.17 ± 0.06 to 0.26 ± 0.05. The total number of polycystic ovaries in these women decreased from 20 during valproate medication to 11 a year after replacing valproate with lamotrigine.

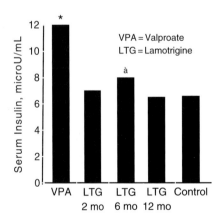 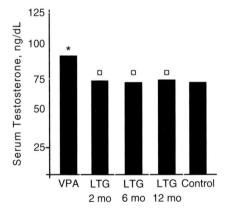

*$P<.05$ compared with control subjects.
à $P<.05$ compared with valproate.

$P<.01$ compared with valproate.
￿$P<.001$ compared with valproate.

Fig. 1. Effects on circulating testosterone and insulin from switching from valproate (VPA) to lamotrigine (LTG). *$p < 0.05$ compared with control subjects; †$p < 0.01$ compared with valproate; ‡$p < 0.05$ compared with valproate; §$p < 0.001$ compared with valproate. Adapted from Isorjarvi et al. *(17)*.

These results appeared to be supported by a multicenter, open-label, cross-sectional study of women with epilepsy on lamotrigine monotherapy (n = 119) with those on valproate monotherapy (n = 103) for greater than 5 years *(18)*. These researchers found that mean total serum testosterone and androstenedione levels were higher ($p < 0.02$) in the valproate group compared with the lamotrigine group at baseline. However, while statistically significant, the levels did not approach a clinically elevated threshold (Fig. 2). The majority of subjects had regular menstrual cycles: lamotrigine patients (87%) and valproate patients (77%). Further, the prevalence of anovulation did not differ between lamotrigine and valproate. Mean HDL cholesterol levels were higher ($p < 0.01$) with lamotrigine compared with valproate as were low-density lipoprotein (LDL) and total cholesterol levels ($p < 0.05$). Mean total insulin levels did not significantly differ between the groups; however, mean weight in valproate patients increased by 3.7 kg over the course of the study.

Other groups have found less convincing evidence of the link between AEDs and PCOS symptoms. Luef et al. *(19,20)* published the results of two trials assessing the frequency of PCOS symptoms in women receiving pharmacologic treatment for epilepsy. The first trial included 43 women who had taken an AED for at least 2 years. Of the 43 women, 22 had been treated with valproate and 21 had taken other AEDs. The authors report that polycystic ovaries, regardless of symptoms, were observed on ultrasound examination in five (23%) of the patients receiving valproate and six (29%) receiving other AEDs. However, actual expression of PCOS (as defined by NIH criteria) occurred in only two (9%) women treated with valproate and one (5%) treated with other AEDs. Levels of DHEA, but not testosterone, were significantly higher in the valproate group than in the group taking other AEDs *(20)*. Although follicle-stimulating hormone (FSH) levels were slightly lower in the valproate group, there were no statistically significant differences between the two groups with respect to LH levels. Menstrual abnormalities were reported in five patients treated with valproate and seven treated with other AEDs. Within the valproate group, 45% of women were overweight compared with 38% of those receiving other AEDs. However, the differences between the two groups with respect to mean weight, waist-to-hip ratio, and abdominal circumference were not statistically significant.

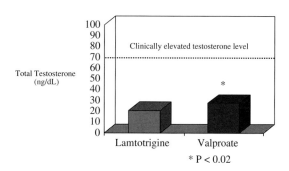

Fig. 2. Mean serum total testosterone levels in women with epilepsy: valproate users versus lamotrigine users. Though women on valproate have statistically higher mean values, these are along the lower ends of normal for women and do not approach clinically meaningful thresholds. Adapted from *(18)*.

A second trial assessed 105 women who had received an AED for 2 or more years *(19)*. Menstrual irregularities occurred in 23% of women receiving valproate and 32% of those receiving carbamazepine. Hirsutism was clinically evident in three women treated with valproate and two treated with carbamazepine. While the percentages of women diagnosed with PCOS were roughly equal in the two groups (valproate, 25% and carbamazepine, 28%), valproate was associated with higher body weight and body mass index (BMI) values. Further, laboratory values for postprandial glucose, insulin, pro-insulin, and C-peptide were significantly higher in the valproate group.

3. PCOS AND BIPOLAR DISEASE

As in epilepsy, reproductive disorders have been noted to be more common in women with bipolar disorder. Also as in epilepsy, it is unusual to study women in a drug naïve state, as treatment is indicated to prevent exacerbations of the underlying disease and is almost always administered at first presentation. Thus, there are usually confounding effects of medication to be considered when studying this population. AEDs such as valproate and carbamazepine are often employed in the treatment of bipolar disorder. It also has been reported that women with bipolar disorder have an increased prevalence of menstrual abnormalities, independent of treatment *(21)*. As a result, several investigators have assessed women with bipolar disorder to examine whether there is an increased prevalence of PCOS.

Rasgon et al. *(22)* presented a preliminary study evaluating the clinical presentation and reproductive hormone levels of 22 women with bipolar disorder. All patients were receiving valproate monotherapy ($n = 10$), lithium monotherapy ($n = 10$), or a lithium–valproate combination ($n = 2$). Women previously diagnosed with PCOS were excluded from the study. Menstrual abnormalities were reported in all lithium-treated patients, 60% of those receiving valproate, and both of the patients on combination therapy. In four patients, menstrual dysfunction preceded diagnosis of bipolar disorder. There were no differences in BMI, hirsutism, or hormone levels among the treatment groups. The investigators concluded that among women with bipolar disorder, there was no association between PCOS and treatment with either valproate or lithium.

O'Donovan et al. *(23)* conducted a two-part study of women with bipolar disorder. In the first phase, 17 patients receiving valproate and 15 patients who were not currently taking the drug were compared with 22 controls who had no history of psychiatric illness. Menstrual irregularities were reported in 47% of patients treated with valproate, 13% of those not taking valproate, and none of the controls. There were no differences among groups with respect to BMI. In the second phase of the study, seven of the eight valproate-treated women who had reported menstrual irregularities underwent further ovarian and hormonal assessments. Two women in the group were overweight. Clinical evidence of hirsutism was present in five women, two of whom reported that the symptom appeared after initiation of valproate. All seven women exhibited hyperandrogenism. Elevated LH/FSH ratios were present in four and five had PCOS as determined by ultrasound. However, none had abnormal FSH or DHEA levels. The investigators concluded that all seven hyperandrogenic women had PCOS and predicted a PCOS prevalence of 41% for all valproate-treated women in the first phase of the study. Not all women in the initial phase were evaluated for PCOS; therefore, it is difficult to accept this conclusion without further verification.

Recently, Akdeniz et al. *(24)* presented a cross-sectional study comparing repro-ductive endocrine and metabolic abnormalities in epileptic women taking valproate with those in women receiving valproate for bipolar disorder. The study included a comparison group of women with bipolar disorder who were receiving lithium and excluded concomitant use of other psychotropics known to cause adverse endocrine or metabolic effects. Women who in the past 6 months had received hormonal or psychotropic medication that could have altered the menstrual cycle or affected carbo-hydrate or lipid metabolism were likewise excluded.

A total of 45 women participated: 15 were taking valproate for epilepsy, another 15 were on valproate for bipolar disorder, and the remaining women were taking lithium for bipolar disorder. Among patients receiving valproate, those being treated for epilepsy had a significantly longer duration of exposure to the drug than those being treated for bipolar disorder; five patients with epilepsy and one with bipolar disorder had begun treatment prior to age 20. However, mean valproate dosages and serum levels were significantly higher in patients with bipolar disorder. Seven (47%) patients with epilepsy reported menstrual disturbances compared with three (20%) of those with bipolar disorder. Of the patients taking valproate, all but one reported onset of menstrual abnormalities after valproate treatment was initiated. None of the patients in the lithium group reported menstrual disturbances.

Clinical hirsutism was evident in one patient taking lithium for bipolar disorder and in four patients taking valproate for epilepsy but in none of the patients who were taking valproate for bipolar disorder. Laboratory tests demonstrated that total testosterone levels were significantly higher in both valproate groups than in the lithium group ($p < 0.05$). The patients taking valproate for epilepsy had significantly lower FSH levels and a higher LH : FSH ratio than patients in either of the other two groups ($p < 0.01$). Fasting glucose levels were significantly higher in both valproate (VPA) groups than in the lithium group. There were no significant differences with respect to fasting lipid profiles.

This study suggests that valproate is associated with development of increased testosterone levels in women who have either bipolar disorder or epilepsy. Women with epilepsy who were treated with valproate demonstrated evidence of hyperandrogenism more frequently than women with bipolar disorder, suggesting that epilepsy itself may increase the likelihood of the development of hyperandrogenism.

A recent multicenter study by Joffe et al. *(25)* of 300 women with bipolar represents the best study to date of the effects of medication on reproductive abnormalities to date. While subjects were on medication at the time of study, a retrospective cohort was constructed out of these data to determine the relationship between medication exposure and development of menstrual and reproductive abnormalities. Three hundred women 18 to 45 years old with bipolar disorder were evaluated for PCOS. A comparison was made between the incidence of hyperandrogenism (hirsutism, acne, male-pattern alopecia, and elevated androgens) with oligomenorrhea that developed while taking valproate versus other anti-convulsants (lamotrigine, topiramate, gabapentin, carba-mazepine, and oxcarbazepine) and lithium. Medication and menstrual cycle histories were obtained, and hyperandrogenism was assessed.

Among 230 women who could be evaluated, oligomenorrhea with hyperandrogenism developed in 9 (10.5%) of 86 women on valproate and in 2 (1.4%) of 144 women on

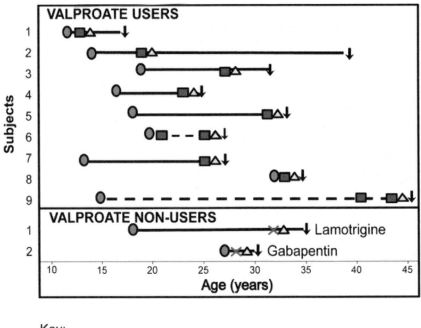

Key:

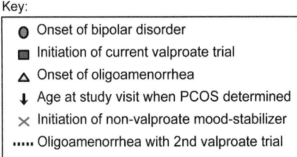

Fig. 3. Temporal relationship between diagnosis of bipolar disorder, initiation of valproate or a nonvalproate mood stabilizer, and onset of oligoamenorrhea, as well as clinical characteristics supporting the diagnosis of polycystic ovarian syndrome for subjects who developed new-onset oligoamenorrhea with hyperandrogenism on valproate or a nonvalproate mood stabilizer. Hyperandrogenism was determined by the presence of hirsutism, acne, or biochemical based on total or calculated free testosterone levels. Adapted from *(25)*.

a nonvalproate anti-convulsant or lithium [relative risk 7.5, 95% confidence interval (CI) = 1.7–34.1, p = 0.002] (Fig. 3). Although the number of subjects developing oligomenorrhea was relatively small, oligomenorrhea always began within 12 months of valproate use (Fig. 3) and was also associated with weight gain while on the drug. This study concluded that valproate is associated with new-onset oligomenorrhea with hyperandrogenism. As with epilepsy, prospective studies are needed to elucidate risk factors for development of PCOS on valproate. Although this study is subject to recall bias, it does support the concept that valproate in selected women, possibly those with a predisposition to PCOS and/or those with weight gain, may lead to the development of PCOS stigmata.

Obviously, a randomized controlled trial in drug naïve women who present with bipolar disease or epilepsy would be the ideal study. However, these studies are difficult to conduct as the presentation of both epilepsy and bipolar disorder is often acute, and immediate intervention is required in most cases. Frequently, they are on some form of maintenance therapy by the time they are referred for specialist care by a neurologist or psychiatrist.

Based on the above studies, it appears that women with epilepsy and bipolar disorder—especially those receiving valproate and, possibly, carbamazepine—have a higher incidence of menstrual abnormalities than their nonepileptic counterparts. Currently, the data are insufficient to determine whether

- epilepsy by itself results in significant menstrual abnormalities that may progress to PCOS or
- AEDs, especially valproate, indirectly cause changes in the menstrual cycle, leading to PCOS.

4. ARE ORAL CONTRACEPTIVE PILLS PROTECTIVE?

Because the hormonal changes of PCOS, including unopposed estrogen, progesterone deficiency, and elevated androgens, can further exacerbate seizure frequency in epilepsy and also potentially mood in bipolar, it is important to examine the effects of AEDs against the backdrop of relatively constant and relatively normal hormonal states. Adjuvant use of the oral contraceptive pill offers a useful model for study. Betts et al. (26) presented a study designed to assess the association between AEDs and ovarian function. Of 105 women with epilepsy, 54 were taking valproate and had never taken another AED and 51 were taking either lamotrigine or carbamazepine and had never taken another AED. The control group consisted of 50 women without epilepsy. Blood samples were collected between days 2 and 6 of the menstrual cycle for FSH, LH, testosterone, and prolactin levels. Concomitant use of oral contraceptive (OCs) was recorded, and all women underwent magnetic resonance imaging to identify the presence of polycystic ovaries.

Women with epilepsy had a significantly higher prevalence of polycystic ovaries (42%) than women without epilepsy (6%). A higher prevalence of PCOS was found in women being treated with valproate than in those treated with lamotrigine or carba-mazepine. However, OC users had a significantly lower prevalence of PCOS (17%) than those who did not take OCs (50%), suggesting that OCs may protect epileptic women taking valproate from the development of symptoms related to PCOS such as hirsutism and oligomenorrhea. Interestingly, OC use did *not* appear to protect nonepileptic women against PCOS. In the absence of OCs, women taking valproate were significantly more likely to have elevated LH and testosterone levels than either normal controls or epileptic women treated with lamotrigine or carbamazepine.

Valproate-treated women younger than 25 years of age were particularly likely to have elevated testosterone levels, suggesting that valproate is most likely to cause (or exacerbate) PCOS in younger women, especially those not taking OCs. The investigators speculated that valproate is associated with a higher prevalence of PCOS than other AEDs, because it is the only one that increases insulin resistance, a key metabolic feature in the development of the syndrome.

5. VALPROATE-ASSOCIATED PCOS: CURRENT THEORIES

There are several proposed theories relating to valproate-associated PCOS:

- Valproate (especially in women who have gained weight) may lead to adverse metabolic changes such as hyperinsulinemia and decreased levels of insulin-like growth factor binding protein-1, resulting in a hyperandrogenic state and polycystic ovaries *(27)*.
- Valproate may interfere with the hepatic metabolism of sex steroids potentiating a hyperandrogenic state. For instance in a porcine model, valproate inhibited hepatic conversion of testosterone to estrogen *(28)*. These abnormal sex steroid levels in turn may decrease FSH levels and directly induce polycystic ovaries.
- Valproate may directly affect gonadotropin secretion leading to increased LH pulsatility and amplitude although this has not been noted in small studies of women with PCOS *(29)* or in normal premenopausal women *(30)*. However, the interaction with epilepsy may be necessary for this effect to manifest.
- Valproate may directly stimulate the ovary to produce excess androgens. The best evidence for this comes from human thecal cell cultures in which valproate further augments androgen production in women with PCOS, as well as transforms normal thecal cells into PCOS-like thecal cells (Figs 4 and 5) *(31)*. Other investigators have suggested similar effects but only at supraphysiological levels unlikely to be achieved in human subjects *(32)*.

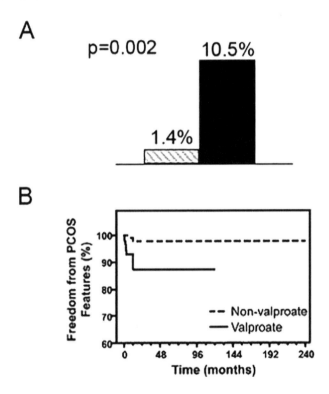

Fig. 4. (**A**) Proportion of 86 valproate users (dark bar) and 144 valproate nonusers (striped bar) who developed new-onset oligomenorrhea with hyperandrogenism and (**B**) Kaplan–Meier survival curve indicating the number of months until onset of new-onset oligomenorrhea with hyperandrogenism developing on valproate (solid line) and nonvalproate (dashed line) mood stabilizers (log-rank χ^2= 108.1, $p < 0.001$). Adapted from *(25)*.

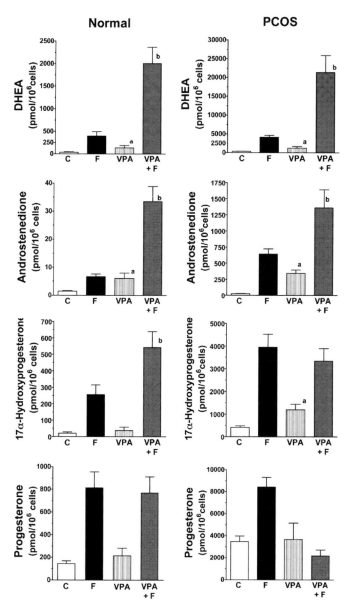

Fig. 5. The effects of valproate (VPA) on steroid biosynthesis in normal and polycystic ovary syndrome (PCOS) theca cells. To compare the effect of VPA treatment on overall steroid biosynthesis, normal and PCOS theca cells, VPA-stimulated DHEA, 4A, 17OHP4, and P4 biosynthesis were examined. Fourth-passage theca cells isolated from normal and PCOS women were treated in the presence or absence (C) of 20 µM forskolin (F) with and without VPA (500 µM). After 72 h of treatment, the media were collected, and DHEA, 4A, 17OHP4, and P4 production was evaluated by RIA, and the data were normalized to cell number. Results are presented as the mean ± SEM of steroid levels from triplicate theca cell cultures from five independent normal and four independent PCOS patients. DHEA, 4A, and 17OHP4 production was increased in response to VPA treatment under basal- (a, $p < 0.05$) and forskolin-stimulated conditions (b, $p < 0.05$). Adapted from *(31)*.

6. CONCLUSION

Despite the lack of clarity, clinicians should be aware of the link between epilepsy and PCOS and prospectively screen epileptic women of childbearing age for reproductive and metabolic abnormalities. Polycystic ovary syndrome is a multidimensional metabolic syndrome involving hyperinsulinemia, glucose dysregulation, hyperlipidemia, and obesity as well as chronic anovulation, hyperandrogenism, and abnormal ovarian morphology. However, the prevalence of PCOS is higher in certain subgroups, such as women with epilepsy and, possibly, bipolar disorder. In addition, studies suggest that AEDs, particularly valproate, may heighten a woman's risk for developing PCOS while OC use may be protective in certain instances. Further prospective studies are needed to better quantify the effects of treatment as well as the underlying disorder itself on development of the PCOS phenotype.

REFERENCES

1. Sam S, Dunaif A. Polycystic ovary syndrome: syndrome XX? *Trends Endocrinol Metab* 2003;14(8):365–70.
2. Legro RS, Spielman R, Urbanek M, Driscoll D, Strauss JFr, Dunaif A. Phenotype and genotype in polycystic ovary syndrome. *Recent Prog in Horm Res* 1998; 53:217–56.
3. Rotterdam ESHRE/ASRM-Sponsored PCOS Consensus Workshop Group. Revised 2003 consensus on diagnostic criteria and long-term health risks related to polycystic ovary syndrome. *Fertil Steril* 2004;81(1):19–25.
4. Rotterdam ESHRE/ASRM-Sponsored PCOS Consensus Workshop Group. Revised 2003 consensus on diagnostic criteria and long-term health risks related to polycystic ovary syndrome (PCOS). *Hum Reprod* 2004;19(1):41–7.
5. Wallace H, Shorvon S, Tallis R. Age-specific incidence and prevalence rates of treated epilepsy in an unselected population of 2,052,922 and age-specific fertility rates of women with epilepsy. *Lancet* 1998;352(9145):1970–3.
6. Herzog AG, Coleman AE, Jacobs AR, et al. Interictal EEG discharges, reproductive hormones, and menstrual disorders in epilepsy. *Ann Neurol* 2003;54(5):625–37.
7. Herzog AG, Friedman MN. Menstrual cycle interval and ovulation in women with localization-related epilepsy. *Neurology* 2001;57(11):2133–5.
8. Svalheim S, Tauboll E, Bjornenak T, et al. Do women with epilepsy have increased frequency of menstrual disturbances? *Seizure* 2003;12(8):529–33.
9. Morrell MJ, Giudice L, Flynn KL, et al. Predictors of ovulatory failure in women with epilepsy. *Ann Neurol* 2002;52(6):704–11.
10. Herzog AG. Menstrual disorders in women with epilepsy. *Neurology* 2006;66(6 Suppl 3):S23–8.
11. Herzog AG, Seibel MM, Schomer DL, Vaitukaitis JL, Geschwind N. Reproductive endocrine disorders in women with partial seizures of temporal lobe origin. *Arch Neurol* 1986;43(4):341–6.
12. Drislane FW, Coleman AE, Schomer DL, et al. Altered pulsatile secretion of luteinizing hormone in women with epilepsy. *Neurology* 1994;44(2):306–10.
13. Herzog AG. Intermittent progesterone therapy and frequency of complex partial seizures in women with menstrual disorders. *Neurology* 1986;36(12):1607–10.
14. Isojarvi JI, Laatikainen TJ, Pakarinen AJ, Juntunen KT, Myllyla VV. Polycystic ovaries and hyperandrogenism in women taking valproate for epilepsy. *N Engl J Med* 1993;329:1383–8.
15. Isojarvi JI, Laatikainen TJ, Pakarinen AJ, Juntunen KT, Myllyla VV. Menstrual disorders in women with epilepsy receiving carbamazepine. *Epilepsia* 1995;36(7):676–81.

16. Zawadski JK, Dunaif A. Diagnostic criteria for polycystic ovary syndrome; towards a rational approach. In: A D, JR G, F H, GR M, eds. *Polycystic Ovary Syndrome*. Boston, MA: Blackwell Scientific; 1992:377–84.

17. Isojarvi JI, Rattya J, Myllyla VV, et al. Valproate, lamotrigine, and insulin-mediated risks in women with epilepsy. *Ann Neurol* 1998;43:446–51.

18. Morrell MJ, Isojarvi J, Taylor AE, et al. Higher androgens and weight gain with valproate compared with lamotrigine for epilepsy. *Epilepsy Res* 2003;54(2–3):189–99.

19. Luef G, Abraham I, Haslinger M, et al. Polycystic ovaries, obesity and insulin resistance in women with epilepsy. A comparative study of carbamazepine and valproic acid in 105 women. *J Neurol* 2002;249(7):835–41.

20. Luef G, Abraham I, Trinka E, et al. Hyperandrogenism, postprandial hyperinsulinism and the risk of PCOS in a cross sectional study of women with epilepsy treated with valproate. *Epilepsy Res* 2002;48(1–2):91–102.

21. Matsunaga H, Sarai M. Elevated serum LH and androgens in affective disorder related to the menstrual cycle: with reference to polycystic ovary syndrome. *Jpn J Psychiatry Neurol* 1993;47:825–42.

22. Rasgon NL, Altshuler LL, Gudeman D, et al. Medication status and polycystic ovary syndrome in women with bipolar disorder: a preliminary report. *J Clin Psychiatry* 2000;61(3):173–8.

23. O'Donovan C, Kusumakar V, Graves GR, Bird DC. Menstrual abnormalities and polycystic ovary syndrome in women taking valproate for bipolar mood disorder. *J Clin Psychiatry* 2002;63(4):322–30.

24. Akdeniz F, Taneli F, Noyan A, Yuncu Z, Vahip S. Valproate-associated reproductive and metabolic abnormalities: are epileptic women at greater risk than bipolar women? *Prog Neuropsychopharmacol Biol Psychiatry* 2003;27(1):115–21.

25. Joffe H, Cohen LS, Suppes T, et al. Valproate is associated with new-onset oligoamenorrhea with hyperandrogenism in women with bipolar disorder. *Biol Psychiatry* 2006;59(11):1078–86.

26. Betts T, Yarrow H, Dutton N, Greenhill L, Rolfe T. A study of anticonvulsant medication on ovarian function in a group of women with epilepsy who have only ever taken one anticonvulsant compared with a group of women without epilepsy. *Seizure* 2003;12(6):323–9.

27. Soares JC. Valproate treatment and the risk of hyperandrogenism and polycystic ovaries. *Bipolar Disorders* 2000;2(1):37–41.

28. Tauboll E, Gregoraszczuk EL, Kolodziej A, Kajta M, Ropstad E. Valproate inhibits the conversion of testosterone to estradiol and acts as an apoptotic agent in growing porcine ovarian follicular cells. *Epilepsia* 2003;44(8):1014–21.

29. Popovic V, Spremovic S. The effect of sodium valproate on luteinizing hormone secretion in women with polycystic ovary disease. *J Endocrinol Invest* 1995;18:104–8.

30. Popovic V, Spremovic-Radjenovic S, Eric-Marinkovic J, Grossman A. Effect of sodium valproate on luteinizing hormone secretion in pre- and postmenopausal women and its modulation by naloxone infusion. *J Clin Endocrinol Metab* 1996;81(7):2520–4.

31. Nelson-DeGrave VL, Wickenheisser JK, Cockrell JE, et al. Valproate potentiates androgen biosynthesis in human ovarian theca cells. *Endocrinology* 2004;145(2):799–808.

32. Fluck CE, Yaworsky DC, Miller WL. Effects of anticonvulsants on human p450c17 (17alpha-hydroxylase/17,20 lyase) and 3beta-hydroxysteroid dehydrogenase type 2. *Epilepsia* 2005;46(3):444–8.

10 Recommendations for the Early Recognition and Prevention of Polycystic Ovary Syndrome

R. Jeffrey Chang, MD

CONTENTS

1 EARLY RECOGNITION
2 LABORATORY EVALUATION
3 PREVENTION

Summary

The symptoms of polycystic ovary syndrome (PCOS) commonly occur during or soon after the onset of puberty, which may preclude early recognition of the disorder, because the clinical expression of gonadal activation with pubertal development may bear close resemblance to that of PCOS. The single-most important finding is that of progressive hirsutism. Chronic anovulation is less reliable unless the pattern of menstrual irregularity persists beyond 2–3 years. Obesity does not appear to be an etiology for PCOS but may hasten the onset by virtue of associated insulin resistance and compensatory hyperinsulinemia. Efforts to minimize the clinical features of PCOS in young adolescent girls depend on early diagnosis and timely suppression of excess ovarian androgen production.

Key Words: PCOS; adolescence; hirsutism; irregular bleeding; obesity; acne; insulin; ovary; oral contraceptive.

1. EARLY RECOGNITION

1.1. Onset of PCOS

Polycystic ovary syndrome (PCOS) is a multi-system reproductive metabolic disorder associated primarily with excessive ovarian androgen production and chronic anovulation, which are responsible for hyperandrogenism and irregular menstruation, respectively. Though the clinical features of PCOS may vary in order of appearance and degree of severity, most women with PCOS commonly date the onset of symptoms to the peripubertal period or during early adolescence. In many instances, PCOS is not recognized until adulthood because of a lack of diagnosis by the physician or a failure

From: *Contemporary Endocrinology: Polycystic Ovary Syndrome*
Edited by: A. Dunaif, R. J. Chang, S. Franks, and R. S. Legro © Humana Press, Totowa, NJ

to seek medical attention by the patient. Because the symptoms of PCOS emerge insidiously coincident with changes that accompany normal pubertal development, subtle features may not be realized in the early stages, which may account for the failure to identify the disorder in young girls resulting in delayed treatment.

The events of normal puberty include acceleration of growth in height, breast budding and enlargement, appearance of sexual hair, and menstrual bleeding *(1)*. This process is gradual and may require several years before the process is completed. In particular, the normal transition into regular menstrual function is marked by irregular bleeding as a result of anovulation, which may persist for 1–3 years *(2)*. Because the emergence of PCOS commonly can be traced to the events of puberty this disorder may be related to an abnormal expression of those factors that initiate and regulate the process of puberty.

1.2. Hirsutism

In women with PCOS, the most characteristic clinical feature is excessive hair growth. Generally, the increase in hair occurs with the onset of puberty and is steadily progressive. A common initial site of increased hair growth is along the side of the face, which may extend to the chin and neck region. This early distribution may also be accompanied by hair along the upper lip as well, which can be difficult to distinguish from hair growth as a result of normal adrenarche. This pattern of hirsutism invariably is accompanied by extension of pubic hair growth toward the umbilicus and may resemble a male escutcheon. Given the rather pernicious prevalence of PCOS, 4–12%, even modest evidence of increased hair growth warrants consideration of the diagnosis in early adolescence *(3,4)*. Initially, the hair is lightly pigmented and thin. However, in the presence of persistent hyperandrogenemia, the hair will become more abundant and soon appears darkly pigmented and thick. As the condition progresses, older adolescent girls may exhibit excessive hair in the pubic region, abdomen, chest, and extremities. It is important to note that hair growth on the upper lip or mild hirsutism does not necessarily constitute hyperandrogenism. However, persistence and a progressive increase in hair growth should be considered evidence of excess androgen production and possibly PCOS.

Excessive hair may be found on the extremities, abdominal flank, and back although these areas are not considered specific sites of sexual hair growth. Prolonged exposure to abnormally high androgens may lead to mild virilizing signs such as temporal balding, a change in body habitus, lowered voice, and clitoromegaly. However, the latter feature is not usually seen in PCOS. In PCOS, the gradual progression of hirsutism contrasts to the rapid rate of hair growth experienced by individuals with androgen-producing neoplasms.

Girls with premature pubarche, defined as hair growth in the pubic region before the age of 8 years, are at increased risk for functional ovarian hyperandrogenism and PCOS following puberty *(5)*. This is particularly true of premature pubarchal girls who subsequently are oligomenorrheic compared to those with regular cycles. Moreover, if these individuals exhibit hyperandrogenism and hyperinsulinemia, it has been reported that there is a corresponding reduction in birth weight *(5)*. This relationship may subserve a possible mechanism for PCOS in this population. In a study of paired discordant weight siblings who achieved similar weight in childhood, dehydroepiandrosterone sulfate

(DHEA-S) levels were higher in those of low birth weight compared to those born with normal weight *(6)*. If as proposed, fetal growth modulates adrenarche, then greater DHEA-S production may reflect an exaggerated adrenarche in these children. The resultant increased androgen pool may set in motion a cycle of altered hypothalamic–pituitary–ovarian function characteristic of PCOS.

It has been well documented that adolescent girls with PCOS have increased levels of circulating androgens as well as elevated luteinizing hormone (LH) levels and increased LH to follicle-stimulating hormone (FSH) ratios *(7)*. Previous studies have shown that hyperandrogenic girls with likely PCOS exhibited changes in gonadotropin secretion patterns that were similar to those found in adult PCOS *(8)*. Increased concentrations of serum LH were accompanied by an increase in pulse frequency and amplitude, which were significantly greater than those of normal controls. In addition, mean serum levels of testosterone and androstenedione were elevated.

1.3. Irregular Bleeding

Because the duration of menstrual irregularity that accompanies normal puberty may be variable, to base the diagnosis of PCOS on menstrual history in young girls is ill-advised. Little is known about mechanisms that determine the initiation of ovarian activity at puberty and the duration required to achieve regular ovulatory menstruation. However, the intervening interval of chronic anovulation is associated with prolonged estrogen secretion, which in the absence of progesterone production may lead to excessive endometrial proliferation. As growth of the endometrium extends beyond available blood supply, the superficial layers begin to slough, giving rise to breakthrough bleeding until a stable endometrial layer is reestablished. Conversely, the pattern of chronic estrogen secretion is characterized by intermittent increases and decreases in circulating levels. In the case of a decline in serum estradiol, endometrial support is compromised and withdrawal bleeding may occur. In PCOS, the basis for chronic anovulation appears to be linked, at least in part, to a lack of FSH or FSH bioactivity. Whether a similar mechanism underlies postmenarchal anovulation is not known. Nevertheless, the irregular bleeding patterns among adolescent girls with PCOS and postmenarchal girls are indistinguishable.

Among nonhirsute adolescent girls with irregular bleeding, it has been estimated that approximately 50% of oligomenorrheic individuals have increased serum LH levels associated with mild elevations of circulating androgens *(9)*. These individuals also demonstrated an increased rate of LH pulse frequency, which suggested a diagnosis of PCOS. In a long-term follow-up study of oligomenorrheic girls, those with normal serum LH values eventually developed regular ovulatory function compared to more than half of those with elevated LH levels in which the gonadotropin abnormalities persisted along with hyperandrogenism *(10)*. The data suggested that oligomenorrhea in early adolescence with mild hyperandrogenemia may be associated with an endocrinological phenotype of PCOS in the absence of excessive hair growth. Recently, we have conducted preliminary studies of LH secretion in obese oligomenorrheic girls without either hirsutism or elevated androgen levels. The pattern of LH pulse frequency in eight of nine oligomenorrheic girls was strikingly similar compared to LH secretion in adolescent PCOS girls and distinctly greater that the rate of LH release in normal adolescents *(11)*. The implication of increased LH pulse frequency in obese girls is not readily apparent although the potential for increased androgen production with increased bioactivity exists. Whether this LH secretion pattern in these individuals is linked to the neuroendocrine abnormality found in PCOS remains to be determined.

1.4. Obesity

Previously, it has been reported that in PCOS women, the prevalence of obesity was a little more than 50% of cases *(12)*. However, with the recognition of increasing obesity worldwide, there is a growing impression that the incidence may be greater, at least in the USA, than that previously described. Characteristically, there is an increase in the upper body or central distribution of fat that gives rise to an increased waist-to-hip ratio as compared to obese women without PCOS *(13)*. This pattern of fat distribution has been termed android obesity and is evident in young girls who develop the disorder. Notably, there is a preponderance of visceral fat compared to peripheral fat not unlike the distribution of adipose tissue in individuals with insulin resistance. In contrast, girls with gynecoid obesity generally have an enhanced accumulation of normal fat in the hips, buttocks, and thighs. As a result the waist-to-hip ratio in these individuals is usually less than one.

The notion that adolescent girls with PCOS may be predisposed to obesity has not been addressed. Similar to studies in obese women without androgen excess, obese PCOS women tend to have great difficulty in achieving significant and permanent weight loss despite dietary regimens and exercise. In these women, it has been shown that postprandial thermogenesis may be reduced, thereby contributing, at least in part, to weight gain *(14)*. However, resting energy expenditure in PCOS was equivalent to that of normal weight-matched controls, which suggested a relative disparity of increased caloric intake and decreased total energy expenditure *(15)*. Comparable studies in adolescent girls with PCOS have not been performed.

The presence of obesity may serve to stimulate or amplify the functional abnormalities that are associated with PCOS. In late pubertal girls, a relationship between obesity and androgen secretion has been previously reported *(16)*. In addition, an association between body mass index (BMI) and serum testosterone has been observed in premenarchal adolescents. It has been recently demonstrated in peripubertal girls that overweight individuals exhibit significantly greater hyperandrogenemia compared to normal-weight girls, which is consistent with the notion that obesity facilitates androgen excess *(17)*. In particular, this association was shown in a sub-cohort of overweight, early pubertal girls with hyperandrogenemia being more pronounced. In this study, increased serum insulin and LH were found to contribute to hyperandrogenemia, but these abnormalities did not completely account for excess androgen production.

Obesity is negatively related to sex hormone-binding globulin (SHBG), which results in increased androgen bioactivity and enhances hyperandrogenism in PCOS. That hyperandrogenemia is linked to inappropriate gonadotropin secretion in PCOS women underscores this issue. Excessive weight gain and obesity is also associated with insulin resistance and compensatory hyperinsulinemia, which is independent of PCOS *(13)*. Serum insulin is inversely correlated to SHBG concentrations, which may increase the clinical impact of hyperandrogenism in affected women. Correspondingly, the effects of chronic unopposed estrogen secretion are also magnified by increased bioavailable estradiol. These reproductive metabolic abnormalities may contribute to the broader recognized risks of obesity that likely create potential long-term health consequences for young individuals with PCOS.

1.5. Insulin Resistance

It has been well documented that women with PCOS exhibit insulin resistance with compensatory hyperinsulinemia *(13)*. The prevalence of insulin resistance in PCOS has been reported to range between 20 and 40% *(18)*. That insulin resistance is common in obesity may account, in part, for the rather wide prevalence. However, independent of obesity, the presence of a defect in insulin action in PCOS women has been clearly established *(13)*. Generally, insulin resistance is mild although glucose intolerance and subsequent diabetes has been reported to be as high as 31 and 7.5% in affected women, respectively. Evidence suggests that insulin resistance may worsen the clinical manifestations of PCOS. Administration of insulin-lowering drugs has been shown to improve insulin sensitivity, reduce androgen levels, and restore ovulation in some but not all patients with this disorder *(19,20)*. Insulin resistance may also contribute to metabolic dysfunction in PCOS, including an increased likelihood of lipid abnormalities.

The clinical recognition of insulin resistance in PCOS derives from associated physical manifestations. In particular, obesity and acanthosis nigricans are both markers for insulin resistance, such that in the presence of these findings, insulin resistance may be strongly suspected unless proven otherwise. A family history of type 2 diabetes is also helpful but much less specific. By comparison, identification of insulin resistance by laboratory testing has been difficult as most patients exhibit normal fasting blood glucose levels, and increased circulating insulin levels are not common. As a result, effective and convenient screening tests to determine evidence-based therapeutic modalities have been limited.

1.6. Ovarian Morphology

Depiction of the ovary by ultrasound imaging has assumed a role in the diagnosis of PCOS relevant to the classical features of hyperandrogenism and chronic anovulation. This is particularly true of women with hirsutism and regular menstrual function. Despite the observation that an estimated 20% of normal women have PCO, confirmation by ultrasound in hirsute women is diagnostic for the disorder. However, the utility of ultrasonography in the early detection of PCOS in young girls is commonly limited by *(1)* the necessity of an abdominal versus vaginal approach and *(2)* the difficulty of securing adequate imaging in obese girls. In lean and nonobese adolescent girls with hirsutism and oligomenorrhea, it has been demonstrated that ultrasound imaging may be used for the detection of PCO, which are morphologically similar to those described in adult women *(21)*. In contrast, the results of ovarian imaging by us in obese PCOS girls have been of poor quality, which frequently has precluded accurate interpretation. Nevertheless, the critical features of PCOS, hyperandrogenism, and chronic anovulation remain reliable indices of the disorder. In a study of obese adolescent girls with hirsutism and oligomenorrhea with poor resolution of ovarian imaging by transabdominal ultrasound, we were able to demonstrate classical PCO morphology by magnetic resonance imaging *(22)*.

1.7. Acne

Acne may also be encountered in adolescent girls with PCOS. Excessive sebum production is the precipitating factor for the formation of acne lesions. In normal girls, acne is commonly observed during the onset of puberty as the size and activity of sebaceous glands increase secondary to rising adrenal androgen production. With the advance of puberty, circulating androgen levels increase further as ovarian steroidogenesis becomes activated. Androgens not only increase sebum production but also cause the abnormal follicular epithelial cell desquamation that is required for the formation of the comedone. The presence of acne has been correlated with increased levels of DHEA and DHEA-S, whereas the relationship with serum testosterone and androstenedione has been inconsistent *(23)*. Although there is a high incidence of acne in PCOS adolescents and adults, this clinical feature is not among the criteria for the diagnosis.

2. LABORATORY EVALUATION

It is apparent from the foregoing discussion that the early recognition of PCOS in adolescent girls is predicted on clinical features, the most notable being evidence of hyperandrogenism. Any laboratory assessment performed must be based on the degree to which a diagnosis of PCOS is suspected. In a young adolescent girl, the appearance of mild hair growth on the upper lip alone does not merit an evaluation. Moreover, mild hirsutism may not necessarily warrant laboratory testing based on the premise that screening serum testosterone and DHEAS levels serve to eliminate the possibility of an androgen-producing neoplasm, a condition that usually is evident from the rapid onset and severity of symptoms. Determination of 17-hydroxyprogesterone is useful as a screening test for the detection of congenital adrenal hyperplasia (CAH) due to 21-hydroxylase deficiency. However, should the situation indicate the need for laboratory evaluation, then the minimum testing includes measurement of serum total testosterone, DHEAS, and 17-hydroxyprogesterone. Threshold values beyond which a neoplasm should be considered are 200 ng/dl for testosterone and 7000 ng/dl for DHEA-S. If circulating concentrations exceed these levels, then imaging studies such as ultrasound and MR are warranted to locate the lesion. The threshold concentration of basal 17-hydroxyprogesterone is 2 ng/ml. A value above 2 ng/ml should be repeated to ensure that the sample was obtained at random in anovulatory individuals or during the follicular phase in women with regular menstrual cycle. Persistent values in excess of 2 ng/ml warrant further evaluation by an ACTH stimulation test. Women with Cushing's syndrome may also present with a clinical picture consistent with PCOS. The optimal screening test is a 24-h urinary free cortisol. Values that exceed the upper normal limit by three to fourfold are highly suggestive of the diagnosis.

The observation that women with PCOS are insulin resistant and have compensatory hyperinsulinemia raises the question of whether assessment of glucose metabolism and insulin secretion should be evaluated in these patients. Unfortunately, at the present time, the ability to determine insulin resistance is limited by tests that lack sensitivity or are impractical for implementation. Based on fasting levels of glucose and insulin, a variety of indices have been designed to establish insulin resistance *(24–26)*. Although a reasonable correlation exists between each model and provocative glucose tolerance tests, normal values do not preclude the presence of insulin resistance. However, the fasting level of glucose may be used to distinguish glucose intolerance or diabetes, and an elevated fasting insulin level will confer insulin resistance. An oral glucose tolerance test may also be done to rule out diabetes.

As part of the assessment of oligomenorrhea due to anovulation, measurements of prolactin and thyroid stimulating hormone (TSH) may be desirable. In addition, in the presence of obesity, a lipid profile is recommended.

3. PREVENTION

Based on early recognition of PCOS, efforts may be expended to limit or forestall the onset or progression of clinical symptomatology. In addition, treatment may be instituted in an attempt to prevent or restrict the long-term consequences of PCOS, namely diabetes and its related complications, including cardiovascular disease. Currently, the most effective modalities appear to be life-style modification and ovarian suppression by oral contraceptives. There is no known cure for this disorder although in some individuals the disorder may be self-limiting as suggested by a perceived amelioration of abnormalities in later reproductive life commensurate with declining ovarian function *(27)*.

3.1. Life-Style Modification

The influence of obesity on endocrine metabolic and reproductive function in adult PCOS women is conveyed by responses to weight reduction efforts. In anovulatory PCOS women achieving significant weight loss, resumption of ovulatory function has been reported to occur in 35–90% of cases *(28)*. In addition, reduction in hair growth, skin oiliness, and acne has also been reported. The clinical improvement associated with an energy imbalance achieved by reduced intake has been accompanied by decreases in serum androgens, lipids, and fasting insulin. In particular, decreased BMI has been correlated with improved insulin sensitivity, which suggests that the detrimental effects of obesity may be mediated, in part, through insulin resistance. Interestingly, the degree of weight loss required to effect these changes has been variable and as little as 2–5% reduction over a 6-month interval may result in clinical and biochemical benefit *(29)*. Increased physical activity also appears to enhance the advantages of reduced intake in adults with PCOS. That the decrease in body weight was modest suggests weight loss need not be large in light of a persistent life-style modification that may bear on favorable outcomes.

Reports of the effects of life-style intervention on clinical symptomatology in adolescent PCOS girls are lacking. Despite the encouraging results of recent studies performed in adults, initiating and maintaining these programs as a community activity requires an enormous amount of self commitment, energy, and personal expense. Long-term follow-up in life-style modification therapies are needed in the adolescent PCOS population to determine ultimate efficacy (see Chapter 16).

3.2. Oral Contraceptives

Identification of PCOS with mild symptoms affords the best opportunity to limit the progression of clinical features by ovarian suppression using oral contraceptives, particularly in the case of young adolescent girls. Administration of combination estrogen–progestin formulations effectively lower serum androgen levels and thus minimize the major stimulus for hair growth. In addition, estrogen has been shown to increase circulating levels of SHBG, which results in decreased serum-free T concentrations. Progestins have been reported to inhibit 5α-reductase activity, antagonize the androgen receptor, and increase the metabolic clearance rate of both T and DHT (30). This modality of treatment also has the advantage of instituting regular cyclic withdrawal bleeding and providing sufficient progestin to prevent excessive endometrial proliferation and hyperplasia. Generally, in a young population, OCs are well tolerated although intolerance to the medication may be experienced by some. Additional side effects include an increased risk for thrombophlebitis and gall bladder disease. Although some OCs containing progestins with low androgenic potential have been advocated, studies that compare clinical efficacy among various preparations have not been performed.

In the presence of obesity, the effectiveness of OC therapy administration may be less effective than that observed in nonobese PCOS women. A poor therapeutic response in obese individuals with PCOS may warrant consideration of supplementation with an anti-androgen. Whether combined OCs and an antiandrogenic agent might prove to be more effective than either therapy alone in obese PCOS women has not been examined carefully.

3.3. Anti-Androgens

In many instances, anti-androgenic agents have been used in conjunction with oral contraceptives to maximize clinical benefit. Spironolactone is an aldosterone antagonist which, along with its major metabolite canrenone, competes for testosterone-binding sites, thereby exerting a direct anti-androgenic effect at the pilosebaceous unit (31). In addition, spironolactone appears to interfere with cytochrome P450, thereby inhibiting steroid enzyme action and resultant androgen production. Because this medication opposes the action of aldosterone, serum potassium levels may increase and therefore should be monitored. Other anti-androgens include flutamide and finasteride. Flutamide competes for the androgen receptor, whereas finasteride inhibits 5α-reductase. Both agents have been shown to be effective for the treatment of hirsutism (32). In a few cases, flutamide has been associated with liver toxicity. Clinical studies have determined that these compounds exhibit comparable effectiveness in reducing hair growth (33). An isolated role for anti-androgen in the prevention of PCOS symptoms has not been established (see Chapter 18).

3.4. Insulin-Lowering Drugs

Insulin-lowering drugs have been shown to improve insulin sensitivity in PCOS women with insulin resistance, which warrants their consideration in the management of this disorder. However, reduction of serum androgen levels in response to treatment has been inconsistent (34,35). Metformin, a biguanide, increases insulin sensitivity in the liver to reduce gluconeogenesis and hyperinsulinemia. In a prospective randomized trial, metformin administration to individuals at risk for diabetes lowered the incidence of disease compared to an untreated group, which demonstrated a preventative benefit of treatment (36). However, in the same study, individuals subjected to life-style intervention displayed the greatest reduction in diabetes risk. These results suggest that metformin may provide some protection for obese adolescent girls with respect to the development of diabetes. However, the utility of metformin in minimizing PCOS symptoms in young girls remains to be determined.

Clinical studies have shown that administration of metformin to PCOS women resulted in decreased androgen levels, increased rates of spontaneous ovulation, and enhanced ovulatory responses to clomiphene (37). Recent studies have shown that metformin may have direct effects on ovarian steroidogenesis independent of insulin action. Incubation of human ovarian theca-like tumor cells with metformin inhibited the mRNA expression of steroidogenic regulatory protein and 17α-hydroxylase, whereas no effect was detected for 3β-hydroxysteroid dehydrogenase (3β-HSD) or cholesterol side chain cleavage (38). In contrast, metformin was not associated with changes in 17α-hydroxylase or 3βHSD in studies of yeast cells (39). The disparity between results may reflect differences in the cell systems employed. Side effects of metformin include gastrointestinal symptoms that are dose-related and tend to resolve after several weeks. In addition, precautionary temporal withdrawal of metformin is advised in patients undergoing radiological procedures involving intravascular iodinated contrast materials and surgery.

Thiazolidinediones comprise another group of insulin-lowering drugs that include rosiglitazone and pioglitazone. These drugs act by binding to perioxisome proliferation activator receptor gamma that forms a heterodimer with retinoic acid receptor and binds to a promoter to increase the expression of genes that regulate glucose homeostasis. It has been well documented that thiazolidinediones decrease androgen levels in women with PCOS (34). In addition, in a large multi-center clinical trial, it was shown that improved insulin sensitivity was associated with resumption of ovulation following long-term treatment with troglitazone (19). This effect was dose-dependent as determined by the rate of ovulation and the length of time required to achieve ovulation. Similar to metformin, thiazolidinediones have also been shown to have direct effect on steroidogenesis. In studies using yeast, the steroidogenic enzymes, 17α-hydroxylase and 3βHSD, were inhibited by troglitazone and to a lesser extent rosiglitazone and pioglitazone (39). Similar results have been achieved in human granulosa cells (40). However, studies to determine whether troglitazone influences aromatase enzyme have not produced consistent results in human granulosa cells (41). Liver toxicity was associated with first generation drugs of this class of compounds. However, both rosiglitazone and pioglitazone have been virtually devoid of liver effects. Nevertheless, thiazolidinediones should not be initiated in patients with evidence of liver disease. The experience with thiazolidinedione use in adolescents and child is minimal with few individuals studied.

REFERENCES

1. Marshall WA, Tanner JM. Variations in pattern of pubertal changes in girls. *Arch Dis Child* 1969;44:291–303.
2. Apter D, Vihko R. Premenarcheal endocrine changes in relation to age at menarche. *Clin Endocrinol (Oxf)* 1985;22:753–760.
3. Knochenhauer ES, Key TJ, Kahsar-Miller M, et al. Prevalence of the polycystic ovary syndrome in unselected black and white women of the southeastern United States: a prospective study. *J Clin Endocrinol Metab* 1998;83:3078–3082.

4. Diamanti-Kandarakis E, Kouli CR, Bergiele AT, et al. A survey of the polycystic ovary syndrome in the Greek island of Lesbos: hormonal and metabolic profile. *J Clin Endocrinol Metab* 1999;84: 4006–4011.

5. Ibanez L, Potau N, Francois I, et al. Precocious pubarche, hyperinsulinism, and ovarian hyperandrogenism in girls: relation to reduced fetal growth. *J Clin Endocrinol Metab* 1998;83:3558–3562.

6. Francois I, de Zegher F. Adrenarche and fetal growth. *Pediatr Res* 1997;41:440–442.

7. van Hooff MH, Voorhorst FJ, Kaptein MB, et al. Polycystic ovaries in adolescents and the relationship with menstrual cycle patterns, luteinizing hormone, androgens, and insulin. *Fertil Steril* 2000;74: 49–58.

8. Apter D, Butzow T, Laughlin GA, et al. Accelerated 24-hour luteinizing hormone pulsatile activity in adolescent girls with ovarian hyperandrogenism: relevance to the developmental phase of polycystic ovarian syndrome. *J Clin Endocrinol Metab* 1994;79:119–125.

9. van Hooff MH, Voorhorst FJ, Kaptein MB, et al. Endocrine features of polycystic ovary syndrome in a random population sample of 14–16 year old adolescents. *Hum Reprod* 1999;14:2223–2229.

10. Venturoli S, Porcu E, Fabbri R, et al. Longitudinal evaluation of the different gonadotropin pulsatile patterns in anovulatory cycles of young girls. *J Clin Endocrinol Metab* 1992;74:836–841.

11. Yoo RY, Dewan A, Basu R, et al. Common alterations of increased LH pulse frequency in obese oligomenorrheic girls without hyperandrogenism and age- and weight-matched girls with adolescent PCOS. *Fertil Steril* 2006;85:1049–1056.

12. Goldzieher JW, Green JA. The polycystic ovary. I. Clinical and histologic features. *J Clin Endocrinol Metab* 1962;50:113–116.

13. Dunaif A, Graf M. Insulin administration alters gonadal steroid metabolism independent of changes in gonadotropin secretion in insulin-resistant women with the polycystic ovary syndrome. *J Clin Invest* 1989;83:23–29.

14. Robinson S, Chan SP, Spacey S, et al. Postprandial thermogenesis is reduced in polycystic ovary syndrome and is associated with increased insulin resistance. *Clin Endocrinol (Oxf)* 1992;36: 537–543.

15. Segal KR, Dunaif A. Resting metabolic rate and postprandial thermogenesis in polycystic ovarian syndrome. *Int J Obes* 1990;14:559–567.

16. Wabitsch M, Hauner H, Heinze E, et al. Body fat distribution and steroid hormone concentrations in obese adolescent girls before and after weight reduction. *J Clin Endocrinol Metab* 1995;80: 3469–3475.

17. McCartney CR, Prendergast KA, Chhabra S, et al. Hyperandrogenism in obese peripubertal girls: a potential factor in the genesis of polycystic ovary syndrome. *J Clin Endocrinol Metab* in press.

18. Ehrmann DA, Barnes RB, Rosenfield RL, et al. Prevalence of impaired glucose tolerance and diabetes in women with polycystic ovary syndrome. *Diabetes Care* 1999;22:141–146.

19. Azziz R, Ehrmann D, Legro RS, et al. Troglitazone improves ovulation and hirsutism in the polycystic ovary syndrome: A multicenter, double blind, placebo-controlled trial. *J Clin Endocrinol Metab* 2001;86:1626–1632.

20. Pasquali R, Gambineri A, Biscotti D, et al. The effect of long-term treatment with Metformin added to hypocaloric diet on body composition, fat distribution, and androgen and insulin levels in abdominally obese women with and without the polycystic ovary syndrome. *J Clin Endocrinol Metab* 2000;85:2767–2774.

21. van Hooff MH, Voorhorst FJ, Kaptein MB, et al. Polycystic ovaries in adolescents and the relationship with menstrual cycle patterns, luteinizing hormone, androgens, and insulin. *Fertil Steril* 2000;74: 49–58.

22. Yoo RY, Sirlin C, Gottschalk M, et al. Ovarian imaging by magnetic resonance in obese adolescent females with polycystic ovary syndrome. *Fertil Steril* 2005;84:985–995.

23. Falsetti L, Gambera A, Andrico S, et al. Acne and hirsutism in polycystic ovary syndrome: clinical, endocrine-metabolic and ultrasonographic differences. *Gynecol Endocrinol* 2002;16:275–284.

24. Legro RS, Finegood D, Dunaif A. A fasting glucose to insulin ratio is a useful measure of insulin sensitivity in women with polycystic ovary syndrome. *J Clin Endocrinol Metab* 1998;83:2694–2698.

25. Matthews DR, Hosker JP, Rudenski AS, et al. Homeostasis model assessment: insulin resistance and beta-cell function from fasting plasma glucose and insulin concentrations in man. *Diabetologia* 1985;28:412–419.

26. Katz A, Nambi SS, Mather K, et al. Quantitative insulin sensitivity check index: a simple, accurate method for assessing insulin sensitivity in humans. *J Clin Endocrinol Metab* 2000;85:2402–2410.

27. Elting MW, Kwee J, Korsen TJ, et al. Aging women with polycystic ovary syndrome who achieve regular menstrual cycles have a smaller follicle cohort than those who continue to have irregular cycles. *Fertil Steril* 2003;79:1154–1160.

28. Kiddy DS, Hamilton-Fairley D, Bush A, et al. Improvement in endocrine and ovarian function during dietary treatment of obese women with polycystic ovary syndrome. *Clin Endocrinol* 1992;36:105–111.

29. Huber-Buchholz MM, Carey DGP, et al. Restoration of reproductive potential by lifestyle modification in obese polycystic ovary syndrome: role of insulin sensitivity and luteinizing hormone. *J Clin Endocrinol Metab* 1999;84:1470–1474.

30. Nolten WE, Sholiton LJ, Srivastava LS et al. The effects of diethylstilbestrol and medroxyprogesterone acetate on kinetics and production of testosterone and dihyrdrotestosterone in patients with prostatic carcinoma. *J Clin Endocrinol Metab* 1976;43:1226–1233.

31. Cumming DC, Yang JC, Rebar RW, et al. Treatment of hirsutism with spironolactone. *JAMA* 1982;247:1295–1298.

32. Muderris, II, Bayram F, Guven M. A prospective, randomized trial comparing flutamide (250 mg/d) and finasteride (5 mg/d) in the treatment of hirsutism. *Fertil Steril* 2000;73:984–987.

33. Venturoli S, Marescalchi O, Colombo FM, et al. A prospective randomized trial comparing low dose flutamide, finasteride, ketoconazole, and cyproterone acetate-estrogen regimens in the treatment of hirsutism. *J Clin Endocrinol Metab* 1999;84:1304–1310.

34. Dunaif A, Scott D, Finegood D, et al. The insulin-sensitizing agent Troglitazone improves metabolic and reproductive abnormalities in the polycystic ovary syndrome. *J Clin Endocrinol Metab* 1996;81:3299–3306.

35. Ehrmann DA, Cavaghan MK, Imperial J, et al. Effects of metformin on insulin secretion, insulin action, and ovarian steroidogenesis in women with polycystic ovary syndrome. *J Clin Endocrinol Metab* 1997;82:524–530.

36. The Diabetes Prevention Program Research Group. Role of insulin secretion and sensitivity in the evolution of type 2 diabetes in the diabetes prevention program. *Diabetes* 2005;54:2404–2414.

37. Nestler JE, Jakubowicz DJ. Decreases in ovarian cytochrome P450c17 alpha activity and serum free testosterone after reduction of insulin secretion in polycystic ovary syndrome. *N Engl J Med* 1996;335:617–623.

38. Attia GR, Rainey WE, Carr BR. Metformin directly inhibits androgen production in human thecal cells. *Fertil Steril* 2001;76:517–524.

39. Arlt W, Auchus RJ, Miller WL. Thiazolidinediones but not metformin directly inhibit the steroidogenic enzymes P450c17 and 3β-hydroxysteroid dehydrogenase. *J Biol Chem* 2001;276:16767–16771.

40. Gasic S, Nagamani M, Green A, et al. Troglitazone is a competitive inhibitor of 3β-hydroxysteroid dehydrogenase enzyme in the ovary. *Am J Obstet Gynecol* 2001;184:575–579.

41. Mu Y-M, Yanase T, Nishi Y, et al. Insulin sensitizer, troglitazone, directly inhibits aromatase activity in human ovarian granulosa cells. *Biochem Biophys Res Commun* 2000;271:710–713.

11 Insulin Action and Secretion in Polycystic Ovary Syndrome

Julia Warren-Ulanch, MD,
and Silva A. Arslanian, MD

CONTENTS

1 INTRODUCTION
2 INSULIN RESISTANCE IN PCOS
3 INSULIN SECRETION IN PCOS
4 IN VITRO INSULIN ACTION IN PCOS
5 PCOS-ASSOCIATED CO-MORBIDITIES OF INSULIN
  RESISTANCE
6 THERAPEUTIC APPROACHES TARGETING INSULIN
  SENSITIZATION
7 CONCLUSION AND FUTURE DIRECTION

Summary

Polycystic ovary syndrome (PCOS) is a common, heterogeneous disorder comprised of hyperandrogenism and anovulation. Although insulin action and secretion are neither necessary nor sufficient for the definition of PCOS, they are both disordered in this setting. Numerous studies have described hyperinsulinism and insulin resistance in both adults and adolescents. Those findings led to more experiments designed to further define the mechanism on a tissue, cellular, and even molecular level. In a time of obesity epidemic, the metabolic consequences of PCOS cannot be overlooked. The importance of complications and associations such as type 2 diabetes, metabolic syndrome, sleep apnea, fatty liver disease (FLD), and early cardiovascular dysfunction underscores the need for appropriate treatment.

Key Words: Insulin action, Insulin secretion, PCOS, adolescents.

1. INTRODUCTION

Polycystic ovary syndrome (PCOS) is a common disorder not only of premenopausal women but also of adolescent girls. It is a heterogeneous disorder characterized by oligo-anovulation and hyperandrogenemia, which in most patients is of combined

From: *Contemporary Endocrinology: Polycystic Ovary Syndrome*
Edited by: A. Dunaif, R. J. Chang, S. Franks, and R. S. Legro © Humana Press, Totowa, NJ

ovarian and adrenal origin. Associated clinical features include hyperandrogenic symptoms and signs such as hirsutism, acne, and menstrual irregularity with or without the presence of ovarian cysts. Obesity, insulin resistance, and the metabolic syndrome are common *(1–3)*.

Hyperinsulinemia and peripheral insulin resistance are the central features of the metabolic disorder which is now recognized to be typical of PCOS. This chapter will review the evidence that insulin resistance is an integral part of the syndrome and is present early in the course of the disorder. Because rates of type 2 diabetes are high in women with PCOS, the important role of β-cell function and its relationship to insulin resistance will be discussed. Lastly, recent evidence for the heightened risk of the metabolic syndrome in these patients will be presented.

2. INSULIN RESISTANCE IN PCOS

2.1. Definition of Insulin Resistance and Methods of Measurement

Over 40 years ago, Yalow and Berson defined insulin resistance as "a state in which greater than normal amounts of insulin are required to elicit a quantitatively normal response" *(4)*. Since then, several definitions have been put forward including the 1998 American Diabetes Association Consensus Panel on Insulin Resistance that defined it as "an impaired biological response to either exogenous or endogenous insulin" *(5)*. Normal glucose homeostasis is a function of the balance between insulin sensitivity (liver, muscle, and adipocytes) and insulin secretion by the pancretic β-cell. While most discussions of insulin resistance center on the glucose–insulin relationship because of its clinical relevance, insulin resistance is not confined to glucose metabolism only. Insulin resistance applies to any of its biological actions, including suppression of lipolysis and proteolysis, stimulation of protein synthesis, vascular endothelial function, gene expression, and mitogenesis. In PCOS, insulin resistance is selective and tissue specific. Although there is profound resistance to insulin action on both carbohydrate and lipid metabolism, there appears to be preserved or enhanced mitogenic activity in fibroblasts, skeletal muscle and granulosa cells from women with PCOS *(6–9)*.

Various approaches have been used to evaluate in vivo insulin sensitivity *(10)*. These include the gold-standard research tool of the glucose–insulin clamp technique, the minimal model frequently sampled intravenous glucose tolerance test (FSIGT), the oral glucose tolerance test (OGTT), and the surrogate estimates of fasting insulin or glucose to insulin ratio. An important observation to make is that there is no universally-accepted, clinically useful, numeric expression that defines insulin resistance. Moreover, there is no well-defined cut point differentiating normal from abnormal *(11)*. The latter has significant bearing since not infrequently clinicians base treatment decisions on arbitrary insulin levels.

2.2. In vivo Insulin Action in Adult Women with PCOS

In 1921, Archard and Thiers first reported a relationship between hyperandrogenism and insulin metabolism in their description of "diabetes des femmes à barbe" *(12)*. In 1980, Burghen and colleagues described strong correlations between plasma insulin concentrations and testosterone and androstenedione in obese women with PCOS *(13)*. They suggested that hyperinsulinemia might have etiologic significance. Since then, increasing evidence supports a central role of insulin resistance and/or compensatory hyperinsulinemia in the syndrome's pathogenesis *(14)*. Adult women, whether of obese or normal weight, have profound insulin resistance *(8)*. This insulin resistance is manifested as fasting or stimulated hyperinsulinemia and decreased insulin-stimulated glucose uptake during euglycemic clamp experiments *(15)* and decreased insulin sensitivity index during FSIGT *(16)*. Moreover, several investigators have demonstrated that hyperinsulinemia, insulin resistance, and insulin secretion are heritable traits in first-degree family members of women with PCOS *(17–19)*. The question that follows is whether hyperandrogenism causes insulin resistance or hyperinsulinemia causes hyperandrogenism. Clinical and experimental observations negate the former. Severity of hyperinsulinemia does not improve with bilateral oophorectomy despite elimination of hyperandrogenism *(20)* nor with long-acting GnRH agonist therapy *(21)*. Antiandrogen therapy with cyproterone acetate lowers circulatory androgens but does not improve hyperinsulinemia *(22)*. At the moment, there is consensus that hyperinsulinemia leads to hyperandrogenemia *(8,23–26)*. This is based on observations that correction or suppression of hyperinsulinemia through weight loss, diazoxide or insulin sensitizers lowers androgen levels and improves ovulatory function with induction of fertility *(25,27–34)*. Furthermore, alteration in D-chiro-inositol, a mediator of insulin action, is present in women with PCOS *(35)*, and administration of D-chiro-inositol to women with PCOS improves ovulatory function and lowers androgenemia *(36,37)*.

It is commonly believed that insulin resistance/hyperinsulinemia may contribute to hyperandrogenemia through multiple ways. In vitro and in vivo studies suggest that insulin, through its own receptor or through insulin-like growth factor (IGF)-1 receptors, synergizes with LH to promote androgen production by thecal cells. Insulin inhibits hepatic synthesis of sex hormone-binding globulin (SHBG), thereby increasing the free androgen pool; insulin may directly influence hypothalamic dysregulation favoring the secretion of LH; and insulin increases adrenal androgen production by enhancing adrenal sensitivity to ACTH *(14,38)*. Additionally, insulin may stimulate cytochrome P450-c17α enzyme ovarian androgens and adrenal steroidogenesis by augmenting activity of *(31,39)*. The contradiction though is how insulin action on ovarian and/or adrenal steroidogenesis is preserved when there is profound resistance to insulin action in skeletal muscle and adipose tissue. Based on clinical and experimental data, it is proposed that women develop PCOS in part because of an intrinsic, selective, and tissue-specific increase in insulin sensitivity in the ovarian androgenic pathway, that is, ovarian hypersensitivity to insulin. In most women with PCOS, the severity of the ovarian hypersensitivity is such that the concomitant development of insulin resistance and hyperinsulinemia is necessary for phenotypic expression of the syndrome *(40)*. The increasing cases of PCOS in women against the backdrop of the obesity epidemic makes such a theory attractive but in need of testing and confirmation.

2.3. In vivo Insulin Action: Studies in Pediatric PCOS

2.3.1. PCOS in Youth

Despite the original description of PCOS by Stein and Leventhal in 1935, it was not until 1980 when Yen postulated that PCOS is a disorder that begins at menarche and whose characteristics are not changed by age *(41,42)*. Moreover, it was proposed that the physiological hormonal and metabolic changes during puberty, particularly increasing insulin levels and IGF-1, may act as inducing factors in the development of PCOS in susceptible subjects *(43)*. Both normal puberty and PCOS have in common hyperpulsatile gonadotropin secretion, hyperactive ovarian and adrenal androgen production, insulin resistance/hyperinsulinemia, and consequent low SHBG and IGF-BP_1 *(44,45)*. In this scenario of puberty triggering PCOS in predisposed girls, insulin resistance/hyperinsulinism appears to play a major role. Several lines of evidence, epidemiological, and clinical research demonstrate that normal physiological puberty is characterized by a transient insulin resistance that recovers with completion of puberty *(46)*. This translates to around 30% decline in in vivo insulin sensitivity in adolescents compared with prepubertal children. The most likely cause for pubertal insulin resistance is the doubling of GH secretion during puberty *(46)*.

It is also proposed that premature pubarche (PP) (the appearance of pubic or axillary hair before 8 years of age in girls) might be a precursor of PCOS *(47)*. Girls with PP are reported to have lower insulin sensitivity, hyperinsulinemia, low SHBG, and low IGF BP-1 *(48–50)*. However, it may very well be that obesity, whether total body or abdominal, is the culprit in girls with PP since not all girls with PP will progress to a clinical picture of PCOS *(1)*.

2.3.2. COS and Insulin Resistance in Adolescents

Very few studies in pediatrics have investigated insulin sensitivity and secretion in adolescents with PCOS. In one study, adolescents with PCOS had higher fasting and stimulated insulin responses to intravenous glucose tolerance test than a control group. However, the PCOS group was significantly heavier *(44)*. In another study of obese hyperandrogenic adolescents, there was hepatic insulin resistance, but peripheral insulin sensitivity was not evaluated *(51)*. In yet another study, serum insulin levels during an OGTT were higher in adolescents with a history of PP, but insulin sensitivity estimated from OGTT was not different *(52)*. Comparison between nonobese and obese adolescents with PCOS demonstrated higher fasting insulin, proinsulin, and insulin area under the curve during OGTT and lower insulin sensitivity index in the obese group *(53)*. Similarly, adolescents with menstrual irregularities and hormonal characteristics of PCOS had higher insulin area under the curve during OGTT than adolescents with regular menstrual cycles *(54)*. We evaluated in vivo insulin sensitivity with the glucose–insulin clamp technique in obese adolescents with PCOS compared with equally obese otherwise normal peers. The two groups were matched for percent body fat and for visceral adiposity assessed with CT scan. Adolescents with PCOS had evidence of hepatic insulin resistance with fasting insulin concentrations twice as high as the obese control group. Insulin-stimulated glucose metabolism and insulin sensitivity was approximately 50% lower in PCOS girls (Fig. 1). This decrease in insulin sensitivity was accompanied with compensatory fasting and stimulated hyperinsulinemia *(55)*.

2.4. Relationship Between Insulin Sensitivity and Insulin Secretion

Glucose homeostasis is maintained through a delicate balance between insulin secretion by the β cells and insulin action in insulin-sensitive tissues. This relationship between insulin sensitivity and acute insulin release in response to glucose is governed by a negative-feedback loop and is best described by a hyperbolic function *(56)*. Thus,

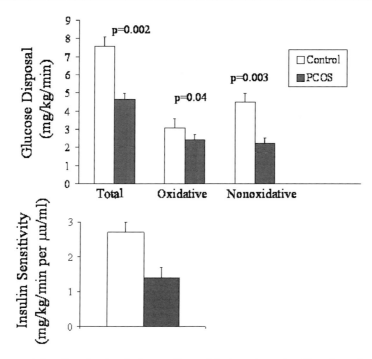

Fig. 1. Upper panel: insulin-stimulated glucose disposal during a hyperinsulinemic euglycemic clamp in obese PCOS girls vs matched obese control girls. Lower panel: insulin sensitivity in PCOS versus obese control girls. Reproduced with permission *(55)*. See insert for color figure.

for a given level of glucose tolerance, the product of insulin sensitivity and β-cell function, termed glucose disposition index, is a constant. When insulin sensitivity decreases, insulin secretion must increase for glucose tolerance to remain constant. If this compensatory increase in insulin secretion is incomplete, then deterioration in glucose tolerance will occur (Fig. 2) *(57)*. Another implication of this hyperbolic relationship is that, although insulin responses may be identical in two groups of individuals, if insulin sensitivity is different, then glucose tolerance may differ between

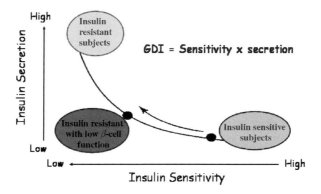

Fig. 2. The hyperbolic relationship between insulin sensitivity and secretion. GDI, glucose disposition index. Reproduced with permission *(5)*.

the groups. Thus, β-cell function should be assessed relative to insulin sensitivity. Individuals at risk of developing type 2 diabetes will have poorer β-cell function than controls with similar degrees of insulin resistance.

3. INSULIN SECRETION IN PCOS

3.1. In vivo Insulin Secretion in Adult Women with PCOS

The reported prevalence of impaired glucose tolerance (IGT) in PCOS women ranges from 15.7% in Mediterranean women to 37% in US women to 47% in Taiwanese women and that of diabetes from 2–10% *(58–61)*. As glucose homeostasis is determined by the balance between insulin resistance and insulin secretion, several investigators have assessed β-cell function in women with PCOS. In these women, the presence of family history of type 2 diabetes was associated with inadequate β-cell compensation for the degree of insulin resistance *(62)*. Both obese and nonobese PCOS women were found to have β-cell dysfunction manifested as decreased glucose disposition index measured with FSIGT *(63)*. However, some of the women had IGT or type 2 diabetes. Thus, abnormalities in β-cell compensation for insulin resistance in PCOS women appear to be present when there is a family history of type 2 diabetes or abnormalities in glucose metabolism. In the absence of the latter, the typical pattern is one of compensatory hyperinsulinemia *(59)*.

3.2. In vivo Insulin Secretion and Glucose Metabolism in Adolescents with PCOS

We sought to investigate the roles of insulin resistance and insulin secretion in the pathogenesis of glucose intolerance in adolescents with PCOS. A group of adolescent girls with PCOS and IGT, diagnosed by OGTT, were compared to a group with normal glucose tolerance. Insulin sensitivity was assessed with a hyperinsulinemic–euglycemic clamp and insulin secretion with a hyperglycemic clamp. Adolescents with PCOS and IGT had significantly higher hepatic glucose production, approximately 40% lower first-phase insulin secretion but no impairment in second-phase insulin. There were no differences in insulin sensitivity between the two groups. Glucose disposition index was 50% lower in the IGT group indicative of β-cell dysfunction (Fig. 3) *(64)*. These metabolic abnormalities are known precursors of type 2 diabetes, and their presence early in the course of PCOS in these adolescents heralds progression to type 2 diabetes. Two adolescents converted from normal glucose tolerance to IGT within a very short period of 6–9 months. In one of these girls who were studied longitudinally over a 5-year period, severe insulin resistance was the preexisting abnormality, but it was the marked decline in insulin secretion that led to T2DM *(65)*. Moreover, the surrogate estimates of insulin sensitivity using fasting glucose and insulin concentrations were not reliable indices in reflecting the longitudinal changes in in vivo insulin sensitivity. Although insulin sensitivity with the hyperinsulinemic–euglycemic clamp decreased by 40% at the time of type 2 diabetes compared with the prior NGT state, both fasting glucose/insulin ratio and HOMA insulin sensitivity showed a paradoxical increase. This is due to the high fasting glucose and low insulin levels at the time of diabetes resulting in an erroneously elevated ratio. Similarly, despite 40% lower first-phase insulin levels in adolescents with IGT, fasting insulin levels were indistinguishable between IGT and NGT groups *(64)*. Thus, the validity and usefulness of fasting indices

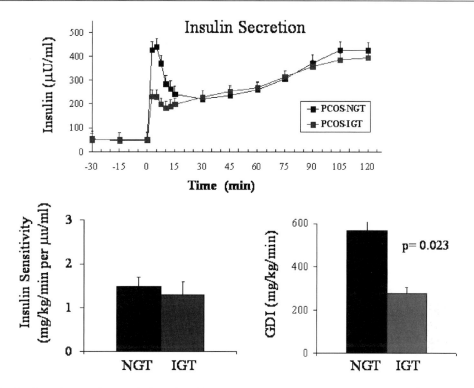

Fig. 3. First-phase and second-phase insulin secretion during a hyperglycemic clamp (upper panel), insulin sensitivity (left lower panel), and glucose disposition index (GDI) (right lower panel) in PCOS adolescents with impaired (IGT) versus normal (NGT) glucose tolerance. Adapted and modified with permission *(64)*. See insert for color figure.

as estimates of insulin sensitivity and secretion should be investigated particularly when using longitudinal interventions that impact fasting glucose and insulin levels.

In adult women with PCOS, the conversion risk from IGT to type 2 diabetes is around 2% per year, whereas conversion from NGT to IGT is more pronounced at 16% per year *(58)*. Moreover, the presence of a family history of type 2 diabetes significantly increases the risk of diabetes *(59)*. Therefore, in adolescents with PCOS and family history of type 2 diabetes, screening for abnormalities in glucose tolerance should be performed. As fasting glucose missed 58% of diabetes in women with PCOS, a 2-h OGTT is recommended when the index of suspicion for abnormal glucose metabolism is high and until such time when data are available in adolescent girls *(66)*. Periodically, re-screening for diabetes should be performed because of worsening glucose tolerance over time, but the interval for this is left to the discretion of the clinician because of lack of data.

4. IN VITRO INSULIN ACTION IN PCOS

In vivo dynamics are important to explore whole-organism effects, but in vitro experiments clarify the cellular and molecular mechanisms responsible for the observations. While the specific molecular mechanisms of insulin resistance in PCOS are discussed elsewhere in this book, it is important, within the context of this chapter, to understand that insulin has multiple actions upon binding to the cell and different roles depending on tissue type. Here, we organize what is known about in vitro insulin action in PCOS by tissue type. Many of these studies were initially done in skin fibroblasts (6,67,68), but we will focus on the more pertinent organs (Table 1).

4.1. Ovary

It has been well documented that although PCOS is an insulin-resistant state, the ovary remains sensitive to insulin (69) at both physiological levels (70–72) and hyperinsulinemic states (70,71). Although the relationship between insulin and the ovary is not intuitive, insulin has been demonstrated to play an important role in normal ovarian growth, folliculogenesis, and steroidogenesis (73). However, androgen production is increased in the presence of physiological levels of insulin in cells from PCOS versus normal healthy women (74). In fact, both baseline and stimulated levels of steroids and steroidogenic enzymes are higher in theca cells cultured from PCOS compared with normal women (75). Through a series of elegant experiments using antibodies to block portions of the signaling cascade, it has been determined that insulin acts through its own receptor (74,76). This is true for both estradiol and progesterone synthesis in granulosa cells (76) and testosterone synthesis in theca cells (74). However, tyrosine autophosphorylation of the insulin receptor is decreased in the ovaries of women with

Table 1
In Vitro Insulin Action in Polycystic Ovary Syndrome (PCOS)

Tissue type	Ovary	Skeletal muscle	Endothelium	Adipocyte
Normal role of insulin	Ovarian growth Folliculogenesis Steroidogenesis	Glucose uptake suppresses glycogenolysis growth	Increase NO vasodilation	Glucose uptake inhibition of lipolysis
In PCOS	↑ Steroidogenesis Basal Stimulated ↓ Tyr auto-P ↑ StAR activity ↑ CYP17 ↑ cAMP (PKA activity) ↑ StAR expression and promotion ↓ glucose uptake ↑ Progesterone ↓ MEK 1/2 and ERK 1/2 ↑ CYP17 mRNA ↑ DHEA	↑ Ser-P of insulin receptor ↑ Ser-P of IRS-1 ↑ MEK1/2 and ERK 1/2 ↑ Ser-P IRS-1	[In states of insulin resistance not studied in PCOS] ↓ NO production	? poor insulin binding ↓ Sensitivity to glucose transport ↓ Maximal glucose transport ↓ Sensitivity to inhibition of lipolysis (normal maximal suppression of lipolysis)

PCOS compared with the normal population *(77)*. Inositolglycans, rather than typical insulin receptor substrates (IRSs), conduct the signal for thecal testosterone synthesis, a pathway unique to insulin *(74)*. Therefore, insulin is synergistic with LH-induced steroidogenesis in PCOS *(69)*, and insulin sensitization of normal women does not affect hormone levels *(78)*.

Activity of the first step in steroidogenesis, the steroidogenic acute regulatory protein (StAR), is increased by insulin *(79)*. In combination, LH and insulin increase the expression of StAR and CYP17, key steroidogenic genes *(80)*. Two mechanisms of this synergy are increased expression by co-binding to the StAR promoter *(79)* and insulin-augmented LH-stimulated cAMP levels. Cyclic AMP-dependent protein kinase A is then a key regulator of StAR expression *(79)*.

Two studies have examined the effects of insulin and LH concentrations on granulosa cells from women with PCOS versus controls *(81,82)*. Both noted decreased insulin-stimulated glucose utilization but insulin augmentation of LH-stimulated progesterone synthesis *(81,82)*. These findings suggest the insulin-resistance of PCOS is pathway specific and explains both the hyperinsulinism and the hyperandrogenism *(82)*.

When this phenomenon was dissected further, investigators found decreased activity of certain pathways of insulin signaling, namely mitogen-activated/extracellular signal-regulated kinase (MEK)1/2 and extracellular signal-regulated kinase (ERK)1/2, in PCOS compared with control subjects *(83)*. This alteration led to higher levels of CYP17mRNA and dehydroepiandrosterone (DHEA). Interestingly, these abnormalities were present even after these cells had been propagated in the absence of insulin. Therefore, these in vitro experiments support the notion of an intrinsic ovarian steroidogenic abnormality as the etiology of PCOS, in a minority of which, could be severe enough to result in PCOS in the absence of hyperinsulinemia *(40,83)*.

4.2. Skeletal Muscle

Insulin action in skeletal muscle is altered at three places along the cascade: the receptor *(67)*, IRS-1 phosphorylation *(84)*, and molecules along MAPKinase pathway *(7)*. Although the discovery of insulin receptor serine phosphorylation was demonstrated in skin fibroblasts *(6)*, this abnormal process also occurs in skeletal muscle *(67)*. Resolution of this deviant phosphorylation after in vitro propagation *(84)* is consistent with a serine kinase extrinsic to the insulin receptor *(68)*. However, insulin signaling remains altered, with constitutively increased levels of phosphorylation at the Ser[312] site of IRS-1 *(84)*. Results from these studies led investigators to further analyze the role of serine phosphorylation of both the insulin receptor and the IRS-1 in the insulin resistance specific to PCOS *(7)*.

Studies closely evaluating insulin signaling in cultured myoblasts from both PCOS and control women have found components of the mitogenic pathway, namely, the extracellular signal-regulated kinase (ERK)1/2 and mitogen-activated/extracellular signal-regulated kinase (MEK)1/2, had increased baseline and insulin-stimulated phosphorylation *(7)*. When inhibited, the inactive form of IRS-1 was reduced, thereby allowing active IRS-1 to conduct the metabolic signal. This specificity of insulin resistance in myotubes from PCOS is different from that seen in T2DM, thereby supporting the notion of a unique mechanism of insulin resistance in PCOS *(84,85)*. However, the details of the interactions between ERK1/2 and IRS-1 remain unknown *(7)*. It has been proposed that this increased mitogenic signaling is the etiology of resistance to metabolic signaling *(7)*. However, the increased mitogenic signaling is also insulin-mediated and is worsened in states of hyperinsulinemia, creating a vicious cycle. Interestingly, these same components of the mitogenic pathway are less active in the theca cells in PCOS *(83)*. Which is the chicken and which is the egg? Rather, selective insulin resistance, that is, through the metabolic pathway, similar to that seen in adipocytes *(86)* and skeletal muscle *(87)* in T2DM is a more likely explanation. In women with PCOS, even though in vivo insulin-stimulated glucose uptake is decreased, this is not demonstrated in myotubes cultured from them, suggesting there remain humoral factors of insulin resistance that deserve further investigation *(84)*.

4.3. Endothelium

Physiological levels of insulin increase nitric oxide (NO), a powerful vasodilator *(88,89)*. However, this vasodilatory effect is lost in those resistant to the metabolic actions of insulin *(90)*. The association between insulin-resistant states, such as type 2 diabetes mellitus and metabolic syndrome, is well founded. It has not yet been described in PCOS, and the specific mechanism, in any population, has not been studied. Blockage of the metabolic pathways of insulin signaling (and thus NO production) in vascular endothelium increased traffic through the prenyltransferase pathways, which led to increased concentrations of adhesion molecules VCAM-1 and E-selectin, molecules associated with endothelial dysfunction *(91)*. This particularly interesting study helps to make the association between selective insulin defects and endothelial dysfunction, one of the consequences of insulin resistance.

4.4. Adipocyte

In the setting of PCOS, the dyslipidemic pattern of low HDL and high TG associate more closely with insulin resistance than with BMI *(92)*. This pattern, among other characteristics, is similar between PCOS and the metabolic syndrome. The role of insulin in the adipocyte is glucose uptake and inhibition of lipolysis, so where is the defect? Studies of insulin binding to adipocytes of PCOS women have mixed results, with some showing normal *(85,93)* and others demonstrating decreased binding *(94)*. These studies included small numbers of subjects and need further exploration.

Sensitivity for glucose transport has also been controversial, with some showing similar results between PCOS and non-PCOS controls *(95)*, and others demonstrating resistance to glucose transport *(93,94)*. However, maximal insulin effect on glucose uptake was low in both studies *(93,95)*, and was attributed to poor ability of the IRS molecule to autophosphorylate *(93)*.

The maximal suppression of lipolysis is not different in PCOS, but adipocytes from PCOS women required almost three times as much insulin to initiate suppression of lipolysis *(96)*. Treatment with the adenosine receptor agonist N6-phenylisopropyl adenosine normalized insulin sensitivity in PCOS cells for both glucose transport and lipolysis, suggesting that the post-receptor binding defect is early in the signaling pathway that is common for both actions *(96)*.

Subcutaneous *(97)*, but not visceral *(98)*, adipocytes are resistant to catecholamine-stimulated lipolysis *(97)*. This phenomenon is explained by two defects in the lipolytic cascade, lower β2 adrenoceptor density and lower enzymatic of the protein kinase, hormone-sensitive lipase complex *(97)*. Although diet-induced weight reduction improved both insulin- and catecholamine-mediated actions on lipolysis *(99)*, neither defect was improved with treatment with an oral contraceptive *(97,99)*.

Because abdominal adiposity is linked to insulin resistance even in the earliest stages of PCOS *(100)*, it is possible that defects in adipose tissue metabolism are key to the pathophysiology of insulin-resistant disorders such as PCOS and metabolic syndrome. It has been thought that the increased abdominal (visceral) adiposity, with its proximity to the liver, is causative of hyperinsulinemia, dyslipidemia, glucose intolerance, and insulin resistance even as early as adolescence *(100)*. Therefore, this finding of increased lipolysis in visceral fat may be an early defect in PCOS *(98)*.

5. PCOS-ASSOCIATED CO-MORBIDITIES OF INSULIN RESISTANCE

5.1. Type 2 Diabetes

As stated above, it is well established that both adult women and adolescents with PCOS are at increased risk for IGT and type 2 diabetes *(66,101)*. A diagnosis of PCOS confers a 5- to 10-fold increased risk of developing type 2 diabetes *(102)*. Young women with PCOS were evaluated for IGT using a 3-h, 75-g OGTT *(103)*. Using the 1997 Guidelines of the ADA, 35% were diagnosed with IGT (2-h post-load >140 but <200 mg/dl), 10% already had type 2 diabetes (≥200 mg/dl), and 45% had normal glucose tolerance (<140 mg/dl) *(103)*. Of those with T2DM, 83% had a significant family history of diabetes compared with only 31% of those with normal glucose tolerance *(103)*. Also, those with DM were more obese, with average BMI of 41 versus 33.4 kg/m2 *(103)*. Levels of total and free testosterone were higher in both IGT (107 ng/dl, 35 pg/ml) and T2DM (115 ng/dl, 41 pg/ml) than in those with normal glucose tolerance (79 ng/dl, 24 pg/ml). So, obesity and degree of androgenemia, as well as genetics/family history all play a significant role in glucose tolerance *(103)*. In a small study of 27 adolescents with PCOS, both lean and obese, the rate of IGT was 30% and that of undiagnosed diabetes 3.7% *(102)*. Another study *(64)* demonstrated that the metabolic precursors of type 2 diabetes, severe insulin resistance, deficiency in first phase insulin secretion, and increased hepatic glucose production are present early in the course of PCOS in adolescents. These are important, but cross-sectional data. To study the incidence of IGT or diabetes, a subset of 25 nondiabetic women were followed. Although approximately two-thirds remained unchanged or improved, 10% worsened over an approximately 3-year follow-up time *(103)*. Therefore, periodic screening of adolescents with PCOS using OGTT is recommended to detect these abnormalities in glucose metabolism without unnecessary delay *(102,104)*. In fact, the progression from normal glucose tolerance to type 2 diabetes in high-risk adolescents with PCOS could be as fast as 5 years *(65)*.

5.2. Metabolic Syndrome

Insulin resistance is considered the culprit of the metabolic syndrome: central obesity, glucose intolerance, dyslipidemia, and hypertension *(105–108)*. The metabolic syndrome has been associated with development of type 2 diabetes and cardiovascular disease (CVD) *(109)*. As PCOS has been noted to be associated with insulin resistance both in adults (see above) and in adolescents *(64,102)*, it has also been found to be associated with metabolic syndrome. A few studies in adults *(110,111)* demonstrate that the prevalence of the metabolic syndrome in PCOS is double that of the general population. This finding persists even after controlling for obesity *(112)*. There is no consensus on diagnostic criteria for the metabolic syndrome in adolescents *(113)*. However, investigators have used variations of the adult criteria to assess the prevalence in youth. In a study of 49 adolescent girls with PCOS and 165 age- and ethnic-matched, but not weight- or BMI-matched NHANES control girls, the prevalence of metabolic syndrome as defined by two different sets of criteria *(114)* was 37 and 47%, respectively *(2)*. After allowances were made for BMI, girls with PCOS had a 4.5 times greater risk of having metabolic syndrome than the NHANES control girls *(2)*. The authors concluded that while adiposity could explain some of the increased risk to develop the metabolic syndrome, more of the variance was explained by hyper-androgenism, with odds increasing fourfold by each increasing quartile of unbound testosterone *(2)*. Clearly, more studies are needed both to clarify the best definition of metabolic syndrome in adolescents and to determine the etiology of the increased risk seen in adolescents with PCOS.

A recent study evaluating 368 PCOS women for metabolic syndrome found that approximately 33% of nondiabetic women with PCOS have metabolic syndrome in their thirties and forties *(3)*. This is more than fourfold higher than rates in 20 year olds, and twice that seen in 30 year olds per NHANES data *(108)*. Needless to say, the rate depends on criteria used to define both metabolic syndrome and the characteristics of the PCOS subjects *(3)*. For instance, a study of lean Czech women with PCOS determined the rate of metabolic syndrome (as defined by NCEP criteria) *(115)* to be similar to the control population at 1.6% *(116)*. However, if a modification is made to the definition of metabolic syndrome, such as substitution of BMI > 32 kg/m^2 for waist circumference >88 cm, the prevalence is 23% in PCOS *(111)*. Furthermore, PCOS women with BMI in the highest quartile have an approximate 14-fold increase in the metabolic syndrome than those in the lowest BMI quartile *(3)*. Fasting insulin levels were almost twice as high in PCOS women with the syndrome *(3)*. The authors emphasize that while treatment for insulin resistance in PCOS is important, the long-term effect on development of either the metabolic syndrome or type 2 diabetes remains unknown *(3)*. However, as the second main concern of the metabolic syndrome is increased risk of CVD, let us explore the association between PCOS and CVD.

5.3. CVD Risk and Outcomes

Whether or not the rate of cardiovascular events in PCOS is increased remains contro-versial *(117,118)*. Investigators began making observations of an association between PCOS and CVD risk factors such as insulin resistance *(13)*, hypertension, dyslipidemia, and upper body obesity as early as the 1980s *(119)*. Then, throughout the 1990s, some studies found increased cardiovascular risk in PCOS *(120–123)*. In fact, one study found a greater than sevenfold higher risk of myocardial infarction in women with PCOS *(124)*. On the other hand, one UK study with 30 year follow-up data on more than 700 women with PCOS demonstrated that there was no increased rate of cardiovas-cular death than what would be expected *(117)*. This is an important but contradictory finding and could be due to the definition of PCOS in Europe compared with the USA, where the presence of polycystic ovaries in USA is not a diagnostic criterion.

Adolescents with PCOS have a prevalence of hypertension of 27% compared with 1% of a control population *(2)*. They also demonstrate lack of diurnal blood pressure variation *(64)*. Many markers of vascular dysfunction have been documented in young adults with PCOS *(125–131)*. One study of coronary flow reserve found no difference in coronary flow reserve between lean, young women with and without PCOS *(132)*. However, this technique was validated in an older (average age of 53), high-risk population *(133)*. More sensitive markers, such as coronary artery calcification *(134)* and carotid intima-media thickness, have been found to be higher in PCOS than in controls *(127,129,135)*. Impairment in flow-mediated vasodilation was also observed in both obese *(136)* and lean *(129)* women with PCOS than in BMI-matched controls. Although this early marker has been shown to be useful in older subjects *(137)*, the predictive value in young patients with PCOS has yet to be determined.

5.4. Sleep Apnea

Obstructive sleep apnea (OSA) is characterized by multiple episodes of airway obstruction, either partial or complete, during sleep. Prevalence rates in women range from 0.6 to 5.5% in the general population *(138,139)*. The most significant risk factors are male gender and obesity *(140)*. More recent studies identified an association between OSA and insulin resistance *(138,141)*. The insulin resistance, obesity, and hyperandrogenemia of PCOS seemed to beg the question of prevalence of OSA in this population, and indeed, studies of PCOS women have determined the prevalence of OSA to range from 17 to 75% *(138,139,142,143)*. This wide range, likely due to methods used to determine presence of OSA, is nonetheless at least threefold higher than the control populations.

The characteristics of the relationship between OSA and PCOS remain controversial. Although one study found the apnea-hypopnea index (AHI) to closely correlate with testosterone levels *(139)*, many more point to the relationship between sleep disordered breathing and insulin resistance. Men *(144,145)* and women *(144)* with OSA are more insulin resistant than age- and BMI-matched controls. This fact and that treatment of OSA with CPAP improved insulin sensitivity in obese diabetics *(146)* seem to imply that OSA is the cause and insulin resistance is the effect. Indeed, sleep-disordered breathing scores positively correlate with fasting insulin levels *(138,143)* and hyper-insulinemic response to OGTT *(143)* in the PCOS population. This is similar to the associations found in other groups between sleep-disordered breathing and components of the metabolic syndrome: glucose intolerance, insulin resistance, diabetes, hypertension, and dyslipidemia *(141,147,148)*. While longitudinal studies are needed to more clearly define which is cause and which is effect, theories to support this relationship abound.

Different reasons for cause/effect relationship between sleep-disordered breathing and insulin resistance include increased sympathetic activity *(146,149)*, increased abdominal adiposity, inflammation *(145)*, and hypoxia *(144)*. Studies evaluating for sleep-disordered breathing at the time of PCOS diagnosis, as well as longitudinal studies evaluating the effect of treatment of sleep-disordered breathing with CPAP on insulin resistance in PCOS will help illuminate this intriguing topic further.

5.5. *Fatty Liver Disease*

Fatty liver disease (FLD), a diagnosis of exclusion, is the excess accumulation of adipocytes in the liver *(150)*. Clinically, this is detected as abnormal liver enzymes (transaminases) or abnormal imaging. The prevalence of FLD (defined as otherwise unexplained elevations of hepatic enzymes) in the general population is 4.6% *(151)*. Recent studies have linked FLD to insulin resistance *(152–155)*. Depending on the definition of elevated liver enzymes, prevalence rates of FLD based on this criteria in women with PCOS are 7–30% *(156–158)*. When ultrasound was used to evaluate for hepatic steatosis in those with elevated transaminases, 55% were affected *(157)*. Thirty-eight percent of women with PCOS had FLD using the NHANES criteria *(151)* of transaminases greater than 31 IU/l *(158)*. Thirty percent of women with PCOS had levels greater than 40 IU/l *(156,158)*, and 15% had liver enzymes greater than 60 IU/l *(158)*. However, some investigators are even suggesting that levels as low as 19 IU/l should be used, which would elevate the prevalence of FLD amongst those with PCOS even higher *(158)*. Even with the most conservative definition, the rate is still threefold higher than the general population and is both significant and concerning *(158)*.

When using imaging (16/29), 50–100% were determined to have hepatic steatosis *(157,158)*. During follow-up, 55% experienced resolution of their FLD either spontaneously or after treatment with therapeutic lifestyle, metformin, or gastric bypass surgery *(158)*. Those with FLD (21%) had a liver biopsy demonstrating steatohepatitis and fibrosis *(158)*. However, one subject normalized her aminotransferases and had documented improvement in the level of biopsy-proven steatosis and fibrosis after therapeutic lifestyle changes *(158)*.

Interestingly, the biochemical parameters of the metabolic syndrome were positive in the majority of these six women with documented hepatic fibrosis: five had triglycerides in excess of 150 mg/dl, all six had low HDL, and the two for whom OGTT data were available showed evidence of IGT *(158)*. In NHANES III subjects with triglycerides exceeding 200 mg/dl, the risk for FLD was three times higher than those with triglyceride levels 200 mg/dl and lower *(159)*, and almost twice as high in those with HDL lesser than 35mg/dl *(159)*.

FLD is not usually diagnosed until after the age of 40 *(160)*, but this study, with an average subject age of 29, demonstrated early onset of FLD and fibrosis in PCOS *(158)*. Early evaluation for FLD in patients with PCOS should be considered, especially in the existence of elevated triglycerides, depressed HDL, and insulin resistance *(158)*. Also, treatments geared toward increasing insulin sensitivity: therapeutic lifestyle changes, metformin, and gastric bypass, all led to improvements in liver transaminases, steatosis, and fibrosis *(158)*.

6. THERAPEUTIC APPROACHES TARGETING INSULIN SENSITIZATION

Because insulin resistance/hyperinsulinism plays an important role in the pathophysiology of PCOS, its clinical and metabolic manifestations and its co-morbidities, therapeutic strategies targeting insulin resistance have been promoted. There is sufficient evidence in adult women with PCOS to justify the use of insulin sensitizers for the management of short-term (fertility and hyperandrogenism) as well as long-term (type 2 diabetes, metabolic syndrome, and CVD) manifestations of the syndrome *(25,27)*.

The most commonly used and investigated insulin sensitizer is metformin. The majority of the randomized controlled trials support the usefulness of metformin in improving ovulation and pregnancy rate and outcome in women with PCOS *(25,27)*. Additional insulin sensitizers that have been tested and shown to be beneficial are pioglitazone, rosiglitazone, and troglitazone, the latter was banned by FDA for liver toxicity *(161–163)*. Although oral contraceptives are the traditional therapy for the treatment of PCOS and they may provide a more reliable control of menstrual irregularities, the concern has been the potential of OCPs to worsen insulin resistance and metabolic complications. This medical quandary will not resolve until there are convincing short- and long-term data regarding the beneficial versus adverse effects of OCPs versus insulin sensitizers *(164)*.

Data regarding the use of insulin sensitizers in adolescents with PCOS are limited. A 3-month open-label trial of metformin (850 mg twice daily) in obese adolescents with PCOS resulted in lowering of free testosterone by approximately 30% and total testosterone by approximately 45%, improvement in in vivo insulin sensitivity with lowering of fasting and stimulated insulin levels, and improvement in glucose tolerance with 57% reversal from IGT to NGT *(165)*. Equally important, however, was the observation that metformin therapy was associated with attenuation of adrenal steroidogenic hyper-responsiveness to ACTH (Fig. 4). In a randomized, placebo-controlled, double blind 12-week trial of obese adolescents with PCOS, metformin significantly lowered total testosterone, increased the likelihood of menses, and improved high-density lipoprotein cholesterol level *(166)*. Similar observations were reported by others in obese and

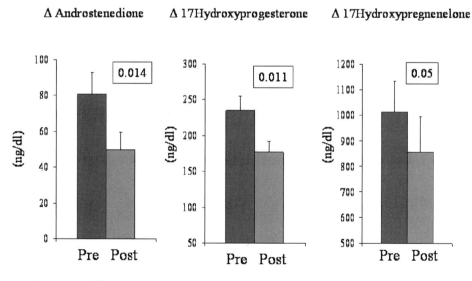

Fig. 4. Change in (Δ) hormone levels (30-min value minus 0-min value) in response to ACTH stimulation pre- and post-metformin treatment in adolescents with PCOS. Adapted with permission *(165)*. See insert for color figure.

nonobese adolescents *(167,168)*. Moreover, there is some suggestion, based on open label trials, that metformin at only 850 mg/day may prevent progression from precocious pubarche to PCOS in normal-weight adolescents at high risk for PCOS *(169)*. In these girls with precocious pubarche and low birth weight, prepubertal initiation of metformin at 425 mg/day appeared to improve hormonal, metabolic, and body composition parameters with no change in testosterone or HOMA insulin sensitivity *(170)*. On the other hand, post-pubertal discontinuation of metformin appears to worsen the hormonal and metabolic profile *(170)*. Even though such results may appear promising, there is an urgent need for carefully designed, double-blind placebo-controlled studies with uniform doses of metformin to provide convincing scientific data about the benefits of metformin in the pediatric age group.

7. CONCLUSION AND FUTURE DIRECTION

PCOS is a common disorder not only of premenopausal women but also of adolescent girls. Premature adrenarche caused by early activation of adrenal androgen production may be a precursor of PCOS during adolescence in some girls, especially those with obesity and insulin resistance/hyperinsulinemia. Hyperinsulinemia is believed to play a pathophysiologic role in stimulating ovarian and adrenal androgen biosynthesis. There is an overall clinical impression that adolescent PCOS is increasing. It is tempting to speculate that the epidemic of obesity afflicting the nation's children is the driving force *(171)*. Insulin resistance and hyperinsulinemia consequent to obesity may trigger or unmask the syndrome in genetically predisposed individuals. Heightened awareness of the condition is a must for the proper diagnosis and appropriate treatment.

Future research should focus on the natural history of hyperandrogenism/PCOS in the pediatric age group. Well-designed, prospective longitudinal cohorts must be studied to trace the childhood origin of PCOS, the early risk factors (physical, metabolic, genetic, and environmental), the co-morbidities associated with PCOS and to identify potential intervention, prevention, and therapeutic strategies that are effective and safe in the long run.

ACKNOWLEDGMENTS

This work was supported by United States Public Health Service grant RO1 HD27503 (SA), K24 HD01357 (SA), MO1-RR00084 General Clinical Research Center, Renziehausen Trust Fund (SA), Bristol Myers-Squibb (SA), Eli-Lilly and Company (SA), and the Endocrine Fellows Foundation (JW-U).

REFERENCES

1. Arslanian S, Witchel SF. Polycystic ovary syndrome in adolescents: is there an epidemic? *Curr Opin Endocrinol Diabetes* 2002;9:32–42.
2. Coviello AD, Legro RS, Dunaif A. Adolescent girls with polycystic ovary syndrome have an increased risk of the metabolic syndrome associated with increasing androgen levels independent of obesity and insulin resistance. *J Clin Endocrinol Metab* 2006;91:492–7.
3. Ehrmann DA, Liljenquist DR, Kasza K, Azziz R, Legro RS, Ghazzi MN. Prevalence and predictors of the metabolic syndrome in women with polycystic ovary syndrome. *J Clin Endocrinol Metab* 2006;91:48–53.

4. Yalow RS, Berson SA. Immunoassay of endogenous plasma insulin in man. *J Clin Invest* 1960;39:1157–75.

5. Arslanian SA. Clamp techniques in paediatrics: what have we learned? *Horm Res* 2005;64 Suppl 3:16–24.

6. Book CB, Dunaif A. Selective insulin resistance in the polycystic ovary syndrome. *J Clin Endocrinol Metab* 1999;84:3110–6.

7. Corbould A, Zhao H, Mirzoeva S, Aird F, Dunaif A. Enhanced mitogenic signaling in skeletal muscle of women with polycystic ovary syndrome. *Diabetes* 2006;55:751–9.

8. Dunaif A. Insulin resistance and the polycystic ovary syndrome: mechanism and implications for pathogenesis. *Endocr Rev* 1997;18:774–800.

9. Wu XK, Zhou SY, Liu JX, et al. Selective ovary resistance to insulin signaling in women with polycystic ovary syndrome. *Fertil Steril* 2003;80:954–65.

10. Arslanian SA, Saad R, F. B. *Insulin Resistance in Youth: Definition and Methods of Measurement*. Nova Science Publishers, Inc. Hauppauge, NY. In: Insulin Resistance children anol Adolescence. Editors: D. Daneman and J. Hamilton pp. 31–56. 2005.

11. Consensus Development Conference on Insulin Resistance. 5–6 November 1997. American Diabetes Association. *Diabetes Care* 1998;21:310–4.

12. Archard M, Thiers M. LeVirilisme Plaire et son association a L'insuffisance glyolytique (diabetes des femmes à barbe). *Bull Acad Natl Med* 1921;86:51–64.

13. Burghen GA, Givens JR, Kitabchi AE. Correlation of hyperandrogenism with hyperinsulinism in polycystic ovarian disease. *J Clin Endocrinol Metab* 1980;50:113–6.

14. De Leo V, la Marca A, Petraglia F. Insulin-lowering agents in the management of polycystic ovary syndrome. *Endocr Rev* 2003;24:633–67.

15. Dunaif A, Segal KR, Futterweit W, Dobrjansky A. Profound peripheral insulin resistance, independent of obesity, in polycystic ovary syndrome. *Diabetes* 1989;38:1165–74.

16. Legro RS, Finegood D, Dunaif A. A fasting glucose to insulin ratio is a useful measure of insulin sensitivity in women with polycystic ovary syndrome. *J Clin Endocrinol Metab* 1998;83:2694–8.

17. Norman RJ, Masters S, Hague W. Hyperinsulinemia is common in family members of women with polycystic ovary syndrome. *Fertil Steril* 1996;66:942–7.

18. Colilla S, Cox NJ, Ehrmann DA. Heritability of insulin secretion and insulin action in women with polycystic ovary syndrome and their first degree relatives. *J Clin Endocrinol Metab* 2001;86: 2027–31.

19. Yildiz BO, Yarali H, Oguz H, Bayraktar M. Glucose intolerance, insulin resistance, and hyperandrogenemia in first degree relatives of women with polycystic ovary syndrome. *J Clin Endocrinol Metab* 2003;88:2031–6.

20. Nagamani M, Van Dinh T, Kelver ME. Hyperinsulinemia in hyperthecosis of the ovaries. *Am J Obstet Gynecol* 1986;154:384–9.

21. Geffner ME, Kaplan SA, Bersch N, Golde DW, Landaw EM, Chang RJ. Persistence of insulin resistance in polycystic ovarian disease after inhibition of ovarian steroid secretion. *Fertil Steril* 1986;45:327–33.

22. Pasquali R, Fabbri R, Venturoli S, Paradisi R, Antenucci D, Melchionda N. Effect of weight loss and antiandrogenic therapy on sex hormone blood levels and insulin resistance in obese patients with polycystic ovaries. *Am J Obstet Gynecol* 1986;154:139–44.

23. Nestler JE. Insulin regulation of human ovarian androgens. *Hum Reprod* 1997;12 Suppl 1:53–62.

24. Nestler JE. Role of hyperinsulinemia in the pathogenesis of the polycystic ovary syndrome, and its clinical implications. *Semin Reprod Endocrinol* 1997;15:111–22.

25. Teede HJ, Meyer C, Norman RJ. Insulin-sensitisers in the treatment of polycystic ovary syndrome. *Expert Opin Pharmacother* 2005;6:2419–27.

26. Utiger RD. Insulin and the polycystic ovary syndrome. *N Engl J Med* 1996;335:657–8.

27. Baillargeon JP. Use of insulin sensitizers in polycystic ovarian syndrome. *Curr Opin Investig Drugs* 2005;6:1012–22.

28. Dunaif A, Scott D, Finegood D, Quintana B, Whitcomb R. The insulin-sensitizing agent troglitazone improves metabolic and reproductive abnormalities in the polycystic ovary syndrome. *J Clin Endocrinol Metab* 1996;81:3299–306.

29. Kiddy DS, Hamilton-Fairley D, Bush A, et al. Improvement in endocrine and ovarian function during dietary treatment of obese women with polycystic ovary syndrome. *Clin Endocrinol (Oxf)* 1992;36:105 11.

30. Nestler JE, Barlascini CO, Matt DW, et al. Suppression of serum insulin by diazoxide reduces serum testosterone levels in obese women with polycystic ovary syndrome. *J Clin Endocrinol Metab* 1989;68:1027–32.

31. Nestler JE, Jakubowicz DJ. Decreases in ovarian cytochrome P450c17 alpha activity and serum free testosterone after reduction of insulin secretion in polycystic ovary syndrome. *N Engl J Med* 1996;335:617–23.

32. Nestler JE, Jakubowicz DJ, Evans WS, Pasquali R. Effects of metformin on spontaneous and clomiphene-induced ovulation in the polycystic ovary syndrome. *N Engl J Med* 1998;338:1876–80.

33. Pasquali R, Gambineri A, Biscotti D, et al. Effect of long-term treatment with metformin added to hypocaloric diet on body composition, fat distribution, and androgen and insulin levels in abdominally obese women with and without the polycystic ovary syndrome. *J Clin Endocrinol Metab* 2000;85:2767–74.

34. Yilmaz M, Biri A, Karakoc A, et al. The effects of rosiglitazone and metformin on insulin resistance and serum androgen levels in obese and lean patients with polycystic ovary syndrome. *J Endocrinol Invest* 2005;28:1003–8.

35. Baillargeon JP, Diamanti-Kandarakis E, Ostlund RE, Jr., Apridonidze T, Iuorno MJ, Nestler JE. Altered D-chiro-inositol urinary clearance in women with polycystic ovary syndrome. *Diabetes Care* 2006;29:300–5.

36. Gerli S, Mignosa M, Di Renzo GC. Effects of inositol on ovarian function and metabolic factors in women with PCOS: a randomized double blind placebo-controlled trial. *Eur Rev Med Pharmacol Sci* 2003;7:151–9.

37. Nestler JE, Jakubowicz DJ, Reamer P, Gunn RD, Allan G. Ovulatory and metabolic effects of D-chiro-inositol in the polycystic ovary syndrome. *N Engl J Med* 1999;340:1314–20.

38. Oberfield SE. Metabolic lessons from the study of young adolescents with polycystic ovary syndrome–is insulin, indeed, the culprit? *J Clin Endocrinol Metab* 2000;85:3520–5.

39. Rosenfield RL, Barnes RB, Cara JF, Lucky AW. Dysregulation of cytochrome P450c 17 alpha as the cause of polycystic ovarian syndrome. *Fertil Steril* 1990;53:785–91.

40. Baillargeon JP, Nestler JE. Commentary: polycystic ovary syndrome: a syndrome of ovarian hypersensitivity to insulin? *J Clin Endocrinol Metab* 2006;91:22–4.

41. Yen SS. The polycystic ovary syndrome. *Clin Endocrinol (Oxf)* 1980;12:177–207.

42. Stein I, Leventhal M. Amenorrhea associated with bilateral polycystic ovaries. *Am J Obstet Gynecol* 1935;29:181–91.

43. Nobels F, Dewailly D. Puberty and polycystic ovarian syndrome: the insulin/insulin-like growth factor I hypothesis. *Fertil Steril* 1992;58:655–66.

44. Apter D, Butzow T, Laughlin GA, Yen SS. Metabolic features of polycystic ovary syndrome are found in adolescent girls with hyperandrogenism. *J Clin Endocrinol Metab* 1995;80:2966–73.

45. Ibanez L, Potau N, Georgopoulos N, Prat N, Gussinye M, Carrascosa A. Growth hormone, insulin-like growth factor-I axis, and insulin secretion in hyperandrogenic adolescents. *Fertil Steril* 1995;64:1113–9.

46. Arslanian S. Type 2 diabetes in children: clinical aspects and risk factors. *Horm Res* 2002;57 Suppl 1:19–28.

47. Ibanez L, Dimartino-Nardi J, Potau N, Saenger P. Premature adrenarche–normal variant or forerunner of adult disease? *Endocr Rev* 2000;21:671–96.

48. Oppenheimer E, Linder B, DiMartino-Nardi J. Decreased insulin sensitivity in prepubertal girls with premature adrenarche and acanthosis nigricans. *J Clin Endocrinol Metab* 1995;80:614–8.

49. Vuguin P, Linder B, Rosenfeld RG, Saenger P, DiMartino-Nardi J. The roles of insulin sensitivity, insulin-like growth factor I (IGF-I), and IGF-binding protein-1 and -3 in the hyperandrogenism of African-American and Caribbean Hispanic girls with premature adrenarche. *J Clin Endocrinol Metab* 1999;84:2037–42.

50. Ibanez L, Potau N, Zampolli M, Rique S, Saenger P, Carrascosa A. Hyperinsulinemia and decreased insulin-like growth factor-binding protein-1 are common features in prepubertal and pubertal girls with a history of premature pubarche. *J Clin Endocrinol Metab* 1997;82:2283–8.

51. Mauras N, Welch S, Rini A, Haymond MW. Ovarian hyperandrogenism is associated with insulin resistance to both peripheral carbohydrate and whole-body protein metabolism in postpubertal young females: a metabolic study. *J Clin Endocrinol Metab* 1998;83:1900–5.

52. Ibanez L, Potau N, Zampolli M, et al. Hyperinsulinemia in postpubertal girls with a history of premature pubarche and functional ovarian hyperandrogenism. *J Clin Endocrinol Metab* 1996;81:1237–43.

53. Silfen ME, Denburg MR, Manibo AM, et al. Early endocrine, metabolic, and sonographic characteristics of polycystic ovary syndrome (PCOS): comparison between nonobese and obese adolescents. *J Clin Endocrinol Metab* 2003;88:4682–8.

54. Fernandes AR, de Sa Rosa e Silva AC, Romao GS, Pata MC, dos Reis RM. Insulin resistance in adolescents with menstrual irregularities. *J Pediatr Adolesc Gynecol* 2005;18:269–74.

55. Lewy VD, Danadian K, Witchel SF, Arslanian S. Early metabolic abnormalities in adolescent girls with polycystic ovarian syndrome. *J Pediatr* 2001;138:38–44.

56. Kahn SE, Prigeon RL, McCulloch DK, et al. Quantification of the relationship between insulin sensitivity and beta-cell function in human subjects. Evidence for a hyperbolic function. *Diabetes* 1993;42:1663–72.

57. Kahn SE. Clinical review 135: The importance of beta-cell failure in the development and progression of type 2 diabetes. *J Clin Endocrinol Metab* 2001;86:4047–58.

58. Legro RS, Chiu P, Kunselman AR, Bentley CM, Dodson WC, Dunaif A. Polycystic ovaries are common in women with hyperandrogenic chronic anovulation but do not predict metabolic or reproductive phenotype. *J Clin Endocrinol Metab* 2005;90:2571–9.

59. Ehrmann DA, Kasza K, Azziz R, Legro RS, Ghazzi MN. Effects of race and family history of type 2 diabetes on metabolic status of women with polycystic ovary syndrome. *J Clin Endocrinol Metab* 2005;90:66–71.

60. Gambineri A, Pelusi C, Manicardi E, et al. Glucose intolerance in a large cohort of mediterranean women with polycystic ovary syndrome: phenotype and associated factors. *Diabetes* 2004;53:2353–8.

61. Lin TC, Yen JM, Gong KB, et al. Abnormal glucose tolerance and insulin resistance in polycystic ovary syndrome amongst the Taiwanese population- not correlated with insulin receptor substrate-1 Gly972Arg/Ala513Pro polymorphism. *BMC Med Genet* 2006;7:36.

62. Ehrmann DA, Sturis J, Byrne MM, Karrison T, Rosenfield RL, Polonsky KS. Insulin secretory defects in polycystic ovary syndrome. Relationship to insulin sensitivity and family history of non-insulin-dependent diabetes mellitus. *J Clin Invest* 1995;96:520–7.

63. Dunaif A, Finegood DT. Beta-cell dysfunction independent of obesity and glucose intolerance in the polycystic ovary syndrome. *J Clin Endocrinol Metab* 1996;81:942–7.

64. Arslanian SA, Lewy VD, Danadian K. Glucose intolerance in obese adolescents with polycystic ovary syndrome: roles of insulin resistance and beta-cell dysfunction and risk of cardiovascular disease. *J Clin Endocrinol Metab* 2001;86:66–71.

65. Saad R, Gungor N, Arslanian S. Progression from normal glucose tolerance to type 2 diabetes in a young girl: longitudinal changes in insulin sensitivity and secretion assessed by the clamp technique and surrogate estimates. *Pediatr Diabetes* 2005;6:95–9.

66. Legro RS, Kunselman AR, Dodson WC, Dunaif A. Prevalence and predictors of risk for type 2 diabetes mellitus and impaired glucose tolerance in polycystic ovary syndrome: a prospective, controlled study in 254 affected women. *J Clin Endocrinol Metab* 1999;84:165–9.

67. Dunaif A, Xia J, Book CB, Schenker E, Tang Z. Excessive insulin receptor serine phosphorylation in cultured fibroblasts and in skeletal muscle. A potential mechanism for insulin resistance in the polycystic ovary syndrome. *J Clin Invest* 1995;96:801–10.

68. Li M, Youngren JF, Dunaif A, et al. Decreased insulin receptor (IR) autophosphorylation in fibroblasts from patients with PCOS: effects of serine kinase inhibitors and IR activators. *J Clin Endocrinol Metab* 2002;87:4088–93.

69. Willis D, Mason H, Gilling-Smith C, Franks S. Modulation by insulin of follicle-stimulating hormone and luteinizing hormone actions in human granulosa cells of normal and polycystic ovaries. *J Clin Endocrinol Metab* 1996;81:302–9.

70. Dunaif A. Insulin resistance and ovarian hyperandrogenism. *Endocrinologist* 1992;2:248–60.

71. Dunaif A, Givens J, Haseltine F, Merriam Ge. *The Polycystic Ovary Syndrome*. Cambridge, MA: Blackwell Scientific; 1992.

72. Nestler JE, Strauss JF, 3rd. Insulin as an effector of human ovarian and adrenal steroid metabolism. *Endocrinol Metab Clin North Am* 1991;20:807–23.

73. Poretsky L, Cataldo NA, Rosenwaks Z, Giudice LC. The insulin-related ovarian regulatory system in health and disease. *Endocr Rev* 1999;20:535–82.

74. Nestler JE, Jakubowicz DJ, de Vargas AF, Brik C, Quintero N, Medina F. Insulin stimulates testosterone biosynthesis by human thecal cells from women with polycystic ovary syndrome by activating its own receptor and using inositolglycan mediators as the signal transduction system. *J Clin Endocrinol Metab* 1998;83:2001–5.

75. Nelson VL, Legro RS, Strauss JF, 3rd, McAllister JM. Augmented androgen production is a stable steroidogenic phenotype of propagated theca cells from polycystic ovaries. *Mol Endocrinol* 1999;13:946–57.

76. Willis D, Franks S. Insulin action in human granulosa cells from normal and polycystic ovaries is mediated by the insulin receptor and not the type-I insulin-like growth factor receptor. *J Clin Endocrinol Metab* 1995;80:3788–90.

77. Moran C, Huerta R, Conway-Myers BA, Hines GA, Azziz R. Altered autophosphorylation of the insulin receptor in the ovary of a woman with polycystic ovary syndrome. *Fertil Steril* 2001;75:625–8.

78. Nestler JE, Singh R, Matt DW, Clore JN, Blackard WG. Suppression of serum insulin level by diazoxide does not alter serum testosterone or sex hormone-binding globulin levels in healthy, nonobese women. *Am J Obstet Gynecol* 1990;163:1243–6.

79. Sekar N, Lavoie HA, Veldhuis JD. Concerted regulation of steroidogenic acute regulatory gene expression by luteinizing hormone and insulin (or insulin-like growth factor I) in primary cultures of porcine granulosa-luteal cells. *Endocrinology* 2000;141:3983–92.

80. Zhang G, Garmey JC, Veldhuis JD. Interactive stimulation by luteinizing hormone and insulin of the steroidogenic acute regulatory (StAR) protein and 17alpha-hydroxylase/17,20-lyase (CYP17) genes in porcine theca cells. *Endocrinology* 2000;141:2735–42.

81. Fedorcsak P, Storeng R, Dale PO, Tanbo T, Abyholm T. Impaired insulin action on granulosa-lutein cells in women with polycystic ovary syndrome and insulin resistance. *Gynecol Endocrinol* 2000;14:327–36.

82. Rice S, Christoforidis N, Gadd C, et al. Impaired insulin-dependent glucose metabolism in granulosa-lutein cells from anovulatory women with polycystic ovaries. *Hum Reprod* 2005;20:373–81.

83. Nelson-Degrave VL, Wickenheisser JK, Hendricks KL, et al. Alterations in mitogen-activated protein kinase and extracellular regulated kinase signaling in theca cells contribute to excessive androgen production in polycystic ovary syndrome. *Mol Endocrinol* 2005;19:379–90.

84. Corbould A, Kim YB, Youngren JF, et al. Insulin resistance in the skeletal muscle of women with PCOS involves intrinsic and acquired defects in insulin signaling. *Am J Physiol Endocrinol Metab* 2005;288:E1047–54.

85. Dunaif A, Segal KR, Shelley DR, Green G, Dobrjansky A, Licholai T. Evidence for distinctive and intrinsic defects in insulin action in polycystic ovary syndrome. *Diabetes* 1992;41:1257–66.

86. Carlson CJ, Koterski S, Sciotti RJ, Poccard GB, Rondinone CM. Enhanced basal activation of mitogen-activated protein kinases in adipocytes from type 2 diabetes: potential role of p38 in the downregulation of GLUT4 expression. *Diabetes* 2003;52:634–41.

87. Bouzakri K, Roques M, Gual P, et al. Reduced activation of phosphatidylinositol-3 kinase and increased serine 636 phosphorylation of insulin receptor substrate-1 in primary culture of skeletal muscle cells from patients with type 2 diabetes. *Diabetes* 2003;52:1319–25.

88. Scherrer U, Randin D, Vollenweider P, Vollenweider L, Nicod P. Nitric oxide release accounts for insulin's vascular effects in humans. *J Clin Invest* 1994;94:2511–5.

89. Steinberg HO, Brechtel G, Johnson A, Fineberg N, Baron AD. Insulin-mediated skeletal muscle vasodilation is nitric oxide dependent. A novel action of insulin to increase nitric oxide release. *J Clin Invest* 1994;94:1172–9.

90. Steinberg HO, Chaker H, Leaming R, Johnson A, Brechtel G, Baron AD. Obesity/insulin resistance is associated with endothelial dysfunction. Implications for the syndrome of insulin resistance. *J Clin Invest* 1996;97:2601–10.

91. Montagnani M, Golovchenko I, Kim I, et al. Inhibition of phosphatidylinositol 3-kinase enhances mitogenic actions of insulin in endothelial cells. *J Biol Chem* 2002;277:1794–9.

92. Robinson S, Henderson AD, Gelding SV, et al. Dyslipidaemia is associated with insulin resistance in women with polycystic ovaries. *Clin Endocrinol (Oxf)* 1996;44:277–84.

93. Ciaraldi TP, el-Roeiy A, Madar Z, Reichart D, Olefsky JM, Yen SS. Cellular mechanisms of insulin resistance in polycystic ovarian syndrome. *J Clin Endocrinol Metab* 1992;75:577–83.

94. Marsden PJ, Murdoch A, Taylor R. Severe impairment of insulin action in adipocytes from amenorrheic subjects with polycystic ovary syndrome. *Metabolism* 1994;43:1536–42.

95. Lystedt E, Westergren H, Brynhildsen J, et al. Subcutaneous adipocytes from obese hyperinsulinemic women with polycystic ovary syndrome exhibit normal insulin sensitivity but reduced maximal insulin responsiveness. *Eur J Endocrinol* 2005;153:831–5.

96. Ciaraldi TP, Morales AJ, Hickman MG, Odom-Ford R, Olefsky JM, Yen SS. Cellular insulin resistance in adipocytes from obese polycystic ovary syndrome subjects involves adenosine modulation of insulin sensitivity. *J Clin Endocrinol Metab* 1997;82:1421–5.

97. Ek I, Arner P, Bergqvist A, Carlstrom K, Wahrenberg H. Impaired adipocyte lipolysis in nonobese women with the polycystic ovary syndrome: a possible link to insulin resistance? *J Clin Endocrinol Metab* 1997;82:1147–53.

98. Ek I, Arner P, Ryden M, et al. A unique defect in the regulation of visceral fat cell lipolysis in the polycystic ovary syndrome as an early link to insulin resistance. *Diabetes* 2002;51:484–92.

99. Wahrenberg H, Ek I, Reynisdottir S, Carlstrom K, Bergqvist A, Arner P. Divergent effects of weight reduction and oral anticonception treatment on adrenergic lipolysis regulation in obese women with the polycystic ovary syndrome. *J Clin Endocrinol Metab* 1999;84:2182–7.

100. Ibanez L, Ong K, de Zegher F, Marcos MV, del Rio L, Dunger DB. Fat distribution in non-obese girls with and without precocious pubarche: central adiposity related to insulinaemia and androgenaemia from prepuberty to postmenarche. *Clin Endocrinol (Oxf)* 2003;58:372–9.

101. Legro RS. Detection of insulin resistance and its treatment in adolescents with polycystic ovary syndrome. *J Pediatr Endocrinol Metab* 2002;15 Suppl 5:1367–78.

102. Palmert MR, Gordon CM, Kartashov AI, Legro RS, Emans SJ, Dunaif A. Screening for abnormal glucose tolerance in adolescents with polycystic ovary syndrome. *J Clin Endocrinol Metab* 2002;87:1017–23.

103. Ehrmann DA, Barnes RB, Rosenfield RL, Cavaghan MK, Imperial J. Prevalence of impaired glucose tolerance and diabetes in women with polycystic ovary syndrome. *Diabetes Care* 1999;22:141–6.

104. Kent SC, Legro RS. Polycystic ovary syndrome in adolescents. *Adolesc Med* 2002;13:73–88, vi.

105. Hedley AA, Ogden CL, Johnson CL, Carroll MD, Curtin LR, Flegal KM. Prevalence of overweight and obesity among US children, adolescents, and adults, 1999–2002. *JAMA* 2004;291:2847–50.

106. Reaven GM, Lithell H, Landsberg L. Hypertension and associated metabolic abnormalities–the role of insulin resistance and the sympathoadrenal system. *N Engl J Med* 1996;334:374–81.

107. Grundy SM. Hypertriglyceridemia, insulin resistance, and the metabolic syndrome. *Am J Cardiol* 1999;83:25F–9F.

108. Ford ES, Giles WH, Dietz WH. Prevalence of the metabolic syndrome among US adults: findings from the third National Health and Nutrition Examination Survey. *JAMA* 2002;287:356–9.

109. Goodarzi MO, Korenman SG. The importance of insulin resistance in polycystic ovary syndrome. *Fertil Steril* 2003;80:255–8.

110. Glueck CJ, Papanna R, Wang P, Goldenberg N, Sieve-Smith L. Incidence and treatment of metabolic syndrome in newly referred women with confirmed polycystic ovarian syndrome. *Metabolism* 2003;52:908–15.

111. Apridonidze T, Essah PA, Iuorno MJ, Nestler JE. Prevalence and characteristics of the metabolic syndrome in women with polycystic ovary syndrome. *J Clin Endocrinol Metab* 2005;90:1929–35.

112. Sam S, Legro RS, Bentley-Lewis R, Dunaif A. Dyslipidemia and metabolic syndrome in the sisters of women with polycystic ovary syndrome. *J Clin Endocrinol Metab* 2005;90:4797–802.

113. Goodman E, Daniels SR, Morrison JA, Huang B, Dolan LM. Contrasting prevalence of and demographic disparities in the World Health Organization and National Cholesterol Education Program Adult Treatment Panel III definitions of metabolic syndrome among adolescents. *J Pediatr* 2004;145:445–51.

114. Cook S, Weitzman M, Auinger P, Nguyen M, Dietz WH. Prevalence of a metabolic syndrome phenotype in adolescents: findings from the third National Health and Nutrition Examination Survey, 1988–1994. *Arch Pediatr Adolesc Med* 2003;157:821–7.

115. National Cholesterol Education Program (NCEP) Expert Panel on Detection, Evaluation, and Treatment of High Blood Cholesterol in Adults (Adult Treatment Panel III). Third report of the National Cholesterol Education Program (NCEP) expert panel on detection, evaluation, and treatment of high blood cholesterol in adults (Adult Treatment Panel III) final report. *Circulation* 2002;106: 3143–421.

116. Vrbikova J, Vondra K, Cibula D, et al. Metabolic syndrome in young Czech women with polycystic ovary syndrome. *Hum Reprod* 2005;20:3328–32.

117. Pierpoint T, McKeigue PM, Isaacs AJ, Wild SH, Jacobs HS. Mortality of women with polycystic ovary syndrome at long-term follow-up. *J Clin Epidemiol* 1998;51:581–6.

118. Wild S, Pierpoint T, McKeigue P, Jacobs H. Cardiovascular disease in women with polycystic ovary syndrome at long-term follow-up: a retrospective cohort study. *Clin Endocrinol (Oxf)* 2000;52: 595–600.

119. Wild RA, Painter PC, Coulson PB, Carruth KB, Ranney GB. Lipoprotein lipid concentrations and cardiovascular risk in women with polycystic ovary syndrome. *J Clin Endocrinol Metab* 1985;61: 946–51.

120. Talbott E, Guzick D, Clerici A, et al. Coronary heart disease risk factors in women with polycystic ovary syndrome. *Arterioscler Thromb Vasc Biol* 1995;15:821–6.

121. Talbott E, Clerici A, Berga SL, et al. Adverse lipid and coronary heart disease risk profiles in young women with polycystic ovary syndrome: results of a case-control study. *J Clin Epidemiol* 1998;51:415–22.

122. Pasquali R, Casimirri F, Cantobelli S, et al. Insulin and androgen relationships with abdominal body fat distribution in women with and without hyperandrogenism. *Horm Res* 1993;39:179–87.

123. Conway GS, Agrawal R, Betteridge DJ, Jacobs HS. Risk factors for coronary artery disease in lean and obese women with the polycystic ovary syndrome. *Clin Endocrinol (Oxf)* 1992;37:119–25.

124. Dahlgren E, Janson PO, Johansson S, Lapidus L, Oden A. Polycystic ovary syndrome and risk for myocardial infarction. Evaluated from a risk factor model based on a prospective population study of women. *Acta Obstet Gynecol Scand* 1992;71:599–604.

125. Tarkun I, Arslan BC, Canturk Z, Turemen E, Sahin T, Duman C. Endothelial dysfunction in young women with polycystic ovary syndrome: relationship with insulin resistance and low-grade chronic inflammation. *J Clin Endocrinol Metab* 2004;89:5592–6.

126. Diamanti-Kandarakis E, Spina G, Kouli C, Migdalis I. Increased endothelin-1 levels in women with polycystic ovary syndrome and the beneficial effect of metformin therapy. *J Clin Endocrinol Metab* 2001;86:4666–73.

127. Lakhani K, Hardiman P, Seifalian AM. Intima-media thickness of elastic and muscular arteries of young women with polycystic ovaries. *Atherosclerosis* 2004;175:353–9.

128. Meyer C, McGrath BP, Cameron J, Kotsopoulos D, Teede HJ. Vascular dysfunction and metabolic parameters in polycystic ovary syndrome. *J Clin Endocrinol Metab* 2005;90:4630–5.

129. Orio F, Jr., Palomba S, Cascella T, et al. Early impairment of endothelial structure and function in young normal-weight women with polycystic ovary syndrome. *J Clin Endocrinol Metab* 2004;89:4588–93.

130. Tarkun I, Canturk Z, Arslan BC, Turemen E, Tarkun P. The plasminogen activator system in young and lean women with polycystic ovary syndrome. *Endocr J* 2004;51:467–72.

131. Vryonidou A, Papatheodorou A, Tavridou A, et al. Association of hyperandrogenemic and metabolic phenotype with carotid intima-media thickness in young women with polycystic ovary syndrome. *J Clin Endocrinol Metab* 2005;90:2740–6.

132. Topcu S, Caliskan M, Ozcimen EE, et al. Do young women with polycystic ovary syndrome show early evidence of preclinical coronary artery disease? *Hum Reprod* 2006;21:930–5.

133. Britten MB, Zeiher AM, Schachinger V. Microvascular dysfunction in angiographically normal or mildly diseased coronary arteries predicts adverse cardiovascular long-term outcome. *Coron Artery Dis* 2004;15:259–64.

134. Christian RC, Dumesic DA, Behrenbeck T, Oberg AL, Sheedy PF, 2nd, Fitzpatrick LA. Prevalence and predictors of coronary artery calcification in women with polycystic ovary syndrome. *J Clin Endocrinol Metab* 2003;88:2562–8.

135. Talbott EO, Guzick DS, Sutton-Tyrrell K, et al. Evidence for association between polycystic ovary syndrome and premature carotid atherosclerosis in middle-aged women. *Arterioscler Thromb Vasc Biol* 2000;20:2414–21.

136. Paradisi G, Steinberg HO, Hempfling A, et al. Polycystic ovary syndrome is associated with endothelial dysfunction. *Circulation* 2001;103:1410–5.

137. O'Leary DH, Polak JF, Kronmal RA, Manolio TA, Burke GL, Wolfson SK, Jr. Carotid-artery intima and media thickness as a risk factor for myocardial infarction and stroke in older adults. Cardiovascular Health Study Collaborative Research Group. *N Engl J Med* 1999;340:14–22.

138. Vgontzas AN, Legro RS, Bixler EO, Grayev A, Kales A, Chrousos GP. Polycystic ovary syndrome is associated with obstructive sleep apnea and daytime sleepiness: role of insulin resistance. *J Clin Endocrinol Metab* 2001;86:517–20.

139. Fogel RB, Malhotra A, Pillar G, Pittman SD, Dunaif A, White DP. Increased prevalence of obstructive sleep apnea syndrome in obese women with polycystic ovary syndrome. *J Clin Endocrinol Metab* 2001;86:1175–80.

140. Sanders M. *Sleep Breathing Disorders.* Philadelphia, PA: W.B Saunders Company; 2000.

141. Ip MS, Lam B, Ng MM, Lam WK, Tsang KW, Lam KS. Obstructive sleep apnea is independently associated with insulin resistance. *Am J Respir Crit Care Med* 2002;165:670–6.

142. Gopal M, Duntley S, Uhles M, Attarian H. The role of obesity in the increased prevalence of obstructive sleep apnea syndrome in patients with polycystic ovarian syndrome. *Sleep Med* 2002;3:401–4.

143. Tasali E, Van Cauter E, Ehrmann DA. Relationships between sleep disordered breathing and glucose metabolism in polycystic ovary syndrome. *J Clin Endocrinol Metab* 2006;91:36–42.

144. Tassone F, Lanfranco F, Gianotti L, et al. Obstructive sleep apnoea syndrome impairs insulin sensitivity independently of anthropometric variables. *Clin Endocrinol (Oxf)* 2003;59:374–9.

145. Vgontzas AN, Papanicolaou DA, Bixler EO, et al. Sleep apnea and daytime sleepiness and fatigue: relation to visceral obesity, insulin resistance, and hypercytokinemia. *J Clin Endocrinol Metab* 2000;85:1151–8.

146. Harsch IA, Schahin SP, Bruckner K, et al. The effect of continuous positive airway pressure treatment on insulin sensitivity in patients with obstructive sleep apnoea syndrome and type 2 diabetes. *Respiration* 2004;71:252–9.

147. Punjabi NM, Shahar E, Redline S, Gottlieb DJ, Givelber R, Resnick HE. Sleep-disordered breathing, glucose intolerance, and insulin resistance: the Sleep Heart Health Study. *Am J Epidemiol* 2004;160:521–30.

148. Svatikova A, Wolk R, Gami AS, Pohanka M, Somers VK. Interactions between obstructive sleep apnea and the metabolic syndrome. *Curr Diab Rep* 2005;5:53–8.

149. Somers VK, Dyken ME, Clary MP, Abboud FM. Sympathetic neural mechanisms in obstructive sleep apnea. *J Clin Invest* 1995;96:1897–904.

150. Clark JM, Brancati FL, Diehl AM. The prevalence and etiology of elevated aminotransferase levels in the United States. *Am J Gastroenterol* 2003;98:960–7.

151. Clark JM, Brancati FL, Diehl AM. The prevalence and etiology of elevated aminotransferase levels in the United States. *Am Journ Gastro* 2003;98:960.

152. Pagano G, Pacini G, Musso G, et al. Nonalcoholic steatohepatitis, insulin resistance, and metabolic syndrome: further evidence for an etiologic association. *Hepatology* 2002;35:367–72.

153. Marchesini G, Brizi M, Bianchi G, et al. Nonalcoholic fatty liver disease: a feature of the metabolic syndrome. *Diabetes* 2001;50:1844–50.

154. Chitturi S, Abeygunasekera S, Farrell GC, et al. NASH and insulin resistance: insulin hypersecretion and specific association with the insulin resistance syndrome. *Hepatology* 2002;35:373–9.

155. Bugianesi E, Manzini P, D'Antico S, et al. Relative contribution of iron burden, HFE mutations, and insulin resistance to fibrosis in nonalcoholic fatty liver. *Hepatology* 2004;39:179–87.

156. Schwimmer JB, Khorram O, Chiu V, Schwimmer WB. Abnormal aminotransferase activity in women with polycystic ovary syndrome. *Fertil Steril* 2005;83:494–7.

157. Kinkhabwala S, Futterweit W. *Nonalcoholic Fatty Liver Disease in Lean, Overweight, and Obese Women with Polycystic Ovary Syndrome.* Poster presentation at 3rd Annual Meeting of the Androgen Excess Society in San Diego, CA (Abstract) 2005.

158. Setji TL, Holland ND, Sanders LL, Pereira KC, Mae Diehl A, Brown AJ. Nonalcoholic steatohepatitis and nonalcoholic fatty liver disease in young women with polycystic ovary syndrome. *J Clin Endocrinol Metab* 2006;91:1741–7.

159. Clark JM, Brancati FL, Diehl AM. Nonalcoholic fatty liver disease. *Gastroenterology* 2002;122: 1649–57.

160. Sheth SG, Gordon FD, Chopra S. Nonalcoholic steatohepatitis. *Ann Intern Med* 1997;126:137–45.

161. Azziz R, Ehrmann D, Legro RS, et al. Troglitazone improves ovulation and hirsutism in the polycystic ovary syndrome: a multicenter, double blind, placebo-controlled trial. *J Clin Endocrinol Metab* 2001;86:1626–32.

162. Garmes HM, Tambascia MA, Zantut-Wittmann DE. Endocrine-metabolic effects of the treatment with pioglitazonein obese patients with polycystic ovary syndrome. *Gynecol Endocrinol* 2005;21:317–23.

163. Rautio K, Tapanainen JS, Ruokonen A, Morin-Papunen LC. Endocrine and metabolic effects of rosiglitazone in overweight women with PCOS: a randomized placebo-controlled study. *Hum Reprod* 2006;21:1400–1407.

164. Diamanti-Kandarakis E, Baillargeon JP, Iuorno MJ, Jakubowicz DJ, Nestler JE. A modern medical quandary: polycystic ovary syndrome, insulin resistance, and oral contraceptive pills. *J Clin Endocrinol Metab* 2003;88:1927–32.

165. Arslanian SA, Lewy V, Danadian K, Saad R. Metformin therapy in obese adolescents with polycystic ovary syndrome and impaired glucose tolerance: amelioration of exaggerated adrenal response to adrenocorticotropin with reduction of insulinemia/insulin resistance. *J Clin Endocrinol Metab* 2002;87:1555–9.

166. Bridger T, MacDonald S, Baltzer F, Rodd C. Randomized placebo-controlled trial of metformin for adolescents with polycystic ovary syndrome. *Arch Pediatr Adolesc Med* 2006;160:241–6.

167. Glueck CJ, Wang P, Fontaine R, Tracy T, Sieve-Smith L. Metformin to restore normal menses in oligo-amenorrheic teenage girls with polycystic ovary syndrome (PCOS). *J Adolesc Health* 2001;29:160–9.

168. Ibanez L, Valls C, Potau N, Marcos MV, de Zegher F. Sensitization to insulin in adolescent girls to normalize hirsutism, hyperandrogenism, oligomenorrhea, dyslipidemia, and hyperinsulinism after precocious pubarche. *J Clin Endocrinol Metab* 2000;85:3526–30.

169. Ibanez L, Ferrer A, Ong K, Amin R, Dunger D, de Zegher F. Insulin sensitization early after menarche prevents progression from precocious pubarche to polycystic ovary syndrome. *J Pediatr* 2004;144:23–9.

170. Ibanez L, de Zegher F. Ethinylestradiol-drospirenone, flutamide-metformin, or both for adolescents and women with hyperinsulinemic hyperandrogenism: opposite effects on adipocytokines and body adiposity. *J Clin Endocrinol Metab* 2004;89:1592–7.

171. McCartney CR, Prendergast KA, Chhabra S, Eagleson CA, Yoo R, Chang RJ, Foster CM, Marshall JC. The Association of Obesity and Hyperandrogenemia during the Pubertal Transition in Girls: Obesity as a Potential Factor in the Genesis of Postpubertal Hyperandrogenism. *J Clin Endocrinol Metab* 2006;91:1714–1722.

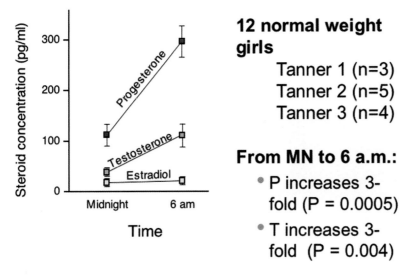

Color Plate 1. Overnight changes in ovarian steroids in normal early pubertal girls (Tanner stages I–III). (Fig. 2, Chapter 7.)

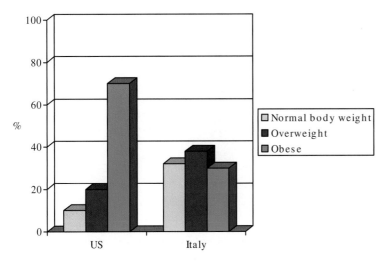

Color Plate 2. Distribution of body weight in US and Italian women with the classic polycystic ovary syndrome (PCOS) phenotype. (Fig. 1, Chapter 8.)

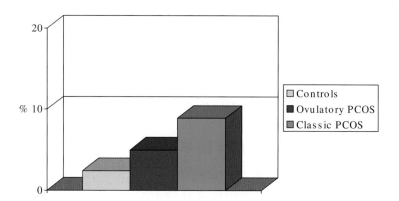

Color Plate 3. Prevalence of the metabolic syndrome in Italian normal women aged 20–39 years and in Italian polycystic ovary syndrome (PCOS) patients with the classic or ovulatory hyperandrogenic phenotype. (Fig. 2, Chapter 8.)

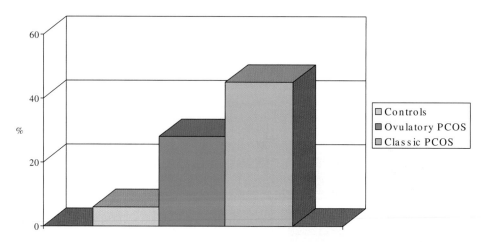

Color Plate 4. Prevalence of the finding of at least one altered cardiovascular risk factor in Italian polycystic ovary syndrome (PCOS) patients with classic or ovulatory hyperandrogenic phenotype. (Fig. 3, Chapter 8.)

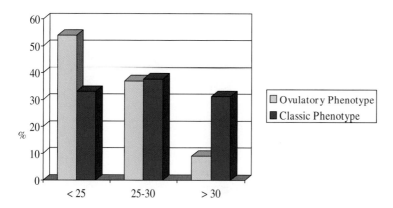

Color Plate 5. Distribution of body weight in Italian polycystic ovary syndrome (PCOS) patients with classic or ovulatory hyperandrogenic phenotype. (Fig. 4, Chapter 8.)

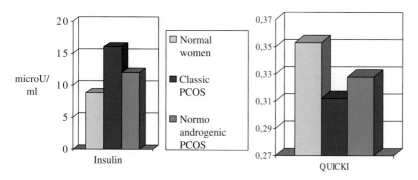

Color Plate 6. Insulin serum levels and insulin sensitivity (by QUICKI) in Italian normal women and in Italian PCOS patients with classic hyperandrogenic or with normoandrogenic phenotype. (Fig. 5, Chapter 8.)

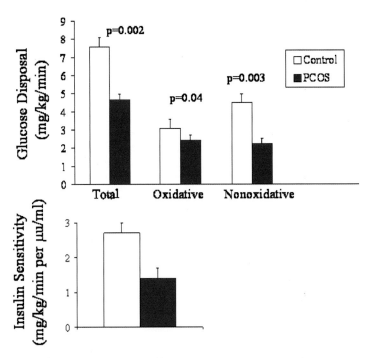

Color Plate 7. Upper panel: insulin-stimulated glucose disposal during a hyperinsulinemic euglycemic clamp in obese PCOS girls vs matched obese control girls. Lower panel: insulin sensitivity in PCOS versus obese control girls. (Fig. 1, Chapter 11; *See* complete caption on p. 163.)

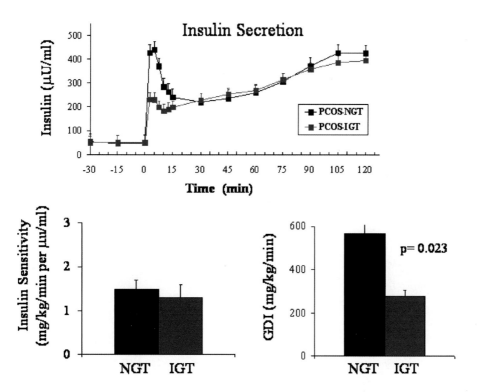

Color Plate 8. First-phase and second-phase insulin secretion during a hyperglycemic clamp (upper panel), insulin sensitivity (left lower panel), and glucose disposition index (GDI) (right lower panel) in PCOS adolescents with impaired (IGT) versus normal (NGT) glucose tolerance. (Fig. 3, Chapter 11; *See* complete caption on p. 165.)

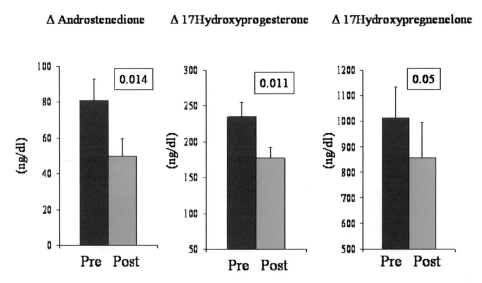

Color Plate 9. Change in (Δ) hormone levels (30-min value minus 0-min value) in response to ACTH stimulation pre- and post-metformin treatment in adolescents with PCOS. (Fig. 4, Chapter 11; *See* complete caption on p. 173.)

12 Polycystic Ovary Syndrome and the Metabolic Syndrome Long-Term Risks

Eva Dahlgren, MD, PhD,
and Per Olof Janson, MD, PhD

CONTENTS

Summary

Polycystic ovary syndrome (PCOS) is a heterogeneous clinical entity defined as the association of hyperandrogenism with chronic anovulation and the appearance of polycystic ovaries on sonography. Infertility is part of the syndrome but could be successfully treated with modern reproductive techniques. Hirsutism can be managed with drugs that suppress ovarian function, increase sex hormone-binding globulin (SHBG) levels and/or blocking androgen receptors or 5-alpha reductase. A topical agent inhibiting ornithine decarboxylase also ameliorates excessive facial terminal hair growth. The causative correlation between PCOS and endometrial cancer is established, and possibly, there is also a link between PCOS and breast cancer. Women with PCOS share many features in common with the metabolic syndrome (MS), in particular. In 1921, Achard and Thiers *(1)* described the bearded diabetic, but it was not until 1980 that more systematic research focussed on the relation between hyperandrogenism and hyperinsulinism *(2)* in obese affected women. The prevalence of type 2 diabetes is substantially increased in women with PCOS. However, despite the increased risk factors, evidence for increased mortality due to cardiovascular disease (CVD) has not been found. Awareness of the deleterious effects of sedentary life style and active promotion of healthy eating habits and physical activity is essential. Promising results have been shown with insulin sensitizers, but long-term follow-up studies are needed.

Key Words: PCOS; metabolic syndrome; morbidity; risk.

From: *Contemporary Endocrinology: Polycystic Ovary Syndrome*
Edited by: A. Dunaif, R. J. Chang, S. Franks, and R. S. Legro © Humana Press, Totowa, NJ

1. INTRODUCTION

Polycystic ovary syndrome (PCOS) is a heterogeneous clinical entity affecting 5–10% of premenopausal women. It is characterized by the association of hyperandrogenism with chronic anovulation and the appearance of polycystic ovaries on sonography, without specific underlying diseases of the adrenal and pituitary glands, and it is frequently associated with insulin resistance. In recent years, increasing attention has been paid to the non-reproductive aspects of PCOS. The long-term impact of the metabolic disturbances associated with the disorder on women's health has focussed considerable interest on follow-up studies and intervention studies. Such studies are, however, so far sparse. This chapter gives a brief review on the long-term implications of PCOS on women's reproductive health, hormonal balance, and clinical expressions such as hirsutism, obesity and anthropometry, bone metabolism, risks of cancer and cardiovascular disease. The discussions on primary prevention based on those issues are at present mostly speculative because of lack of firm evidence.

2. REPRODUCTIVE HEALTH

2.1. Menstruation

According to a retrospective follow-up study in 1992 involving 33 women with PCOS diagnosed by clinical features and histology of wedge resection during 1956–1965, we found no difference from controls in the age of menarche (3). Preoperatively, the women were oligomenorrhoeic in 81% of cases, and after the wedge resection, 61% of them remained oligomenorrhoeic, whereas their periods tended to become regular with time. Twenty-eight percent of the PCOS cohort reported irregular cycles during the entire fertile period. Most of the women who became pregnant resumed regular cycles after the pregnancy. This finding was confirmed in a Dutch follow-up study of ageing women with PCOS (4). Also, in a long-term follow-up, after ovarian drilling of oligomenorrhoeic women with PCOS, a significant increase in the proportion of regular menstrual cycles was found (5). Women with PCOS appeared to enter the menopause later than referents, as assessed by follicle-stimulating hormone (FSH) levels in serum. Thus, when dividing women with PCOS and age- and weight-matched referents into two subgroups according to whether they presented serum FSH values of more or less than 50 U/l, 60% of the referents and 27% of the women with PCOS presented values of more than 50 U/l (3).

2.2. Fecundity

In our follow-up study (3), 75% of the women with PCOS were married, which at that time (1956–1965) was a prerequisite for infertility treatment. Out of the 70% of the PCOS cohort of women who wanted to become pregnant, 24% remained nulliparous compared to 16% among referents. Successful outcomes of the infertile condition of the syndrome was also found by Wild et al. (6), who, in a retrospective cohort follow-up study in the United Kingdom, reported that only 17.5% of women with PCOS remained nulliparous.

Women with PCOS suffering from infertility conceived in 50% of cases after up to six cycles with clomiphene citrate and in 62% of cases after treatment with gonadotrophin or ovarian drilling (5,7,8). Numerous reports have shown increased success rate in assisted reproduction by adding insulin sensitizers to the ovulation-induction treatment *(9,10)*. Studies suggest that there is an increased rate of miscarriage in women with PCOS (30–40%) *(8,11,12)* particularly in women with high serum LH concentrations *(13)*. Abel-Gadir et al. *(14)* found a significantly lower rate of miscarriage in women with PCOS treated with laparoscopic ovarian drilling (21%) compared to women with PCOS subjected to ovulation induction by human menopausal gonadotropin (HMG) or FSH (53 and 40%).

2.3. Hysterectomy

Bleeding irregularities with menorrhagia are indications for hysterectomy worldwide. In our retrospective cohort follow-up study *(3)*, women with PCOS had undergone hysterectomy on benign indications three times more often than the referents (21 vs.7%, $p < 0.05$). An increased incidence of previous hysterectomy in New Zealand in women with PCOS was also reported by Birdsall et al. *(15)*.

3. HIRSUTISM

Almost 70% of women with PCOS have hirsutism *(16)*, varying from growth of some coarse hair on the upper lip and chin to excessive coarse hair on the face, trunk and thighs. In general, the hirsutism develops some years after menarche and is typically exacerbated by weight gain, possibly due to increased serum insulin levels and reduced serum concentrations of sex hormone-binding globulin (SHBG). Hirsutism, which is unrelated to Cushing's disease or ovarian and adrenal tumours, is not a challenge to health in itself, but for most women, it causes serious problems in their social life, threatening their self-esteem and affecting their quality of life. Those women who cannot accept their excessive hair growth will often be subjected to attempts at treatment with anti-androgens and/or oral contraceptives, which reduce the ovarian androgen production and raise serum SHBG levels. In serious cases, destruction of hair follicles with cautery or laser may be employed. It seems reasonable to intervene early in life with anti-androgen treatment to stop further progression of hirsutism. Treatment with oral contraceptives and anti-androgen, i.e. cyproterone acetate or spironolactone, is widely used and usually results in satisfactory control of the growth rate of excessive hair *(17)*. However, such treatment may disturb carbohydrate metabolism, indicating that this type of intervention should be used with caution in obese and insulin-resistant women.

The 5-alpha reductase inhibitor, finasteride, has also been reported to be effective in the treatment of PCOS-associated hirsutism *(18,19)*. There are different opinions about whether treatment with GnRH analogue alone is effective in reducing hirsutism *(20,21)*. Metformin reduces serum testosterone by 20% in women with PCOS, but there is little evidence that it reduces hirsutism *(9,10)*. The topical agent, the orithine decarboxylase inhibitor, eflornithine hydrochloride cream, Vaniqua®, available in the USA and Canada unfortunately not yet available in Europe, has been shown to reduce the growth rate of unwanted hair in the face in 32% of the cases in clinical trials compared to 8% in the placebo group *(22)*.

4. BONE METABOLISM

There has been concern about the bone mineral density in oligomenorrhoeic and amenorrhoeic women with PCOS because osteopenia is a common feature in amenorrhea of hypothalamic origin. However, published data in women with PCOS show a normal *(23,24)* or even supernormal mineralization of the skeleton *(25)* and a positive correlation between androgen levels and bone mineral density *(26)*.

5. RISK OF CANCER

5.1. PCOS and Endometrial Carcinoma

Endometrial cancer in women under 40 years of age is rare, with a reported incidence of 4%. There are numerous reports in the literature on the association of PCOS with the development of endometrial cancer in young women *(27,28)*. Early menarche and late menopause, reduced fecundity, hypertension, diabetes mellitus *(29)*, infertility and obesity *(30)* have been linked to in an increased risk to develop endometrial cancer, in particular among affected younger women, due to unopposed estrogen action and possibly a trophic effect of insulin and insulin-like growth factor-1 on the endometrium *(31–33)*. Coulam et al. investigated 1270 women with chronic anovulation and found a threefold increased risk of endometrial cancer. Ron et al. *(34)* evaluated 2672 women who were treated for infertility up to 20 years before and found a 4.8-fold increased risk of endometrial cancer in the infertility group and a 10.3-fold increased risk in infertile women with chronic anovulation. Brinton et al. *(35)* found, in a case-control study of 405 cases with endometrial cancer and 297 controls, a 7.6-fold increased risk for endometrial cancer among nulliparous with infertility compared to nulliparous without conceiving problems.

In the Gothenburg area, comprising one-fifth of the female population in Sweden, 77 women aged 31–45 years and 99 women aged 46–65 years with endometrial cancer were investigated. When comparing these women with 1746 referents, 39–65 years of age, it was found that increased body mass index, hirsutism and hypertension were significantly more common in both groups of women with endometrial cancer. Nulliparity and infertility were more common among the younger women with endometrial cancer compared to referents, indicating that untreated ovarian dysfunction, such as that found in PCOS, is associated with an increased risk of endometrial cancer *(36,37)*.

5.2. PCOS and Breast Cancer

A number of validated risk factors for breast cancer, such as age, early age of menarche, late menopause, late age at first delivery and nulliparity, are hormone related. Epidemiological studies on the relation between the PCOS and breast cancer have shown conflicting results. Coulam et al. *(31)* showed no increased risk in women with chronic anovulation; however, after stratification by age, the relative risk was 3.6 (95% CI = 1.2–8.3) in the postmenopausal group. Gammon and Thompson *(38)* in a retrospective case-control study of 4730 women with breast cancer and 4688 controls actually found a decreased risk in women who in a self-assessed questionnaire were diagnosed to have PCOS. However, the prevalence of PCOS was 0.49% among cases and 0.94% among controls, which makes the result hard to interpret. In a large prospective study *(39)* designed to examine the development of breast cancer in postmenopausal women, the relative risk for women with PCOS to develop breast cancer was 1.2 (95% CI = 0.7–2). Adjustment for age at menarche, age at menopause, parity, the use of oral contraceptives, body mass index, waist-to-hip ratio (WHT) and family history of breast cancer lowered the RR to 1 (95% CI = 0.6–1.9). The prevalence of PCOS in that study was 1.35%, which is lower than expected.

Sellers et al. *(40)* analyzed data from a prospective study of more than 37,000 women aged 55–69 years. During 4 years of follow-up, 493 new cases of breast cancer were diagnosed. In cases with a positive family history of breast cancer, increased risk to develop the disease was associated with increased WHR (>0.91) (RR = 3.24, nulliparity RR = 2.24 and infertility RR = 2.1). Moseson et al. *(41)* evaluated 354 women with breast cancer and 747 controls and found infertility to be associated with increased risk for the disease (OR = 3.5). Women with signs of hyperandrogenism had an OR of 6.8 for breast cancer. In a retrospective cohort follow-up study in the UK *(42)* on 786 women with a histopathological diagnosis of PCOS in 1930–1979, the standard mortality rate for all neoplasms in the cohort was 0.91 and for breast cancer 1.48 (95% CI = 0.79–2.54).

The interrelationship between hormonal conditions, infertility and breast cancer is complex, but a link between PCOS and breast cancer appears probable *(32,33)*.

5.3. PCOS and Ovarian Carcinoma

Epithelial tumors comprise 90% of all ovarian cancers and no single etiological factor has been found. The inflammatory reaction of ovulation, with the cascade of interleukins and growth factors acting on the ovarian epithelium, has been suggested to be a "risk factor." Nevertheless, infertility and nulliparity are associated with an increased risk for the development of ovarian cancer despite the fact that anovulation should be protective. Harris et al. *(43)* found, in a meta-analysis of 12 case-control studies on ovarian cancer performed during 1956–1986 that included 3000 cases and 10,000 controls, an OR of 2.1 for invasive epithelial ovarian cancer in nulligravid women with a history of female infertility. Rossing et al. *(44)* evaluated the potential neoplastic effect of medical infertility treatment and found in a group of 3837 infertile women the relative risk of ovarian cancer to be 1.9. Schildkraut et al. *(45)* reported a 2.5-fold (95% CI = 1.1–5.9) increased risk of epithelial ovarian cancer among women with PCOS in a population-based, case-control study involving 426 cancer cases and 4081 controls. The association was found to be stronger among women who never used oral contraceptives. In the retrospective cohort follow-up study from the UK, Pierpoint found a standardized mortality rate on ovarian cancer of 0.39 *(42)*. Taken together, these data support the so-called gonadotrophin theory for the development of ovarian cancer. Although more studies are needed to verify the findings of Schildkraut et al. *(45)*, the relative protection afforded by oral contraceptives against ovarian cancer must be taken into consideration when advising women with PCOS with no immediate infertility problem.

6. OBESITY AND ANTHROPOMETRY

In a Swedish study, the average woman has been shown to increase her body weight by 4 kg during the perimenopause *(46)*. In a cohort study *(3)*, a second follow-up was performed after 3 years in the women with PCOS and their referents *(47)*. The women with PCOS decreased in weight, by an average of 2 kg, but retained their upper body obesity, with a constant WHR of 0.81 ± 0.07. In contrast, the referents gained an average of 2 kg but their WHR decreased significantly (0.83 ± 0.08 to 0.78 ± 0.06, $p<0.001$). Thus, women with PCOS appear to remain centrally obese when approaching the menopause. Central-visceral obesity is highly correlated to insulin resistance and atherogenic lipoprotein patterns (48). However, in our and other studies (47,49), aberrations in lipoprotein patterns are less pronounced in older compared to those in younger women with PCOS.

7. THE METABOLIC SYNDROME

The metabolic syndrome (MS) is a cluster of risk factors for the development of CVD. The association between obesity, insulin resistance, deranged lipoproteins and hypertension was first recognized in 1923 (50). MS is characterized by central obesity, elevated levels of triglycerides (TG), low-density lipoprotein (LDL) and very low-density lipoprotein (VLDL) cholesterol and insulin resistance in fat and muscle tissues (51,52). Both men and women with features of the MS have been considered to have an increased risk to develop diabetes mellitus, hypertension and CVD.

7.1. Definitions

7.1.1. THE WHO DEFINITION

The WHO definition (53) requires the presence of impaired glucose tolerance or insulin resistance and at least two of six additional risk factors as described: blood pressure > 140/90 mm Hg, serum TG > 150 mg/dl, high-density lipoprotein cholesterol (<35 mg/dl in men and <39 mg/dl in women), central obesity (WHR males > 0.90 and females > 0.85), body mass index (BMI) > $30 kg/m^2$ and micro-albuminuria (tU-albumin > 20 µg/min).

7.1.2. THE NCEP DEFINITION

The National Cholesterol Education Program's (NCEP) Adult Treatment Panel III 2001 criteria (54) have been increasingly accepted in routine clinical practice and requires three of the following factors: fasting glucose > 110 mg/dl, blood pressure > 130/85 mm Hg or anti-hypertensive treatment, TG > 150mg/dl, HDL cholesterol < 39 mg/dl (men) or <50 mg/dl (women) and girth > 102 cm (men) >88 cm (women). Recently, the American Diabetes Association and the European Association for the Study of Diabetes raised doubt about the utility of the MS diagnosis, because the constellation may not confer more risk for CVD than each of its component parts (55). In a multicenter study, 33.4% of 410 women with PCOS, aged 18–41 years and 368 non-diabetic women met the NCEP's criteria of the MS regardless of racial/ethnic group. There was a positive correlation between the level of free testosterone, BMI and MS. None of the 52 women with a BMI less than 27.0 kg/m^2 had MS (56).

7.2. Insulin Resistance in Women with PCOS

In 1921, Achard and Thiers (1) described the diabetes of bearded women, but it was not until 1980 that more systematic research focussed on the relation between hyperandrogenism and hyperinsulinism (2). In 1980, Burghen et al. (2) described the correlation between hyperandrogenism and hyperinsulinemia in women with PCOS, and in 1983, Chang et al. *(57)* described insulin resistance also in non-obese women with PCOS. In 1987, Dunaif et al. *(58)* reported that women with PCOS were at risk for glucose intolerance. In 1992 Dahlgren et al. *(3)* reported an increased (15%) prevalence of diabetes mellitus in perimenopausal women with PCOS compared to referents 15 versus 2.3%. Legro et al. *(59)* reported a sevenfold increased risk of type 2 diabetes mellitus among young women with PCOS compared to control women of comparable age and weight. Ehrmann et al. *(60)* showed an annual conversion rate from impaired glucose tolerance to type 2 diabetes of 6% in women with PCOS. Norman et al. *(61)* reported that 18% of a cohort of obese women with PCOS aged 20–30 years had abnormal glucose tolerance tests. Seven years later, another 15% of the cohort developed abnormal glucose tolerance tests or type 2 diabetes. The increased risk for glucose intolerance is the result of profound peripheral insulin resistance and pancreatic β-cell dysfunction in women with PCOS *(62,63)*.

It has been shown that weight reduction will normalize hormonal and carbohydrate variables in overweight women with PCOS *(64–68)*. This approach has been shown to be effective on a short-term basis in the treatment of anovulatory infertility. The problem, however, is to achieve a permanent weight reduction. Experience shows that life-style changes with exercise and reduced caloric intake only result in temporary effects. One explanation to why many women with PCOS easily regain weight may be that they have a disorder of energy expenditure characterized by low postprandial thermogenesis *(69)*.

Treatment with insulin-sensitizing drugs (metformin and thiagolodine dioves) has shown promising results in preliminary studies *(70–73)*, improving both metabolic variables and hyperandrogenicity. However, long-term studies are needed to fully assess the role of insulin sensitization therapy in the treatment of PCOS.

7.3. Hypertension

There are conflicting reports as to whether women with PCOS are hypertensive.

Rebuffé-Scrive et al. *(74)* found elevated blood pressure in lean women with PCOS. Dahlgren et al. *(3)* reported an increased prevalence of hypertension in perimenopausal affected women and Holte et al. *(75)* found elevated blood pressure during daytime in younger overweight women with PCOS compared to controls. In a Dutch PCOS population study from 2001, the prevalence of hypertension was increased in women with PCOS compared to controls in women aged 35–44 (8.2 vs. 4.5%) and in women aged 45–54 (28.1 vs. 11.1%) *(76)*. However, this was not confirmed by Zimmermann et al. *(77)* in insulin-resistant women with PCOS.

7.4. Risk for CVD in Women with PCOS

Several studies have reported unfavourable lipoprotein pattern *(78–80)*, more carotid plaques and higher carotid intima-media thickness *(81)* and a predicted increased risk for developing CVD *(82–88)* in women with PCOS. A long-term follow-up study in the UK, however, failed to find an increase in cardiovascular events *(6,42)*. This observation has raised the questions whether women with PCOS, besides having risk factors for CVD, also have protective factors. It has been found that women with PCOS enter menopause later than referents. It has also been found that hyperandrogenism and the dyslipidemia found in younger women with PCOS stabalizes in the menopause while it worsens among the referents *(47,49)*. However, the UK cohort had a mean age of 58 years, and the prevalence of cardiovascular events does not begin to increase in women until the seventh and eight decades *(49)*.

In summary, women with PCOS have a three to sevenfold risk of developing diabetes mellitus; those with obesity, chronic anovulation and/or a family history of type 2 diabetes are at highest risk. They also have a substantially increased risk for MS, but their risk for hypertension is less clear.

REFERENCES

1. Achard MC, Thiers MJ: Le virilisme pilaire et son association a l'Insuffisance glycolytique (diabète des femmes a barbe). *Bulletin Academie National Medicine (Paris)* 1921;86:51–66.
2. Burghen GA, Givens JR, Kitabchi AE. Correlation of hyperandrogenism with hyperinsulinism in polycystic ovarian disease. *J Clin Endocrinol Metab* 1980;50:113–116.
3. Dahlgren E, Johansson S, Lindstedt G, Knutsson F, Odén A, Janson PO, Mattsson LÅ, Crona N, Lundberg PA. Women with polycystic ovary syndrome wedge resected in 1956–65: a long-term follow-up focusing on natural history and circulating hormones. *Fertil Steril* 1992; 57:505–513.
4. Elting MW, Korsen TJM, Rekers-Mombarg LTM, Shoemaker J. Women with polycystic ovary syndrome gain regular menstrual cycles when ageing. *Hum Reprod* 2000;15:24–28.
5. Amer SAK, Gopalan V, Li TC, Ledger WL, Cooke ID. Long term follow-up of patients with polycystic ovarian syndrome after laparoscopic ovarian drilling: clinical outcome. *Hum Reprod* 2002;17:2035–2042.
6. Wild S, Pierpoint T, McKeigue P, Jacobs HS. Cardiovascular disease in women with polycystic ovary syndrome at long-term follow-up:a retrospective cohort study. *Clin Endocrinol* 2000;52:595–600.
7. Balen AH, Braat DD, West C, Patel A, Jacobs HS. Cumulative conception and live birth rates after the treatment of anovulatory infertility: safety and efficacy of ovulation induction in 200 patients. *Hum Reprod* 1994;9:1563–1570.
8. Garcia JE, Jones GS, Wentz AC. The use of clomiphene citrate. *Fertil Steril* 1977;28:707–717.
9. Harborne L, Fleming R, Lyall H, Norman J, Sattar N. Descriptive review of the evidence for the use of metformin in polycystic ovary syndrome. *Lancet* 2003;361:1894–901.
10. Lord JM, Flight IH, Norman RJ. Insulin-sensitising drugs (metformin, troglitazone, rosiglitazone, pioglitazone, D-chiro-inositol) for polycystic ovary syndrome. *Cochrane Database Syst Rev* 2003;3:CD003053.
11. Homburg R, Armar NA, Eshel A, Adams J, Jacobs HS. Influence of serum luteinizing hormone concentrations on ovulation, conception, and early pregnancy loss in polycystic ovary syndrome. *Br Med J* 1988;297:1024–1026.
12. Sagle M, Bishop K, Ridley N, Alexander FM, Michel M, Bonney RC, Beard RW, Franks S. Recurrent early miscarriage and polycystic ovaries. *Br Med J* 1988;297:1027–1028.
13. Regan L, Owen EJ, Jacobs HS. Hyper secretion of luteinising hormone, infertility and miscarriage. *Lancet* 1990;336: 1141–1144.
14. Abel-Gadir A, Mowafi RS, Alnaser HMI, Alrashid AH, Alonezi OM, Shaw RW. Ovarian elctro-cautery versus human gonadotrophins and pure follicle stimulating hormone therapy in treatment of patients with polycystic ovarian disease. *Clin Endocrinol* 1990;33:585–592.
15. Birdsall MA, Farquhar CM, White HD. Association between polycystic ovaries and extent of coronary heart disease in women having cardiac catheterisation. *Ann Int Med* 1997;26:32–35.
16. Legro RS. Polycystic ovary syndrome: current and future treatment paradigms. *Am J Obstet Gynecol* 1998;179;101–108.

17. Spritzer PM, Lisboa KO, Mattiello S, Lhullier F. Spironolactone as a single agent for long-term therapy of hirsute patients. *Clin Endocrinol (Oxf)* 2000 May;52(5):587–594.

18. Petrone A., Civitillo RM, Galante L,Giannotti F, D'Anto V,Rippa G, Tolino A. Usefulness of a 12-month treatment with finasteride in idiopathic and polycystic ovary syndrome-associated hirsutism. *Clin Exp Obstet Gynecol* 1999; 26:213–216.

19. Beigi A, Sobhi A, Zarrinkoub F. Finasteride versus cyproterone acetate-estrogen regimens in the treatment of hirsutism Int *J Gynecol Obstet* 2004; 87,29–33.

20. Falsetti L, Pasinetti E, Ceruti D. Gonadotropin-releasing hormone agonist (GnRH-A) in hirsutism. *Acta Eur Fertil* 1994; 25:303–306.

21. Carmina E, Lobo RA. Gonadotropin-releasing hormone agonist therapy for hirsutism is as effective as high dose cyproterone acetate but results in longer remission. *Hum Reprod* 1997; 12:663–666.

22. Balfour JA, McClellan K. Topical eflornithine. *Am J Clin Dermatol* 2001;2(3):197–201.

23. Dixon JE, Rodin A, Murby B, Chapman MG, Fogelman I. Bone mass in hirsute women with androgen excess. *Clin Endocrinol (Oxf)* 1989;30:271–278.

24. Di Carlo C, Shoham Z, MacDougall J, Patel A, Hall ML, Jacobs HS. Polycystic ovaries as a relative protective factor for bone mineral loss in young women with amenorrhea. *Fertil Steril* 1992;57:314–9.

25. Dagago-Jack S, al-Ali N, Qurttom M. Augmentation of bone mineral density in hirsute women. *J Clin Endocrinol Metab* 1997;82:2821–2825.

26. Adami S, Zamberlan N, Castello R, Tosi F, gatti D, Moghetti P. Effect of hyperandrogenism and menstrual cycle abnormalities on bone mass and bone turnover in young women. *Clin Endocrinol (Oxf)* 1998;48:169–73.

27. Gregorini SD, Lespi PJ, Alvarez GR. Endometrial carcinoma with polycystic ovaries. Report of two cases in women younger than 40 years old. *Medicina (Buonas Aires)* 1977;57:397–402.

28. Hendersen BE, Casagrande JT, Pike MC, Mack T, Rosario I, Duke A. The epidemiology of endometrial cancer in young women. *Br J Cancer* 1983; 47: 749–756.

29. Elwood JM, Cole P, Rothman KJ, Kaplan SD. Epidemiology of endometrial cancer. *J Natl Cancer Inst* 1977;59:1055–60.

30. MacMahon B. Risk factors for endometrial cancer. *Gynecol Oncol* 1974;2:122–129.

31. Coulam CB, Annegers JF, Kranz JS. Chronic anovulation syndrome and associated neoplasia. *Obstet Gynecol* 1983;61:403–407.

32. Meirow D, Schenker JG. The link between female infertility and cancer: epidemiology and possible aetiologies. *Hum Reprod Update* 1996;2:63–75.

33. Balen A. Polycystic ovary syndrome and cancer. *Hum Reprod Update* 2001;7:522–525.

34. Ron E, Lunenfeld B, Menczer J, Blumstein T, Katz L, Oelsner G, Serr D. Cancer incidence in a cohort of infertile women. *Am J Epidemiol* 1987;125:780–790.

35. Brinton LA, Berman ML, Mortel R, Twiggs LB, Barrett RJ, Wilbanks GD, Lannom L, Hoover RN. Reproductive, menstrual, and medical risk factors for endometrial cancer: results from a case-control study. *Am J Obstet Gynecol* 1992:167:1317–1325.

36. Dahlgren E, Friberg LG, Johansson S, Lindstrom B, Oden A, Samsioe G, Janson PO. Endometrial carcinoma; ovarian dysfunction-a risk factor in young women. *J Obstet Gynecol Reprod Biol* 1991;41:143–50.

37. Dahlgren E, Johansson S, Oden A, Lindstrom B, Janson PO. A model for prediction of endometrial canccr. *Acta Obstet Gynecol Scand* 1989;68:507–510.

38. Gammon MD, Thompson WD. Polycystic ovaries and the risk of breast cancer. *Am J Epidemiol* 1991;134:818–824.

39. Anderson KE, Sellers TA, Chen PL, Rich SS, Hong CP, Folsom AR. Association of Stein-Leventhal syndrome with the incidence of postmenopausal breast carcinoma in a large prospective study of women in Iowa. *Cancer* 1997;79:494–499.

40. Sellers TA, Gapstur SM, Potter JD, Kushi LH, Bostick RM, Folsom AR. Association of body fat distribution and family histories of breast and ovarian cancer with risk of postmenopausal breast cancer. *Am J Epidemiol* 1993;138(10):799–803.

41. Moseson M, Koenig KL, Shore RE, Pasternack BS. The influence of medical conditions associated with hormones on the risk of breast cancer. *Int J Epidemiol* 1993; 22:1000–1009.

42. Pierpoint T, McKeigue PM, Isaacs AJ, Wild SH, Jacobs HS. Mortality of women with polycystic ovary syndrome at long-term follow-up. *J Clin Epidemiol* 1998;51:581–586.

43. Harris R, Whittemore AS, Intyre J. Characteristics relating to ovarian cancer risk: collaborative analysis of 12 US case-control studies. III. Epithelial tumors of low malignant potential in white women. Collaborative Ovarian Cancer Group. *Am J Epidemiol* 1992;136:1204–1211.

44. Rossing MA, Daling JR, Weiss NS, Moore DE, Self SG. Ovarian tumors in a cohort of infertile women. *N Engl J Med* 1994;331:771–776.

45. Schildkraut JM, Schwingl PJ, Bastos E, Evanoff A, Hughes C. Epithelial ovarian cancer risk among women with polycystic ovary syndrome. *Obstet Gynecol* 1996;88:554–559.

46. Björkelund C, Hulten B, Lissner L, Rothenberg E, larsson B, Bengtsson C, Steen B, Tibblin G. New height and weight standards for the middle aged and aged. Weight increases more than height. *Lakartidningen* 1997;94:332–335.

47. Dahlgren E, Janson PO, Johansson S, Lapidus L, Lindstedt G, Tengborn L. Hemostatic and metabolic variables in women with polycystic ovary syndrome. *Fertil Steril* 1994;61:455–460.

48. Björntorp P. Hypothesis on visceral fat accumulation:the missing link between psychosocial factors and cardiovascular disease? *Int J Obes* 1991;230:195–201.

49. Legro RS. Polycystic ovary syndrome and cardiovascular disease: a premature association? *Endocr Rev* 2003;24:302–312.

50. Kylin E. Studien über das Hypertonie-Hyperglykämie-Hyperurikämiesyndrom. *Zentralblatt für innere Medizin* 1923;44:105–127.

51. Reaven GM. Role of insulin resistance in human disease. *Diabetes* 1988;37:1595–1607.

52. Reaven GM. Insulin resistance, the insulin resistance syndrome, and cardiovascular disease. *Panminerva Med* 2005;47:201–210.

53. *World health Organization: Definition, Diagnosis, and Classification of Diabetes Mellitus and its Complications: Reports of a WHO consultation.* Geneva, World Health Org., 1999.

54. Expert Panel on the Detection, Evaluation, and Treatment of High Blood Cholesterol in Adults. Executive summary of the third Report of the National Cholesterol Education Program (NCEP) (Adult treatment Panel III). *JAMA* 2001;285:2486–2497.

55. Kahn R, Buse J, Ferrannini E, Stern M. The metabolic syndrome: Time for a critical appraisal joint statement from the American Diabetes Association and the European Association for the study of Diabetes. *Diabetes Care* 2005;28:2289–2304.

56. Ehrmann DA, Liljenquist DR, Kasza K, Azziz R, Legro RS, Ghazzi MN; PCOS/Troglitazone Study Group. Prevalence and predictors of the metabolic syndrome in woman with polycystic ovary syndrome. *J Clin Endocrinol Metab* 2006;91:48–53.

57. Chang RJ, Nakamura RM, Judd HL, Kaplan SA. Insulin resistance in nonobese patients with polycystic ovarian disease. *J Clin Endocrinol Metab* 1983;57:356–359.

58. Dunaif A, Graf M, Mandeli J, Laumas V, Dobrjansky A. Characterization of groups of hyperandrogenic women with acanthosis nigricans, impaired glucose tolerance, and/or hyperinsulinemia. *J Clin Endocrinol Metab* 1987;65:499–507.

59. Legro RS, Kunselman AR, Dodson WC, Dunaif A. Prevalence and predictors of risk for type 2 diabetes mellitus and impaired glucose tolerance in polycystic ovary syndrome: a prospective, controlled study in 254 affected women. *J Clin Endocrinol Metab* 1999;84:165–169.

60. Ehrmann DA, Barnes RB, Rosenfield RL, Cavaghan MK, Imperial J. Prevalence of impaired glucose tolerance and diabetes in women with polycystic ovary syndrome. *Diabetes Care* 1999;22:141–146.

61. Norman RJ, Masters L, Milner CR, Wang JX, Davies MJ. Relative risk of conversion from normo-glycaemia to impaired glucose tolerance or non-insulin dependent diabetes mellitus in polycystic ovarian syndrome. *Hum Reprod* 2001;16:1995–1998.

62. Sam S, Dunaif A. Polycystic ovary syndrome: syndrome XX? *Trends Endocrinol Metab* 2003;14: 365–370.

63. Ehrmann DA. Polycystic ovary syndrome. *N Engl J Med* 2005 24;352(12):1223–36.

64. Pasquali R, Casimirri F, Venturoli S, Paradisi R, Mattioli L, Capelli M, Melchionda N, Labo G. Insulin resistance in patients with polycystic ovaries: its relationship to body weight and androgen levels. *Acta Endocrinol (Copenh)* 1983;104:110–116.

65. Pasquali R, Fabbri R, Venturoli S, Paradisi R, Antenucci D, Melchionda N. Effect of weight loss and antiandrogenic therapy on sex hormone blood levels and insulin resistance in obese patients with polycystic ovaries. *Am J Obstet Gynecol* 1986;154(1):139–144.

66. Kiddy DS, Hamilton-Fairley D, Seppela M, Koistinen R, james VH, Reed MJ, Franks S. Diet-induced changes in sex hormone binding globulin and free testosterone in women with normal or polycystic ovaries: correlation with serum insulin and insulin-like growth factor-I. *Clin Endocrinol (Oxf)* 1989;31:757–763.

67. Holte J, Bergh T, Berne C, Wide L, Lithell H. Restored insulin sensitivity but persistently increased early insulin secretion after weight loss in obese women with polycystic ovary syndrome. *J Clin Endocrinol Metab* 1995;80:2586–2593.

68. Norman RJ, Clark AM. Lifestyle factors in the aetiology and management of polycystic ovary syndrome. In: Kovacs, ed. *Polycystic Ovary Syndrome.* Cambridge Univ Press; The Pitt Building, Trumpington Street, Cambridge, UK 2000.

69. Franks S, Robinson S, Willis DS. Nutrition, insulin and polycystic ovary syndrome. *Rev Reprod* 1996;1:47–53.

70. Velazques E, Acosta A, Mendoza SG. Menstrual cyclicity after metformin therapy in polycystic ovary syndrome. *Obstet Gynecol* 1997;90:392–395.

71. Morin-Papunen LC, Koivunen RM, Ruokonen A, Martikainen HK. Metformin therapy improves the menstrual pattern with minimal endocrine and metabolic effects in women with polycystic ovary syndrome. *Fertil Steril* 1998;69:691–696.

72. Diamanti-Kandarakis E, Kouli C, Tsianateli T, Bergiele A. Therapeutic effects of metformin on insulin resistance and hyperandrogenism in polycystic ovary syndrome. *Eur J Endocrinol* 1998;138:269–274.

73. Nestler JE. Should patients with polycystic ovarian syndrome be treated with metformin?: an enthusiastic endorsement. *Hum Reprod* 2002;17:1950–3.

74. Rebuffé-Scrive M, Cullberg G, Lundberg PA, Lindstedt G, Björntorp P. Anthropo-metric variables and metabolism in polycystic ovarian disease. *Horm Metab Res* 1989;21: 391–397.

75. Holte J, Gennarelli G, Berne C, Bergh T, Lithell H. Elevated ambulatory day-time blood pressure in women with polycystic ovary syndrome: a sign of a pre-hypertensive state? *Hum Reprod* 1996;11: 23–28.

76. Elting MW, Korsens TJ, Bezemer PD, Shoemaker J. Prevalence of diabetes mellitus and, hyper-tension and cardiac complaints in a follow-up study of a Dutch polycystic ovary population. *Hum Reprod* 2001;16:556–560.

77. Zimmermann S, Phillips RA, Dunaif A, Finegood DT, Wilkenfeld C, Ardelian M, Gorlin R, Krakoff LR. Polycystic ovary syndrome: lack of hypertension despite profound insulin resistance. *J Clin Endocrinol Metab* 1992;75:508–513.

78. Mattsson LÅ, Cullberg G, Hamberger L, Samsioe G, Silfverstolpe G. Lipid metabolism in women with polycystic ovary syndrome: possible implications for an increased risk of coronary heart disease. *Fertil Steril* 1984;42:579–584.

79. Wild RA, Applebaum-Bowden D, Demers LM, Bartholomew M, Landis JR, Hazzard WR, Santen RJ. Lipoprotein lipids in women with androgen excess: independent associations with increased insulin and androgen. *Clin Chem* 1990;36:283–9.

80. Robinson S, Henderson AD, Gelding SV, Kiddy D, Niththyananthan R, Bush A, Richmond W, Johnston DG, Franks S. Dyslipidaemia is associated with insulin resistance in women with polycystic ovaries. *Clin Endocrinol (Oxf)* 1996;44:277–284.

81. Talbott EO, Guzick DS, Sutton-Tyrrell K, McHugh-Pemu KP, Zborowski JV, Remsberg KE, Kuller LH. Evidence for association between polycystic ovary syndrome and premature carotid atherosclerosis in middle-aged women. *Arterioscler Thromb Vasc Biol* 2000;20:2414–2421.

82. Ehrmann DA, Liljenquist DR, Kasza K, Azziz R, Legro RS, Mahmoud NG, for the PCOS/Troglitazone Study Group. Prevalence and predictors of the metabolic syndrome in women with polycystic ovary syndrome. *J Clin Endocrinol Metab* 2006;91:48–53.

83. Carmina E, Koyama T, Chang L, Stanczyk FZ, Lobo RA. Does ethnicity influence the prevalence of adrenal hyperandrogenism and insulin resistance in polycystic ovary syndrome? *Am J Obstet Gynecol* 1992;167:1807–1812.

84. Dahlgren E, Johansson S, Lapidus L, Oden A, Janson PO. Polycystic ovary syndrome and risk for myocardial infarction-evaluation from a risk factor model based on a prospective population study of women. *Acta Obstetricia et Gynecologia Scandinavica* 1992;71:599–604.

85. Conway GS, Agrawal R, Betteridge DJ, Jacobs HS. Risk factors for coronary artery disease in lean and obese women with the polycystic ovary syndrome. *Clin Endocrinol (Oxf)* 1992;37:119–125.

86. Palmer JR, Rosenberg L, Shapiro S. Reproductive factors and risk of myocardial infarction. *Am J Epidemiol* 1992;136:408–416.

87. La Veccia C, Decarli A, Franseschi S, Gentile A, Negri E, Parzzini F. Menstrual and reproductive factors and the risk of myocardial infarction in women under fifty-five years of age. *Am J Obstet Gynecol* 1987;157:1108–12.

88. Wild RA, Grubb B, Hartz A, Van Nort JJ, Bachman W, Bartholomew M. Clinical signs of androgen excess as risk factors for coronary artery disease. *Fertil Steril* 1990;54:255–259.

13 Insulin Sensitizers Targeting Metabolic and Reproductive Consequences in Polycystic Ovary Syndrome

Evanthia Diamanti-Kandarakis, MD

Summary

The central importance of insulin resistance in the pathophysiology of polycystic ovary syndrome (PCOS) has been established by pioneering and elegant studies. In addition to the known hormonal and reproductive abnormalities that characterize this syndrome, metabolic disorders, as well as morbidities such as the enhanced risk for type 2 diabetes and increased risk for cardiovascular disease, have also been demonstrated. Current therapeutic approaches justifiably include insulin-sensitizing agents promising to comfort women with PCOS. Management with insulin sensitizers appears to embrace beneficially in a global fashion several aspects of the syndrome and target most of the associated metabolic and reproductive consequences.

Key Words: PCOS; insulin sensitizers; insulin resistance; hyperandrogenemia; metformin; thiazolidinediones; D-chiro-inositol; cardiovascular risk factors; metabolic consequences; reproductive consequences.

1. INTRODUCTION

Polycystic ovary syndrome (PCOS) is an endocrine disorder of unknown aetiology with an enigmatic pathophysiology and variable clinical presentation. This is a complex and heterogeneous disorder characterized by hyperandrogenemia, insulin resistance and chronic anovulation. PCOS is the most common endocrinopathy in women of reproductive age *(1,2)* and is associated with cosmetic, reproductive and long-term

From: *Contemporary Endocrinology: Polycystic Ovary Syndrome*
Edited by: A. Dunaif, R. J. Chang, S. Franks, and R. S. Legro © Humana Press, Totowa, NJ

metabolic abnormalities. Women with PCOS are predisposed to type 2 diabetes (T2D) mellitus and carry an increased risk for cardiovascular disease (CVD). Prospective studies in the USA revealed a 31–35% prevalence of impaired glucose tolerance (IGT) and a 7.5–10% prevalence of T2D in obese PCOS women by their fourth decade *(3,4)*.

These findings may even be present in adolescent *(5)* and in younger women with PCOS, as it has been published recently in a European cohort study from the Mediterranean region *(6)*. A prevalence of 15.7 and 2.5% IGT and T2D, respectively, was demonstrated in this population with PCOS *(6)*. Furthermore, the study has shown an increased conversion rate from normoglycaemia to IGT or to T2D over time in women with this syndrome *(7)*.

In several studies, increased cardiovascular risk factors including hyperinsulinaemia, hypertension *(8,9)* and dyslipidemia *(10)* have been repeatedly demonstrated. The metabolic syndrome has been shown to be several folds more common in the female population suffering from this enigmatic disorder compared with a well-matched normal population *(11)*; however, the prevalence appears to vary according to the nationality and the definitions of these two syndromes *(12)*.

PCOS has been intuitively described like "Syndrome XX" *(13)* to emphasize the association of PCOS with the features of metabolic syndrome. Components of metabolic syndrome such as endothelial dysfunction and low-grade chronic inflammation have been recognized in women with PCOS *((14)–16)*. Data supporting vascular bed impairment are provided by studies demonstrating the presence of endothelial dysfunction *(15–18)*, increased carotid intima media thickness *(19)* and coronary artery calcification *(20)*. Dysfibrinolysis with elevated plasma levels of plasminogen activator inhibitor-1 (PAI-1) *(21,22)* and increased markers of chronic inflammation such as C-reactive protein (CRP) *(18)* have also been found in young women with PCOS. Despite the clustering of cardiovascular risk factors, no increased prevalence of overt CVD has been documented because no prospective longitudinal studies have been conducted.

Reproductive abnormalities, such as menstrual irregularities, anovulation and early pregnancy loss, represent very often the main concern of women with PCOS. Insulin resistance and compensatory hyperinsulinaemia appear to be linked directly and/or indirectly with these reproductive consequences of the multifaceted PCOS *(23)*.

The management of PCOS was mainly symptomatic until the main role of insulin resistance was recognized and the use of insulin sensitizers led to a more aetiological approach of the syndrome. The following chapter will focus on the management of the metabolic and reproductive abnormalities with these new therapeutic tools, the insulin sensitizers. Since 1994, the use of metformin in the management of PCOS has extended our knowledge not only of the pathophysiology of PCOS but broadened therapeutic options in several ways.

However, there are several unanswered questions regarding the clinical use of these drugs. There are no specific criteria for therapeutic application of this group of medications, and there is no agreement for the most appropriate combination of the various therapeutic modalities targeting the metabolic and reproductive consequences of PCOS *(24)*.

2. INSULIN SENSITIZERS TARGETING METABOLIC CONSEQUENCES

There are two classes of insulin-sensitizing agents that have been used in clinical trials for the management of PCOS. Biguanides with metformin and thiazolinediones (TZDs) with troglitazone, and two new agents, rosiglitazone and pioglitazone, for which the data are steadily increasing.

2.1. Carbohydrate Abnormalities and Insulin Resistance

2.1.1. METFORMIN TARGETING METABOLIC CONSEQUENCES

Metformin is a biguanide agent that has been used in the treatment of T2D for several decades. It lowers blood glucose levels by reducing significantly hepatic glucose production and by increasing peripheral glucose utilization (25).

Moreover, metformin appears to enter into the cells and enhance the tyrosine phosphorylation of the intracellular portion of β-subunit of insulin receptor and insulin receptor substrate proteins (IRS) (26). Recently, it has been suggested that IRS genotype may modulate the response to metformin treatment in PCOS women (27).

A number of studies have been published investigating the effect of metformin on insulin resistance in women with PCOS (24,26–29). The first study in 1994 by Velazquez et al. (28) demonstrated that metformin treatment in 26 obese PCOS women for 2 months reduced hyperinsulinaemia, systolic blood pressure and improved hormonal and reproductive abnormalities as well. In another European study conducted in 1998, an increase in insulin sensitivity was confirmed by using the euglycemic clamp, independently of body weight changes, after administration of 1700 mg metformin for 6 months in 13 obese PCOS women (29). A reduction in fasting glucose and insulin levels after treatment with metformin have been reported in both obese and non-obese PCOS women (30,31). A meta-analysis of 13 controlled studies, in different ethnic populations, confirms that metformin has a significant effect in reducing fasting insulin levels with a small reduction of fasting glucose (32). However, in extremely obese PCOS women no beneficial results were found (33), and it has been suggested that metformin in this group of women has no detectable effect on insulin resistance. This finding has been also confirmed, recently, in a randomized, placebo-controlled, double-blind multicenter study 143 women (with BMI 38 kg/m^2) receiving metformin treatment for 6 months (34). These results suggest that severe obesity may be a confounding factor. Another contributing factor to these discrepancies may be the lack of agreement in different methods assessing insulin sensitivity, as mathematical indices do not estimate accurately the insulin resistance in relation to different degree of obesity (35).

In conclusion, metformin has been shown in most (28,29,36) but not all (33) studies to ameliorate the adverse metabolic effects of PCOS over a 2- to 6-month period of treatment. Although longitudinal data are still lacking and metformin is not approved by the US Food and Drug Administration as a primary therapeutic modality in PCOS, its use is steadily gaining grown as a long-term treatment of PCOS. Currently, more than 25 million prescriptions are written for metformin each year. According to the Scott–Levin pharmaceutical database, the diagnosis "polycystic ovaries" accounted for nearly 3% of all prescriptions written for metformin in the year ending April 2003.

That represented an increase of 265% over the prior year, and PCOS remains the most frequent diagnosis for metformin use after diabetes.

2.1.2. THIAZOLIDINEDIONES TARGETING METABOLIC CONSEQUENCES

Thiazolidinediones (TZDs) include troglitazone, rosiglitazone and pioglitazone. These drugs act by enhancing glucose uptake in adipose and muscle tissues. In comparison with metformin which principally decreases hepatic glucose output, TZDs induce a significant increase of peripheral glucose uptake. These medications improve insulin sensitivity and decrease not only circulating insulin but also free fatty acid (FFA) and tumor necrosis factor (TNF)-α release from adipose tissue *(37)*. At the cellular level, they bind and activate the peroxisome proliferator activated receptor (PPAR)-γ and induce transcription of genes involved in glucose and lipid metabolism *(37)*.

Troglitazone was the first of TZDs to become available for treatment of diabetes but was withdrawn from the market as acute liver failure was reported in several cases.

Dunaif, in 1996 *(38)*, was the first who studied the effects of troglitazone on the metabolic profile in women with PCOS. Twenty-five women with PCOS were enrolled in a double-blind randomized 3-month trial of two doses (200 and 400 mg) of troglitazone. Fasting and 2-h post-75-g glucose load insulin levels, as well as integrated insulin responses to the glucose load, decreased significantly while insulin sensitivity, as assessed by a frequently sampled intravenous glucose tolerance test (FSIVGTT), increased significantly.

Azziz et al. *(39)* in the largest prospective double-blind trial, studied four hundred and ten women with PCOS, randomly assigned in placebo or troglitazone, for 44 weeks of treatment and showed that troglitazone improved insulin resistance in PCOS in a dose-related fashion, with a minimum of adverse effects.

Rosiglitazone and pioglitazone have been shown to be effective in improving insulin sensitivity and are a promising alternative in PCOS management, since they have not been incriminated for hepatotoxicity *(40,41)*.

2.1.3. D-CHIRO-INOSITOL TARGETING METABOLIC CONSEQUENCES

Evidence suggests that some actions of insulin are mediated by inositolphosphoglycans (IPG). In PCOS women, there is a defect in tissue availability or utilization of d-chiro-inositol (DCI) that may contribute to the insulin resistance *(42)*. Therefore, administration of DCI, as another insulin-sensitising agent, has also been investigated [Nestler et al. *(43)*]. It has been shown that oral administration of DCI to women with PCOS improved glucose tolerance whereas reduced insulin levels in both obese and lean women with PCOS. The fact that the administration of metformin enhances insulin-stimulated release of DCI–IPG in PCOS women supports the role of DCI–IPG contributing to insulin resistance in the syndrome *(44)*. Currently, there are no data regarding the effect of DCI–IPG on other metabolic or cardiovascular risk factors in PCOS *(45–47)*.

2.1.4. THERAPY TARGETING ON LIPID ABNORMALITIES

Metformin Targeting Lipids.   Metformin has been shown to improve lipid profile, mainly by increasing serum HDL-cholesterol (HDL) concentrations *(48,49)*. On the contrary, other studies have shown either a negligible or no effect on lipids in women with PCOS *(28,33)*. The mechanisms by which metformin improve the lipid profile are not clear.

Metformin treatment even without body weight loss reduces visceral fat, as has been found to reduce waist-to-hip (WHR), marker for visceral obesity *(50)*, and therefore limiting the metabolically most active form of adipose tissue *(51)*.

TZDs targeting Lipids.   In a multicenter, double-blind trial *(52)* of 398 women with PCOS, a 44-week treatment with troglitazone failed to improve abnormal baseline lipid parameters. Insulin sensitivity indices had poor predictive power on lipid parameters, partially explaining the lack of beneficial effect of troglitazone on lipid profile and suggesting the implication of additional factors.

To investigate the effectiveness and safety of pioglitazone (45 mg/day) on clinical and endocrine-metabolic features of PCOS, Romualdi et al. *(40)* studied 18 obese PCOS patients, classified as normoinsulinaemic and hyperinsulinaemic. A trend towards improvement was observed in lipid assessment of both groups. Reported data suggested that there was a selective effect of pioglitazone, partially independent of insulin secretion, on the clinical and hormonal disturbances of PCOS including lipid profile. Conclusions regarding the TZDs effects on lipid or other parameters in PCOS, should been drawn for each one of the TZDs separately, because their effects appear to be mediated by different molecular pathways in various target-tissues.

2.1.5. THERAPY TARGETING ON OTHER METABOLIC CONSEQUENCES: ON CARDIOVASCULAR RISK FACTORS

Metformin Targeting Cardiovascular Risk Factors.   Abnormal vascular function has been shown in PCOS by several investigators, and the syndrome is associated with surrogate cardiovascular markers such as increased serum levels of PAI-1 *(21)*, increased endothelin-1 (ET-1) levels *(15,17)*, elevated serum levels of CRP *(53)*, elevated advanced glycation end-products serum levels (AGEs) *(54)*, endothelial dysfunction *(14,17)* and echocardiographic abnormalities *(55–57)*.

A number of mechanisms could be implicated to link endothelial dysfunction with insulin resistance, including disturbances of subcellular signaling pathways to insulin action or other potential unifying links *(58–60)*. Insulin sensitizers, therefore, have justifiably been administered in PCOS patients with these abnormalities.

In a recent study *(17)*, the administration of 1700 mg metformin daily for 6 months in PCOS women normalized endothelium-dependent vasodilatation (flow-mediated dilatation, FMD) on brachial artery (non-invasive method for endothelial function assessment) and at the same time decreased significantly ET-1 plasma levels. Metformin treatment has been associated with a significant decrease of low-grade chronic inflammatory markers, such as CRP serum concentrations. In a randomized study, Papunen et al. *(61)* demonstrated a significant reduction in serum CRP levels by 31% in non-obese subjects and by 56% in obese subjects following metformin administration. Adhesion molecules (AM) that are independent predictors of coronary heart disease and T2D *(62)* have been also reduced with 6 months of metformin therapy in 62 PCOS patients independently of body weight changes *(63)* in a study conducted by Diamanti-Kandarakis et al.

Recently, AGEs, complex and heterogeneous potent atherogenic molecules *(64)*, and their receptors (RAGE) *(54)* have been found to be elevated in young women with

PCOS. Although the mechanism implicated in this phenomenon is not clear, it could be due to insulin action defects although dietary-exogenous AGEs may also contribute to it (65). Metformin administration, for 6 months, reduced but did not normalize AGEs serum levels compared with pre-treatment levels; this effect of metformin, if confirmed, could be of clinical significance in improving adverse long-term sequelae of the syndrome (66).

TZDs Targeting Cardiovascular Risk Factors. A beneficial effect on reduction of cardiovascular risk factors has been reported also with TZDs. A decrease in PAI-1 levels (67) and an improvement in endothelial-dependent vasodilatation (68) have been observed. Three months treatment with troglitazone restored to control levels endothelium-dependent vasodilation as assessed by an invasive plethysmographic method.

2.1.6. COMBINED STUDIES: COMBINED TREATMENT TARGETING METABOLIC DEFECTS

Metformin and Life Style Modification. The combination of metformin with lifestyle modification has been advocated clinically as a more effective way compared with one drug administration in the management of several aspects of the syndrome, however long-term studies are lacking.

In a recent randomized, 48-week, placebo-controlled trial by Hoeger (69), thirty-eight overweight or obese women with PCOS were randomly assigned to one of the four following groups: metformin, lifestyle modification with placebo, lifestyle modification with metformin, or placebo only. Weight reduction seemed to be enhanced in the guided lifestyle intervention group when metformin was added. Approximately, a 30% weight loss was found in the combined group compared with that in the lifestyle modification group alone. Regarding glucose metabolism, however, either improvement or no deterioration in overall glucose metabolism was noted in all the subjects completing the treatment arms, whereas a deterioration of glucose status occurred in two subjects in the placebo group. This is one of the longest studies of combined therapy of modification in life style and metformin in PCOS women, showing clearly that the combination is a more promising approach in the management of metabolic aspects of the syndrome.

These findings have not been confirmed by a more recent randomized, placebo-controlled, double-blind multicenter study, in which metformin did not enhance weight loss, neither menstrual frequency was improved in severely obese patients with PCOS. This is probably explained by the extreme obesity of patients in the study and the relatively small amount of weight loss (34).

TZDs and Metformin. Studies that compare metformin with TZDs treatment have been conducted and a summary of them is demonstrated in Table 1.

In a recent study, pioglitazone has been compared with metformin in obese PCOS women (70), and it has been shown that pioglitazone is as effective as metformin in improving insulin sensitivity and hyperandrogenemia despite an increase in weight and WHR.

Table 1
Studies comparing metformin with thiazolidinediones

Authors	Nb of PCOS patients	Duration	Medication	BMI	W/H	hirsu-tism	testo levels	Δ₄A levels	menst cycle	ovula-tion	insulin levels	insulin sensi-tivity	Hcy	LDL	HDL	trigly-cerides	Blood pressure
Ortega-Gonzalez et al (2005)	35 Obese	6 months	metf (2250 mg)	↑	↑	↓	↓	↓		↑	↓	↑		↑	↑	↓	
			piogl (30 mg)	↓	↓	↓	↓	↓		↑	↓	↑		↑	↑	↑	
Kilicdag et al (2005)	30 Obese	3 months	metf (1700 mg)	↑								↑	↑	↑	↑	↑	
			rosigl (4 mg)	↑								↑	↑	→	→	↑	
			metf + rosigl														
Baill-argeon et al (2004)	100 non obese normo-insuli-nemic	6 months	metf (850 mg)	↑	→		→		↑	↑	→	↑					→
			rosigl (4 mg)	↓	→		→		↑	↑	↑	↑					→
			metf + rosigl	↑	→		→		↑	↑	→	↑					→
Glueck et al (2003b)	39 Obese (26 resp 13 non resp)	12 months	metf resp (2250 mg)	↓ (wei-ght)			↑	↑	↑		→	↑			↑		→
			metf non-resp	↑			↑	↑	↑		→	↑			↑		↑
		12 months + 10 months	metf non-resp + piogl (45 mg)	↑			↑	↑	↑		→	↑			↓		↑

→: no significant change, ↓: significant decrease, ↑: significant increase
metf: metformin, **piogl:** pioglitazone, **rosigl:** rosiglitazone **resp:** women responders to metformin treatment
non resp: women non responders to metformin treatment **Hcy:** homocystein levels

Interestingly, in women resistant to metformin when pioglitazone was added in a combined therapy, an improvement in insulin resistance and glucose utilization *(71)* was observed.

The combination of both medications may be adding complementary benefits without antagonizing effects, noticeable side effects or changes in safety parameters.

Insulin Sensitizers and Oral Contraceptives. Few studies have evaluated insulin sensitizers in combination with oral contraceptives and/or anti-androgens in insulin-resistant women with PCOS, demonstrating complementary beneficial effects on endocrine and metabolic abnormalities as well as on signs of hyperandrogenism *(72–76)* (Table 2).

2.2. Conclusion

The majority of controlled and uncontrolled studies in different ethnic groups agree that metformin has beneficial effects on insulin resistance and on several cardiovascular risk factors in PCOS, regardless of changes in body weight. The effects of metformin, however, are not present in every woman with the syndrome, and furthermore, there are not known as yet predicting factors of its response. Additionally, the documentation of insulin resistance by different methods does not appear to be a prerequisite for the response to metformin treatment in PCOS. This may be due to the lack of sensitive methods for the detection of insulin resistance *(34)* and because there is evidence that metformin acts via several pathways besides insulin action.

Large long-term trials are needed to confirm the beneficial effects of TZDs on the metabolic abnormalities in PCOS. However, there are two major limitations in using these agents. One is regarding weight gain, which is undesirable in already obese PCOS women, and the second one is that they are pregnancy category C drugs. This potential embryotoxicity would limit their use in women who desire pregnancy. Therefore, TZDs could be used as a second line treatment for management of PCOS, whereas regular monitoring of liver enzyme is required.

3. INSULIN SENSITIZERS AND REPRODUCTIVE CONSEQUENCES

One of the major steps in the management of PCOS, according to accumulating evidence, was the effectiveness of insulin sensitizers and in particular metformin in improving almost all aspects of the reproductive abnormalities observed in the syndrome.

3.1. Metformin

3.1.1. METFORMIN: ON MENSTRUAL CYCLE ABNORMALITIES

The effect of metformin therapy on menstrual cyclicity has been extensively investigated. A significant improvement in menstrual cycle frequency has been reported after metformin administration. Velazquez et al. *(77)* evaluated the effect on menstrual regulation after 6 months treatment in 22 women with PCOS. At the end of this therapy, 21 of 22 women observed an improvement in menstrual frequency with 86% of ovulatory cycles, as assessed by progesterone measurement. In a well-designed double-blind study by Moghetti et al. *(48)*, a small group of PCOS patients was

Table 2
Studies concerning combination of treatments with OCPs

Authors	Nb of PCOS patients	Duration	Medication	BMI	W/H	fat mass	abdominal mass	hirsutism	testo levels	SHBG	insulin sensitivity	IL-6	adiponectine	LDL	HDL	triglycerides
Elter et al (2002)	40 non-obese	4 months	OCP (EE-CA)	↑	↑			↓	↓	↑	↑			↑	↑	↑
			OCP + metf	↓	→			↓	↓	↑	↓			↑	↑	↑
Ibanez et al (2003b)	24 non-obese	3 months	OCP (EE-G)	↑		↑	↑		↓	↑	↑			↑	↓	↑
			OCP + metf + flut (62.5 mg)	↑		→	↑		↓	↑	↑			→	↓	↑
Ibanez et al (2004c)	22 non-obese	9 months	OCP (EE- Dr)	↑		↓	↓	↓	↓	↑	↑	↑	↑	↑	↓	↓
			OCP + metf + flut (62.5 mg)	↑		→	→	↓	↓	↑	↑	→	↓	→	↓	↓
Cibula et al (2005)	28 non-obese	6 months	OCP	↑				↓	↓	↑	↑			↓	↓	↓
			OCP + metf	↑				↓	↓	↑	↑			↑	↓	↑
Mitkov et al (2005)	30 obese	6 months	metf	↑	↑				↓	↓	↓			↑	↑	↑
			metf + OCP (EE- CA)	↑	↑				↓	↓	↓			↑	↑	↑

→: no significant change, ↓: significant decrease, ↑: significant increase
SHBG: sex hormone binding globulin, **IL-6:** interleukin 6
metf: metformin, **flut:** flutamide, **EE:** ethinyl estradiol, **CA:** cyproterone acetate, **G:** gestodene, **Dr:** Drospirenone

randomly assigned to metformin or placebo for 6 months, and the mean frequency of menstrual cycles increased in about 50% of subjects. One of the first questions arising with metformin administration was the variable therapeutic response among different group of PCOS patients even in the same cohorts. To answer this question, the above-mentioned Italian group of investigators divided their patients into "responders" and "no responders" with regard to regulation of their menstruation. Higher Body Mass Index (BMI) index and insulin plasma levels, lower serum androstenedione levels, and less-severe menstrual abnormalities were baseline predictors of clinical efficacy measured by improved menstrual cyclicity. However, in a large randomized study by Fleming et al., subgroup analysis (50) revealed that BMI and insulin concentrations did not predict the ability to establish normal ovarian function, but high SHBG concentrations and lower free-androgen index did. The heterogeneity of the syndrome could be one of the more likely explanations for these variable responses in PCOS women; therefore, the selection criteria for metformin administration have not been established yet. Several other uncontrolled studies have confirmed the effectiveness of metformin in regulation of menstrual cycles supporting its clinical use in these reproductive abnormalities (29,78–82).

3.1.2. Metformin: on Ovulation

The effect of metformin on anovulation was first assessed in a randomized and placebo-controlled trial in response to metformin in an unselected group of women with PCOS. Thirty-four percent ovulated spontaneously compared with (4%) given placebo (35).

Furthermore, it was shown that the interval from start of first ovulation is shorter with metformin than with placebo (30,35,48,50,81,83,84). Interestingly, in several studies, ovulation rate increased with no change in weight, suggesting that metformin effect is independent of weight loss (29,35,48,80,81).

Another group of patients, who seem to benefit from metformin treatment are those with "clomiphene resistant". In the pre-metformin era, the only therapeutic alternative for this group of PCOS patients was gonadotropin therapy for ovulation with the risk of hyperstimulation syndrome. Metformin as an adjuvant therapy to clomiphene, resulted in a more than tenfold increase in ovulation rate (35). A randomized, double-blind, placebo-controlled trial confirmed these results (85). Therefore, metformin alone and later in combination with clomiphene has been proposed as sequential treatment-programme prior gonadotropin therapy use for ovulation induction in infertile women with PCOS (46,86). The addition of metformin has been followed by recruitment of fewer follicles and by lower estradiol levels resulting in a lower risk for multiple pregnancies (87). This therapeutic approach is also less expensive. The combination of clomiphene with metformin could be of particular clinical utility in obese and insulin resistant patients who often exhibit resistance to clomiphene treatment (88).

In patients undergoing in vitro fertilization, metformin administration may contribute to higher rates of fertilization and of successful pregnancies (89). However, Yarali et al., in a randomized placebo-controlled trial of metformin with follicle-stimulating hormone (FSH) in clomiphene-resistant PCOS patients, found that ovulation and pregnancy rates between metformin and placebo group did not differ (90). Although this study suggests that metformin does not influence FSH-induced ovulation, it was limited by a rather small sample size. Further research in this area is needed before making recommendations favoring adjuvant use of metformin with gonadotropin ovulation induction.

3.1.3. METFORMIN AND PREGNANCY

Metformin is the only insulin sensitizer, which has been characterized as a category B agent *(86,91)*. Two retrospective studies *(92,93)* of metformin treatment through the first trimester reported reduced rates of pregnancy loss, although another prospective study did not confirm this result *(94)*. From the current literature no conclusion can be drawn regarding the indication of metformin during pregnancy, and the health providers should handle this issue with the appropriate caution.

Nevertheless, recent experimental data support the beneficial role of metformin in the implantation and intrauterine environment. In PCOS patients treated with metformin, serum glycodelin, a protein, which inhibits endometrial immune response to the embryo *(95)*, is increased several folds compared with placebo *(96)*. In support of the beneficial role in intrauterine environment is the reduction of the resistance index of uterine spiral arteries after metformin treatment, which favors embryo implant and maintenance of pregnancy *(97)*. These data if confirmed with future studies could justify the appropriate timing and duration of metformin treatment during pregnancy. Another major fertility problem is the increased early pregnancy loss rate occurring in these patients. Metformin administration has been associated with an 8.8% early pregnancy loss as compared with 41.9% in the non-treated PCOS women *(93)*; these data have been confirmed in several trials *(29,80,89)*. Decreased PAI activity levels and improvement of impaired fibrinolysis *(98)* post-metformin may play a role to reduce miscarriage rate *(93)*.

Another indication about a possible effect of metformin in follicle maturation process is that its administration in PCOS women results in decreased serum anti-müllerian hormone (AMH) müllerian hormone (AMH) levels *(99)*.

In a recent prospective study *(100)*, it was observed that metformin administration during pregnancy was associated with a tenfold reduction in gestational diabetes (GD). GD developed in 3% women on metformin therapy, as compared with 31% of untreated/placebo-treated women. A significant reduction in body weight in women taking metformin was observed before conception but no BMI changes occurred during pregnancy. However, body weight loss before pregnancy and caloric restriction during pregnancy may have contributed largely to reduced development of GD, confounding the interpretation of these data.

3.2. TZDs: Menstrual Cycle, Ovulation, Ovulation Induction, and Pregnancy

TZDs belong to class C pregnancy drugs, limiting their use as fertility agents. The best data on the effects of troglitazone administration on reproductive function in PCOS come from the multicenter study of PCOS/troglitazone *(101)*. It has been found that the mean rate of ovulation increased in a dose-related fashion in the treatment group compared with that in the placebo group. Interestingly, patients in the highest dose treatment group had 60% ovulation rate and about 5% achieved pregnancy in comparison with placebo *(101)*. Others studies have also confirmed these findings *(38,101–103)*. In clomiphene-resistant patients, troglitazone has also improved menstrual cyclicity and ovulation rate *(102,103)*.

Rosiglitazone compared with metformin administration resulted in a higher rate of menstrual cycles *(104)* and ovulation rate *(105)*. In a prospective uncontrolled study of 24 obese women with PCOS treated with rosiglitazone for 3 months, menstrual cycles were restored in 95% of patients *(106)*.

More recently, Sepilian et al. *(107)* studied 12 obese PCOS patients with BMI > 40 treated with rosiglitazone for 6 months showed spontaneous menstruation in 91% (11 of 12) of patients. In a randomized control trial, rosiglitazone was combined with clomiphene resulting in increased ovulation rate *(108)*. These studies indicate that rosiglitazone is effective in inducing spontaneous ovulation in obese PCOS patients, a group of patients who appear to be less responsive to the combination with metformin. However, no randomized control trial comparing rosiglitazone to metformin in this population has been performed.

Pioglitazone is the most recent TZDs agent, and studies are very limited at the present time. One randomized controlled trial comparing pioglitazone with placebo in 35 women with PCOS, for 3 months, showed that 41% of women on pioglitazone experienced normalization of menstrual cycles and increased ovulation rate compared with the placebo group *(109)*. Interestingly, the combination of metformin with piogli-tazone appears to be more effective than metformin alone *(110)*.

In conclusion, TZDs appear to have a clinical application in improving ovulation and fertility in PCOS patients, but as they are considered class C pregnancy drugs, should be considered with the appropriate caution in patients who desire pregnancy.

3.3. DCI: Ovulation

In a study conducted by Nestler et al. *(111)*, 19 from 22 (86%) women with PCOS who received DCI for 6–8 weeks ovulated during treatment as compared with only 6 of the 22 women (27%) in the placebo group, implying its beneficial role in ovulatory function. However, these data have to be confirmed with large and long-term studies.

3.4. Conclusions

In PCOS women, the medical management remains a very complex issue because a single therapy for all aspects of the syndrome is not established.

It is indispensable to assess carefully predominant symptoms and risk factors in metabolic and reproductive profile of each woman and consequently individualize the treatment. Based on the pathophysiological role of insulin resistance, by improving insulin sensitivity, an improvement in several interlinked metabolic abnormalities is expected. Insulin-sensitizing agents seem to be a promising therapy.

Metformin could be the treatment of choice in hyperinsulinaemic obese or non-obese women, particularly when they desire pregnancy. Short prospective studies with TZDs either alone or combined with metformin appear to be equally effective. However, large randomized controlled studies are needed to ascertain their safety and efficacy in reducing long-term metabolic aberrations.

One of the major difficulties in medical management of PCOS is that there are not specific diagnostic signs or characteristic phenotypes, which could preclude the response to different therapeutic modalities.

REFERENCES

1. Diamanti-Kandarakis E, Kouli CR, Bergiele AT, Filandra FA, Tsianateli TC, Spina GG, Zapanti ED, Bartzis MI. A survey of the polycystic ovary syndrome in the Greek island of Lesbos: hormonal and metabolic profile. *J Clin Endocrinol Metab* 1999; 84:4006–4011.

2. Asuncion M, Calvo RM, San Millan JL, Sancho J, Avila S, Escobar-Morreale HF. A prospective study of the prevalence of the polycystic ovary syndrome in unselected Caucasian women from Spain. *J Clin Endocrinol Metab* 2000; 85:2434–2438.

3. Legro RS, Kunselman AR, Dodson WC, Dunaif A. Prevalence and predictors of risk for type 2 diabetes mellitus and impaired glucose tolerance in polycystic ovary syndrome: a prospective, controlled study in 254 affected women. *J Clin Endocrinol Metab* 1999; 84:165–169.

4. Ehrmann DA, Barnes RB, Rosenfield RL, Cavaghan MK, Imperial J. Prevalence of impaired glucose tolerance and diabetes in women with polycystic ovary syndrome. *Diabetes Care* 1999; 22:141–146.

5. Palmert MR, Gordon CM, Kartashov AI, Legro RS, Emans SJ, Dunaif A. Screening for abnormal glucose tolerance in adolescents with polycystic ovary syndrome. *J Clin Endocrinol Metab* 2002; 87:1017–1023.

6. Gambineri A, Pelusi C, Manicardi E, Vicennati V, Cacciari M, Morselli-Labate AM, Pagotto U, Pasquali R. Glucose intolerance in a large cohort of mediterranean women with polycystic ovary syndrome: phenotype and associated factors. *Diabetes* 2004; 53:2353–2358.

7. Norman RJ, Masters L, Milner CR, Wang JX, Davies MJ. Relative risk of conversion from normo-glycaemia to impaired glucose tolerance or non-insulin dependent diabetes mellitus in polycystic ovarian syndrome. *Hum Reprod* 2001; 16:1995–1998.

8. Dahlgren E, Janson PO, Johansson S, Lapidus L, Oden A. Polycystic ovary syndrome and risk for myocardial infarction. Evaluated from a risk factor model based on a prospective population study of women. *Acta Obstet Gynecol Scand* 1992; 71:599–604.

9. Wild S, Pierpoint T, McKeigue P, Jacobs H. Cardiovascular disease in women with polycystic ovary syndrome at long-term follow-up: a retrospective cohort study. *Clin Endocrinol (Oxf)* 2000; 52:595–600.

10. Legro RS, Kunselman AR, Dunaif A. Prevalence and predictors of dyslipidemia in women with polycystic ovary syndrome. *Am J Med* 2001; 111:607–613.

11. Apridonidze T, Essah PA, Iuorno MJ, Nestler JE. Prevalaence and characteristics of the metabolic syndrome in women with polycystic ovary syndrome. *J Clin Endocrinol Metab* 2005; 90:1929–1935.

12. Carmina E, Napoli N, Longo RA, Rini GB, Lobo RA. Metabolic syndrome in polycystic ovary syndrome (PCOS): lower prevalence in southern Italy than in the USA and the influence of criteria for the diagnosis of PCOS. *Eur J Endocrinol* 2006; 154:141–145.

13. Sam S, Dunaif A. Polycystic ovary syndrome: syndrome XX? *Trends Endocrinol Metab* 2003; 14:365–370.

14. Paradisi G, Steinberg HO, Hempfling A, Cronin J, Hook G, Shepard MK, Baron AD. Polycystic ovary syndrome is associated with endothelial dysfunction. *Circulation* 2001; 103:1410–1415.

15. Diamanti-Kandarakis E, Spina G, Kouli C, Migdalis I. Increased endothelin-1 levels in women with polycystic ovary syndrome and the beneficial effect of metformin therapy. *J Clin Endocrinol Metab* 2001; 86:4666–4673.

16. Kelly CJ, Speirs A, Gould GW, Petrie JR, Lyall H, Connell JM. Altered vascular function in young women with polycystic ovary syndrome. *J Clin Endocrinol Metab* 2002; 87:742–746.

17. Diamanti-Kandarakis E, Alexandraki K, Protogerou A, Piperi C, Papamichael C, Aessopos A, Lekakis J, Mavrikakis M. Metformin administration improves endothelial function in women with polycystic ovary syndrome. *Eur J Endocrinol* 2005; 152:749–756.

18. Kelly C, Lyall H, Petrie JR, Gould GW, Connell JM, Sattar N. Low grade chronic inflammation in women with polycystic ovarian syndrome. *J Clin Endocrinol Metab* 2001; 8:2453–2455.

19. Talbott EO, Guzick DS, Sutton-Tyrrell K, McHugh-Pemu KP, Zborowski JV, Remsberg KE, Kuller LH. Evidence for association between polycystic ovary syndrome and premature carotid atherosclerosis in middle-aged women. *Arterioscler Thromb Vasc Biol* 2000; 20(11):2414–2421.

20. Christian RC, Dumesic DA, Behrenbeck T, Oberg AL, Sheedy PF 2nd, Fitzpatrick LA. Prevalence and predictors of coronary artery calcification in women with polycystic ovary syndrome. *J Clin Endocrinol Metab* 2003; 88:2562–2568.

21. Kelly C, Lyall H, Petrie JR, Gould GW, Connell JM, Rumley A, Lowe GD, Sattar N. A specific elevation in tissue plasminogen activator antigen in women with polycystic ovarian syndrome. *J Clin Endocrinol Metab* 2002; 87:3287–3290.

22. Diamanti-Kandarakis E, Palioniko G, Alexandraki K, Bergiele A, Koutsouba T, Bartzis M. The prevalence of 4G5G polymorphism of plasminogen activator inhibitor-1 (PAI-1) gene in polycystic ovarian syndrome and its association with plasma PAI-1 levels. *Eur J Endocrinol* 2004; 150:793–798.

23. Dunaif A. Insulin resistance and the polycystic ovary syndrome: mechanism and implications for pathogenesis. *Endocr Rev* 1997; 18:774–800.

24. Baillargeon JP, Jakubowicz DJ, Iuorno MJ, et al. Effects of metformin and rosiglitazone, alone and in combination, in nonobese women with polycystic ovary syndrome and normal indices of insulin sensitivity. *Fertil Steril* 2004; 82:893–902.

25. Marena S, Tagliaferro V, Montegrosso G, Pagano A, Scaglione L, Pagano G. Metabolic effects of metformin addition to chronic glibenclamide treatment in type 2 diabetes. *Diabetes Metab* 1994; 20:15–19.

26. Wiernsperger NF, Bailey CJ. The antihyperglycaemic effect of metformin: therapeutic and cellular mechanisms. *Drugs* 1999; 58 Suppl 1:31–39.

27. Ertunc D, Tok EC, Aktas A, Erdal EM, Dilek S. The importance of IRS-1 Gly972Arg polymorphism in evaluating the response to metformin treatment in polycystic ovary syndrome. *Hum Reprod* 2005; 20:1207–1212.

28. Velazquez EM, Mendoza S, Hamer T, Sosa F, Glueck CJ. Metformin therapy in polycystic ovary syndrome reduces hyperinsulinemia, insulin resistance, hyperandrogenemia, and systolic blood pressure, while facilitating normal menses and pregnancy. *Metabolism* 1994; 43:647–654.

29. Diamanti-Kandarakis E, Kouli C, Tsianateli T, Bergiele A. Therapeutic effects of metformin on insulin resistance and hyperandrogenism in polycystic ovary syndrome. *Eur J Endocrinol* 1998; 138:269–274.

30. Morin-Papunen LC, Vauhkonen I, Koivunen RM, Ruokonen A, Martikainen HK, Tapanainen JS. Endocrine and metabolic effects of metformin versus ethinyl estradiol-cyproterone acetate in obese women with polycystic ovary syndrome: a randomized study. *J Clin Endocrinol Metab* 2000; 85:3161–3168.

31. Maciel GA, Soares Junior JM, Alves da Motta EL, Abi Haidar M, de Lima GR, Baracat EC. Nonobese women with polycystic ovary syndrome respond better than obese women to treatment with metformin. *Fertil Steril* 2004; 81:355–360.

32. Lord JM, Flight IH, Norman RJ. Metformin in polycystic ovary syndrome: systematic review and meta-analysis. *BMJ* 2003; 327:951–953.

33. Ehrmann DA, Cavaghan MK, Imperial J, Sturis J, Rosenfield RL, Polonsky KS. Effects of metformin on insulin secretion, insulin action, and ovarian steroidogenesis in women with polycystic ovary syndrome. *J Clin Endocrinol Metab* 1997; 82:524–530.

34. Tang T, Glanville J, Hayden CJ, White D, Barth JH, Balen AH. Combined lifestyle modification and metformin in obese patients with polycystic ovary syndrome. A randomized, placebo-controlled, double-blind multicentre study. *Hum Reprod* 2006; 21:80–89.

35. Diamanti-Kandarakis E, Kouli C, Alexandraki K, Spina G. Failure of mathematical indices to accurately assess insulin resistance in lean, overweight, or obese women with polycystic ovary syndrome. *J Clin Endocrinol Metab* 2004; 89:1273–1276.

36. Nestler JE, Jakubowicz DJ, Evans WS, Pasquali R. Effects of metformin on spontaneous and clomiphene-induced ovulation in the polycystic ovary syndrome. *N Engl J Med* 1998; 338: 1876–1880.

37. Yki-Jarvinen H. Thiazolidinediones. *N Engl J Med* 2004; 351:1106–1118.

38. Dunaif A, Scott D, Finegood D, Quintana B, Whitcomb R. The insulin-sensitizing agent troglitazone improves metabolic and reproductive abnormalities in the polycystic ovary syndrome. *J Clin Endocrinol Metab* 1996; 81:3299–3306.

39. Azziz R, Ehrmann D, Legro RS, Whitcomb RW, Hanley R, Fereshetian AG, O'Keefe M, Ghazzi MN. PCOS/Troglitazone Study Group. Troglitazone improves ovulation and hirsutism in the polycystic ovary syndrome: a multicenter, double blind, placebo-controlled trial. *J Clin Endocrinol Metab* 2001; 86:1626–1632.

40. Romualdi D, Guido M, Ciampelli M, Giuliani M, Leoni F, Perri C, Lanzone A. Selective effects of pioglitazone on insulin and androgen abnormalities in normo- and hyperinsulinaemic obese patients with polycystic ovary syndrome. *Hum Reprod* 2003; 18:1210–1218.

41. Garmes HM, Tambascia MA, Zantut-Wittmann DE. Endocrine-metabolic effects of the treatment with pioglitazone in obese patients with polycystic ovary syndrome. *Gynecol Endocrinol* 2005; 21:317–323.

42. Baillargeon JP, Diamanti-Kandarakis E, Ostlund R Jr, Apridonidze T, Iuorno M, Nestler JE. Altered D-Chiroinositol urinary clearance in women with polycystic ovary syndrome. *Diabetes Care* 2006; 29(2):300–305.

43. Nestler JE, Jakubowicz DJ, Reamer P, Gunn RD, Allan G. Ovulatory and metabolic effects of D-chiro-inositol in the polycystic ovary syndrome. *N Engl J Med* 1999; 340:1314–1320.

44. Baillargeon JP, Iuorno MJ, Jakubowicz DJ, Apridonidze T, He N, Nestler JE. Metformin therapy increases insulin-stimulated release of D-chiro-inositol-containing inositolphosphoglycan mediator in women with polycystic ovary syndrome. *J Clin Endocrinol Metab* 2004; 89:242–249.

45. de Leo V, La Marca A, Petraglia F. Insulin-lowering agents in the management of polycystic ovary syndrome. *Endocr Rev* 2003; 24:633–667.

46. Nestler JE, Stovall D, Akhter N, Iuorno MJ, Jakubowicz DJ. Strategies for the use of insulin-sensitizing drugs to treat infertility in women with polycystic ovary syndrome. *Fertil Steril* 2002; 77:209–215.

47. Kashyap S, Wells G, Rosenwaks Z. Insulin-sensitizing agents as primary therapy for patients with polycystic ovarian syndrome. *Hum Reprod* 2004; 19:2474–2483.

48. Moghetti P, Castello R, Negri C, Tosi F, Perrone F, Caputo M, Zanolin E, Muggeo M. Metformin effects on clinical features, endocrine and metabolic profiles, and insulin sensitivity in polycystic ovary syndrome: a randomized, double-blind, placebo-controlled 6-month trial, followed by open, long-term clinical evaluation. *J Clin Endocrinol Metab* 2000; 85:139–146.

49. Rautio K, Tapanainen JS, Ruokonen A, Morin-Papunen LC. Effects of metformin and ethinyl estradiol-cyproterone acetate on lipid levels in obese and non-obese women with polycystic ovary syndrome. *Eur J Endocrinol* 2005; 152(2):269–275.

50. Pasquali R, Gambineri A, Biscotti D, Vicennati V, Gagliardi L, Colitta D, Fiorini S, Cognigni GE, Filicori M, Morselli-Labate AM. Effect of long-term treatment with metformin added to hypocaloric diet on body composition, fat distribution, and androgen and insulin levels in abdominally obese women with and without the polycystic ovary syndrome. *J Clin Endocrinol Metab* 2000; 85: 2767–2774.

51. Eisenhardt S, Schwarzmann N, Henschel V, Germeyer A, von Wolff M, Hamann A, Strowitzki T. Early effects of metformin in women with polycystic ovary syndrome (PCOS): A Prospective Randomized Double-Blind Placebo-Controlled Trial. *J Clin Endocrinol Metab* 2005 [Epub ahead of print].

52. Legro RS, Azziz R, Ehrmann D, Fereshetian AG, O'Keefe M, Ghazzi MN. Minimal response of circulating lipids in women with polycystic ovary syndrome to improvement in insulin sensitivity with troglitazone. *J Clin Endocrinol Metab* 2003; 88:5137–5144.

53. Boulman N, Levy Y, Leiba R, Shachar S, Linn R, Zinder O, Blumenfeld Z. Increased C-reactive protein levels in the polycystic ovary syndrome: a marker of cardiovascular disease. *J Clin Endocrinol Metab* 2004; 89:2160–2165.

54. Diamanti-Kandarakis E, Piperi C, Kalofoutis A, Creatsas G. Increased levels of serum advanced glycation end-products in women with polycystic ovary syndrome. *Clin Endocrinol (Oxf)* 2005; 62:37–43.

55. Prelevic GM, Beljic T, Balint-Peric L, Ginsburg J. Cardiac flow velocity in women with the polycystic ovary syndrome. *Clin Endocrinol (Oxf)* 1995; 43:677–681.

56. Tiras MB, Yalcin R, Noyan V, Maral I, Yildirim M, Dortlemez O, Daya S. Alterations in cardiac flow parameters in patients with polycystic ovarian syndrome. *Hum Reprod* 1999; 14: 1949–1952.

57. Yarali H, Yildirir A, Aybar F, Kabakci G, Bukulmez O, Akgul E, Oto A. Diastolic dysfunction and increased serum homocysteine concentrations may contribute to increased cardiovascular risk in patients with polycystic ovary syndrome. *Fertil Steril* 2001; 76:511–516.

58. Wheatcroft SB, Williams IL, Shah AM, Kearney MT. Pathophysiological implications of insulin resistance on vascular endothelial function. *Diabet Med* 2003; 20:255–268.

59. Jiang ZY, Zhou QL, Chatterjee A, Feener EP, Myers MG Jr, White MF, King GL. Endothelin-1 modulates insulin signaling through phosphatidylinositol 3-kinase pathway in vascular smooth muscle cells. *Diabetes* 1999; 48:1120–1130.

60. Harrison DG. Cellular and molecular mechanisms of endothelial cell dysfunction. *J Clin Invest* 1997; 100:2153–2215.

61. Morin-Papunen L, Rautio K, Ruokonen A, Hedberg P, Puukka M, Tapanainen JS. Metformin reduces serum C-reactive protein levels in women with polycystic ovary syndrome. *J Clin Endocrinol Metab* 2003; 88:4649–4654.

62. Roldan V, Marin F, Lip GY, Blann AD. Soluble E-selectin in cardiovascular disease and its risk factor. A review of the literature. *Thromb Haemost* 2003; 90:1007–1020.

63. Diamanti-Kandarakis E, Paterakis T, Alexandraki K, Piperi C, Aessopos A, Katsikis I, Katsilambros N, Kreatsas G, Panidis D. Indices of low-grade chronic inflammation in polycystic ovary syndrome and the beneficial effect of metformin. *Hum Reprod* 2006 [Epub ahead of print].

64. Vlassara H, Bucala R, Striker L. Pathogenic effects of advanced glycosylation: biochemical, biologic, and clinical implications for diabetes and aging. *Lab Invest* 1994; 70:138–151.

65. Diamanti-Kandarakis E, Piperi C, Alexandraki K, Katsilambros N, Kouroupi E, Papailiou J, Lazaridis S, Koulouri E, Kandarakis HA, Douzinas EE, Creatsas G, Kalofoutis A. Short-term effect of orlistat on dietary glycotoxins in healthy women and women with polycystic ovary syndrome. *Metabolism* 2006; 55:494–500.

66. Diamanti-Kandarakis E, Alexandraki K, Piperi C, Aessopos A, Paterakis T, Katsikis I, Panidis D. Effect of metformin administration on plasma advanced glycation end products levels in women with polycystic ovary syndrome. *Metabolism* 2007 Jan; 56(1):129–134.

67. Ehrmann DA, Schneider DJ, Sobel BE, Cavaghan MK, Imperial J, Rosenfield RL, Polonsky KS. Troglitazone improves defects in insulin action, insulin secretion, ovarian steroidogenesis, and fibrinolysis in women with polycystic ovary syndrome. *J Clin Endocrinol Metab* 1997; 82: 2108–2116.

68. Paradisi G, Steinberg HO, Shepard MK, Hook G, Baron AD. Troglitazone therapy improves endothelial function to near normal levels in women with polycystic ovary syndrome. *J Clin Endocrinol Metab* 2003; 88:576–580.

69. Hoeger KM, Kochman L, Wixom N, Craig K, Miller RK, Guzick DS. A randomized, 48-week, placebo-controlled trial of intensive lifestyle modification and/or metformin therapy in overweight women with polycystic ovary syndrome: a pilot study. *Fertil Steril* 2004; 82:421–429.

70. Ortega-Gonzalez C, Luna S, Hernandez L, Crespo G, Aguayo P, Arteaga-Troncoso G, Parra A. Responses of serum androgen and insulin resistance to metformin and pioglitazone in obese, insulin-resistant women with polycystic ovary syndrome. *J Clin Endocrinol Metab* 2005; 90:1360–1365.

71. Glueck CJ, Moreira A, Goldenberg N, Sieve L, Wang P. Pioglitazone and metformin in obese women with polycystic ovary syndrome not optimally responsive to metformin. *Hum Reprod* 2003; 18:1618–1625.

72. Lemay A, Dodin S, Turcot L, Dechene F, Forest JC. Rosiglitazone and ethinyl estradiol/cyproterone acetate as single and combined treatment of overweight women with polycystic ovary syndrome and insulin resistance. *Hum Reprod* 2006; 21:121–128.

73. Lv L, Liu Y, Sun Y, Tan K. Effects of metformin combined with cyproterone acetate on clinical features, endocrine and metabolism of non-obese women with polycystic ovarian syndrome. *J Huazhong Univ Sci Technolog Med Sci* 2005; 25:194–197.

74. Mitkov M, Pehlivanov B, Terzieva D. Combined use of metformin and ethinyl estradiol-cyproterone acetate in polycystic ovary syndrome. *Eur J Obstet Gynecol Reprod Biol* 2005; 118:209–213.

75. Ibanez L, De Zegher F. Flutamide-metformin plus an oral contraceptive (OC) for young women with polycystic ovary syndrome: switch from third- to fourth-generation OC reduces body adiposity. *Hum Reprod* 2004; 19(8):1725–1727.

76. Ibanez L, de Zegher F. Low-dose combination of flutamide, metformin and an oral contraceptive for non-obese, young women with polycystic ovary syndrome. *Hum Reprod* 2003; 18:57–60.

77. Velazquez E, Acosta A, Mendoza SG. Menstrual cyclicity after metformin therapy in polycystic ovary syndrome. *Obstet Gynecol* 1997; 90:392–395.

78. Ibanez L, Valls C, Potau N, Marcos MV, de Zegher F. Sensitization to insulin in adolescent girls to normalize hirsutism, hyperandrogenism, oligomenorrhea, dyslipidemia, and hyperinsulinism after precocious pubarche. *J Clin Endocrinol Metab* 2000; 85: 3526–3530.

79. Pirwany IR, Yates RW, Cameron IT, Fleming R. Effects of the insulin sensitizing drug metformin on ovarian function, follicular growth and ovulation rate in obese women with oligomenorrhoea. *Hum Reprod* 1999; 14:2963–2968.

80. Morin-Papunen LC, Koivunen RM, Ruokonen A, Martikainen HK. Metformin therapy improves the menstrual pattern with minimal endocrine and metabolic effects in women with polycystic ovary syndrome. *Fertil Steril* 1998; 69:691–696.

81. Glueck CJ, Wang P, Fontaine R, Tracy T, Sieve-Smith L. Metformin-induced resumption of normal menses in 39 of 43 (91%) previously amenorrheic women with the polycystic ovary syndrome. *Metabolism* 1999; 48:511–519.

82. Glueck CJ, Wang P, Fontaine R, Tracy T, Sieve-Smith L. Metformin to restore normal menses in oligo-amenorrheic teenage girls with polycystic ovary syndrome (PCOS). *J Adolesc Health* 2001; 29:160–169.

83. Fleming R, Hopkinson ZE, Wallace M, Greer IA, Sattar N. Ovarian function and metabolic factors in women with oligomenorrhea treated with metformin in a randomised double blind placebo-controlled trial. *J Clin Endocrinol Metab* 2002; 87:1–6.

84. Ng EH, Wat NM, Ho PC. Effects of metformin on ovulation rate, hormonal and metabolic profiles in women with clomiphene-resistant polycystic ovaries: a randomized, double-blinded placebo-controlled trial. *Hum Reprod* 2001; 16:1625–1631.

85. Vandermolen DT, Ratts VS, Evans WS, Stovall DW, Kauma SW, Nestler JE. Metformin increases the ovulatory rate and pregnancy rate from clomiphene citrate in patients with polycystic ovary syndrome who are resistant to clomiphene citrate alone. *Fertil Steril* 2001; 75:310–315.

86. Kim LH, Taylor AE, Barbieri RL. Insulin sensitizers and polycystic ovary syndrome: Can a diabetes medication treat infertility? *Fertil Steril* 2000; 73:1097–1098.

87. De Leo V, la Marca A, Ditto A, Morgante G, Cianci A. Effects of metformin on gonadotropin-induced ovulation in women with polycystic ovary syndrome. *Fertil Steril* 1999; 72:282–285.

88. Murakawa H, Hasegawa I, Kurabayashi T, Tanaka K. Polycystic ovary syndrome. Insulin resistance and ovulatory responses to clomiphene citrate. *J Reprod Med* 1999; 44:23–27.

89. Stadtmauer LA, Toma SK, Riehl RM, Talbert LM. Metformin treatment of patients with polycystic ovary syndrome undergoing in vitro fertilization improves outcomes and is associated with modulation of the insulin-like growth factors. *Fertil Steril* 2001; 75:505–509.

90. Yarali H, Yildiz BO, Demirol A, Zeyneloglu HB, Yigit N, Bukulmez O et al. Co-administration of metformin during rFSH treatment in patients with clomiphene citrate-resistant polycystic ovarian syndrome: a prospective randomized trial. *Hum Reprod* 2002; 17:289–294.

91. Denno KM, Sadler TW. Effects of biguanide class oral hypoglycaemic agents on mouse embryogenesis. *Teratology* 1994; 49:260–266.

92. Glueck CJ, Phillips H, Cameron D, Sieve-Smith L, Wang P. Continuing metformin throughout pregnancy in women with polycystic ovary syndrome appears to safely reduce first-trimester spontaneous abortion: a pilot study. *Fertil Steril* 2001; 75:46–52.

93. Jakubowicz DJ, Iuorno MJ, Jakubowicz S, Roberts KA, Nestler JE. Effects of metformin on early pregnancy loss in the polycystic ovary syndrome. *J Clin Endocrinol Metab* 2002; 87:524–529.

94. Heard MJ, Pierce A, Carson SA, Buster JE. Pregnancies following use of metformin for ovulation induction in patients with polycystic ovary syndrome. *Fertil Steril* 2002; 77:669–673.

95. Seppala M, Riittinen L, Julkunen M, Koistinen R, Wahlstrom T, Iino K, Alfthan H, Stenman UH, Huhtala ML. Structural studies, localization in tissue and clinical aspects of human endometrial proteins. *J Reprod Fertil Suppl* 1988; 36:127–141.

96. Jakubowicz DJ, Seppala M, Jakubowicz S, Rodriguez-Armas O, Rivas-Santiago A, Koistinen H, Koistinen R, Nestler JE. Insulin reduction with metformin increases luteal phase serum glycodelin and insulin-like growth factor-binding protein 1 concentrations and enhances uterine vascularity and blood flow in the polycystic ovary syndrome. *J Clin Endocrinol Metab* 2001; 86:1126–1133.

97. Steer CV, Tan SL, Dillon D, Mason BA, Campbell S. Vaginal color Doppler assessment of uterine artery impedance correlates with immunohistochemical markers of endometrial receptivity required for the implantation of an embryo. *Fertil Steril* 1995; 63:101–108.

98. Glueck CJ, Wang P, Fontaine RN, Sieve-Smith L, Tracy T, Moore SK. Plasminogen activator inhibitor activity: an independent risk factor for the high miscarriage rate during pregnancy in women with polycystic ovary syndrome. *Metabolism* 1999; 48:1589–1595.

99. Piltonen T, Morin-Papunen L, Koivunen R, Perheentupa A, Ruokonen A, Tapanainen JS. Serum anti-Mullerian hormone levels remain high until late reproductive age and decrease during metformin therapy in women with polycystic ovary syndrome. *Hum Reprod* 2005; 20:1820–1826.

100. Glueck CJ, Wang P, Kobayashi S, Phillips H, Sieve-Smith L. Metformin therapy throughout pregnancy reduces the development of gestational diabetes in women with polycystic ovary syndrome. *Fertil Steril* 2002; 77:520–525.

101. Azziz R, Ehrmann D, Legro RS, Whitcomb RW, Hanley R, Fereshetian AG, O'Keefe M, Ghazzi MN. Troglitazone improves ovulation and hirsutism in the polycystic ovary syndrome: a multicenter, double blind, placebo-controlled trial. *J Clin Endocrinol Metab* 2001; 86:1626–1632.

102. Hasegawa I, Murakawa H, Suzuki M, Yamamoto Y, Kurabayashi T, Tanaka K. Effect of troglitazone on endocrine and ovulatory performance in women with insulin resistance-related polycystic ovary syndrome. *Fertil Steril* 1999; 71:323–327.

103. Mitwally MF, Kuscu NK, Yalcinkaya TM. High ovulatory rates with use of troglitazone in clomiphene-resistant women with polycystic ovary syndrome. *Hum Reprod* 1999; 14:2700–2703.

104. Yilmaz M, Karakoc A, Toruner FB, Cakir N, Tiras B, Ayvaz G, Arslan M. The effects of rosigli-tazone and metformin on menstrual cyclicity and hirsutism in polycystic ovary syndrome. *Gynecol Endocrinol* 2005; 21:154–160.

105. Zheng Z, Li M, Lin Y, Ma Y. Effect of rosiglitazone on insulin resistance and hyperandrogenism in polycystic ovary syndrome. *Zhonghua Fu Chan Ke Za Zhi* 2002; 37:271–273.

106. Belli SH, Graffigna MN, Oneto A, Otero P, Schurman L, Levalle OA. Effect of rosiglitazone on insulin resistance, growth factors, and reproductive disturbances in women with polycystic ovary syndrome. *Fertil Steril* 2004; 81:624–629.

107. Sepilian V, Nagamani M. Effects of rosiglitazone in obese women with polycystic ovary syndrome and severe insulin resistance. *J Clin Endocrinol Metab* 2005; 90:60–65.

108. Ghazeeri G, Kutteh WH, Bryer-Ash M, Haas D, Ke RW. Effect of rosiglitazone on spontaneous and clomiphene citrate-induced ovulation in women with polycystic ovary syndrome. *Fertil Steril* 2003; 79:562–566.

109. Brettenthaler N, De Geyter C, Huber PR, Keller U. Effect of the insulin sensitizer pioglitazone on insulin resistance, hyperandrogenism, and ovulatory dysfunction in women with polycystic ovary syndrome. *J Clin Endocrinol Metab* 2004; 89:3835–3840.

110. Glueck CJ, Moreira A, Goldenberg N, Sieve L, Wang P. Pioglitazone and metformin in obese women with polycystic ovary syndrome not optimally responsive to metformin. *Hum Reprod* 2003; 18:1618–1625.

111. Nestler JE, Jakubowicz DJ, Reamer P, Gunn RD, Allan G. Ovulatory and metabolic effects of D-chiro-inositol in the polycystic ovary syndrome. *N Engl J Med* 1999; 340:1314–1320.

14 Mechanisms and Treatment of Obesity in Polycystic Ovary Syndrome

Renato Pasquali, MD,
and Alessandra Gambineri, MD

CONTENTS

Summary

The polycystic ovary syndrome (PCOS), one of the most common causes of infertility because of anovulation, affects 4–7% of women. Intriguingly, obesity has an important pathophysiological impact on PCOS, and obese PCOS women are characterized by worsened endocrine and metabolic profiles and poorer fertility. Although it is believed that obesity simply emphasizes most common alterations such as hyperandrogenism and the insulin-resistant state, it is nonetheless likely that the obesity–PCOS phenotype represents a heterogeneous group of women with different pathophysiological events. In our opinion, this represents an exciting area for future research. Whatever the mechanisms, treatment with lifestyle interventional programs has clearly demonstrated its efficacy in obese PCOS women. Unfortunately, this approach is probably underestimated by many physicians. This is probably because of the well-known and considerable difficulties in the management of obesity and related disorders. The recognition that many benefits can be achieved even in the short term may however improve patient compliance. In fact,

From: *Contemporary Endocrinology: Polycystic Ovary Syndrome*
Edited by: A. Dunaif, R. J. Chang, S. Franks, and R. S. Legro © Humana Press, Totowa, NJ

in many patients, there is no need to achieve an impressive weight loss to improve menses, ovulation, and therefore fertility. There is however the need for lifestyle interventional programs targeted to women affected by PCOS. The long story of metformin in PCOS seems to demonstrate that by reducing insulin a great benefit can be achieved regardless of minor changes in body weight. These and others represent excellent opportunities for future research in the field of PCOS.

Key Words: Obesity, insulin resistance, body fat distribution, life style intervention, metformin fertility, polycystic ovary syndrome

1. INTRODUCTION

The polycystic ovary syndrome (PCOS), one of the most common causes of infertility because of anovulation, affects 4–7% of women *(1)*. The pathophysiology of PCOS may have a genetic component although it can be suggested that the main factors responsible for the increasing prevalence of PCOS are related to the influence of the environment, including dietary habits, behavior, and other still undefined factors *(1)*. The clinical features of PCOS are heterogeneous and may change throughout the lifespan, starting from adolescence to postmenopausal age *(1,2)*. This is largely dependent on the influence of obesity and metabolic alterations, including an insulin-resistant state and the metabolic syndrome, which consistently affect most women with PCOS *(3)*. This represents an important factor in the evaluation of PCOS throughout life, and implies that PCOS by itself may not be a hyperandrogenic disorder exclusively restricted and relevant to young and fertile aged women, but may also have some health implications later in life. Whereas in young women with PCOS, hyperandrogenism and menstrual irregularities represent the major complaints, symptoms related to androgen excess, oligo- or amenorrhea, and particularly infertility, represent the major complaints of adult PCOS women during the reproductive age. Obesity has an important impact on the progression and severity of these manifestations in proportion to its degree, particularly in the presence of the abdominal phenotype *(3)*, which renders affected women more susceptible to develop type 2 diabetes mellitus (T2DM), with some differences in the prevalence rates between countries and, potentially, in favoring the development of cardiovascular diseases (CVDs) *(1)*. This chapter focuses on *(1)* the prevalence of obesity in women with PCOS across the world, *(2)* the influence of obesity on the PCOS phenotype, *(3)* the pathophysiological role of obesity on PCOS; and *(4)* the beneficial effect of weight loss on the hormonal and metabolic abnormalities, on menses, and ovulation and fertility rates in obese PCOS women.

2. EPIDEMIOLOGY OF PCOS

All studies performed to date on the prevalence of PCOS in the general population applied the 1990 NIH criteria for diagnosis, which included oligo/amenorrhea and either biochemical or clinical evidence of androgen excess *(4)*. The prevalence of PCOS in the general population is over 6% according to the major epidemiological studies published so far *(5–9)*. These studies were performed in three European and two North-American cohorts, with a total of 1253 women. While the populations included in these studies were different in ethnicity (Caucasians, European, and Black and White Americans) as well as recruitment criteria for the studies (pre-employment check-up, blood donors, or women accepting an invitation to participate in a free medical examination), the

Table 1
Rates of Obesity in Studies Examining the Prevalence of Polycystic Ovary Syndrome (PCOS)

Authors	Country and ethnicity	Number of subjects investigated	Prevalence of women with PCOS[b]	Subjects with overweight or obesity
Michelmore (5)	European (ethnicity undefined)	230	8–26%[a]	NA
Knochenhauer (4)	USA (Blacks and Whites)	277	3.4% Blacks; 4.7% Whites	40% Blacks; 50% Whites
Diamanti-Kandarakis (6)	European (Caucasians)	192	6.8%	NA
Asuncion (7)	European (Caucasians)	154	6.5%	40%
Azziz (8)	USA (Blacks and Whites)	400	6.6%	66%

NA= not available.

[a]Prevalence rate varied according to the criteria used among the following: PCO at ultrasound plus one additional features including high testosterone (>3 nmol/L), high LH (>10 IU/L), menstrual irregularities, acne, hirsutism, BMI > 25.

[b]NIH criteria.

prevalence rates proved remarkably similar, at least in these four studies. In the study by Michelmore et al. (5), who investigated volunteer young women, aged 18–25 years, invited to participate in "a study of women's health issues", the prevalence rate varied from 8 to 26%, probably because of the less stringent criteria the authors used, that is polycystic ovaries at ultrasound plus one additional feature including high testosterone (>3 nmol/L), high LH (>10 IU/L), menstrual irregularities, acne, hirsutism, and body mass index (BMI) > 25 (Table 1). Differences in the prevalence rate with respect to other studies are likely to depend on the population, on criteria for inclusion and those chosen to define the PCOS phenotype. Despite this, it should be emphasized that much larger cross-sectional and prospective studies are needed, including adequate representation of young peri-pubertal girls, young and adult fertile women, and, finally, postmenopausal women. In fact, there is emerging evidence that PCOS may also be detected after the menopause, although its clinical features and accompanying metabolic and possibly cardiovascular comorbidities are still largely undefined (2). Excess testosterone levels are in fact recognized as a potential risk factor for CVDs throughout the lifespan (10). Moreover, an increased prevalence of PCOS has been reported for women who present with gestational diabetes and T2DM (11).

3. EPIDEMIOLOGY OF OBESITY

We are facing a worldwide public health emergency because of the increasing epidemic of obesity and related disorders (12). The problem of overweight and obesity has achieved global recognition only in the last 10–15 years. Recent estimates of the prevalence of obesity, based on BMI measurement in appropriate population samples, show that its increasing prevalence is recognized worldwide, with few exceptions. Women are generally found to have a higher BMI than men, probably for biological reasons as well as environmental factors *(12)*. The International Obesity Task Force estimates that at least 1.1 billion adults are currently overweight, including 312 million who are obese, and that with the new Asian BMI criteria, the number is even higher *(13)*. Most importantly, there is emerging evidence that overweight is increasing not only in adults but in children too, where prevalence rates of more than 10% affected individuals have been reported, particularly in western countries.

4. PREVALENCE OF OBESITY IN PCOS

More than 2400 years ago, Hippocrates wrote that "corpulence is not only a disease itself, but the harbinger of others" *(14)*. The price of obesity is represented in fact by a long list of comorbidities and social, psychological, and demographic problems. Obese women are characterized by similar comorbidities to men, particularly T2DM and CVDs *(15)*. On the contrary, they also have some specific problems, including fertility-related disorders and some hormone-dependent forms of cancer *(16,17)*. Again, Hippocrates described the association between fatness and infertility: "The girls get amazingly flabby and podgy … fatness and flabbiness are to blame. The womb is unable to receive the semen and they menstruate infrequently and little" *(14)*. We hypothesize that the increasing epidemic of obesity may be a factor responsible for the worldwide increased incidence of young women attending endocrinological or gynecological clinics because of menstrual irregularities, clinical hyperandrogenism, and infertility problems, features that suggest a PCOS phenotype. If this pessimistic scenario were to happen, we could expect an increasing rate of problems affecting PCOS women.

The association between obesity and alterations of reproductive function in women was recognized a long time ago. In Stein and Leventhal's original description *(18)*, obesity, together with hirsutism and infertility, represented one of the characteristics of the syndrome that eventually bore their names. Much later, Rogers and Mitchell *(19)* demonstrated that 43% of women affected by various menstrual disorders, infertility, and recurrent miscarriages, all features of the PCOS phenotype, were also overweight or obese. Furthermore, Hartz and colleagues *(20)* showed that the presence of anovulatory cycles, oligomenorrhea, and hirsutism, separately or in association with one another, was significantly higher in obese than in normal-weight women. In adolescent and young women, the age of onset of obesity and that of menstrual irregularities are significantly correlated *(21)*. There are also data indicating that the association with menstrual disorders may be more frequent in girls with onset of excess body weight during puberty than in those who were obese during infancy. These findings have been substantially confirmed in a large study performed in approximately 6,000 women by Lake et al. *(22)*, who found that obesity in childhood and the early twenties increased the risk of menstrual problems. It is therefore likely that overweight and obesity do contribute to a significant proportion of menstrual disorders in young women. Although all the aforementioned studies did not focus on a specific PCOS phenotype, it nonetheless clearly appears that menstrual disorders, oligo-anovulation, infertility, and clinical signs of androgen excess are key features in the definition of PCOS *(4,23)*, it is likely that most of the women investigated in these studies had PCOS.

The prevalence of obesity in PCOS appears to be much larger that that expected in the general population. Although the cause of this association remains unknown, a recent comprehensive review by Ehrmann *(1)* reported an estimated prevalence rate for more than 30% of cases and, in some series, a percentage as high as 75%. In the few epidemiological articles cited above, we observed that the prevalence of overweight or obesity among PCOS women ranged from 4 to 66% (Table 1). We recently reported the prevalence of underweight, normal-weight, overweight, and obesity in a large unselected cohort of 320 consecutive women with well-defined PCOS (according to the NIH criteria) attending our outpatient endocrinology clinic, and we found that 18% were overweight (BMI 25–29.9) and 43% were obese (BMI $\geq$ 30) *(24)*.

5. THE ABDOMINAL OBESITY PHENOTYPE IS PREVALENT IN PCOS WOMEN

Obesity tends to be abdominal in its distribution in PCOS women, and even lean effected women may have a fat distribution favoring visceral depots, particularly in the abdomen *(3)*. This is not unexpected, as androgens have an important role in the regulation of fat metabolism, differentiation, and morphology, through specific receptors whose distribution and characteristics vary according to different fat localization *(25)*. Importantly, stimulation with androgens seems to up-regulate the expression of their own receptors *(26)*. Androgens stimulate lipolysis in adipose tissue and when administered chronically, they induce an antiadipogenic effect, at least in primary cultured preadipocytes *(25)*. In isolated cultured differentiated adipocytes from omental and abdominal subcutaneous fat taken from overweight or obese individuals, it has been demonstrated that, in physiological concentrations, testosterone caused a depot-specific reduction of catecholamine-stimulated lipolysis in subcutaneous fat cells, probably because of reduced protein expression of ß3-adrenoreceptors and hormone sensitive lipase (HSL) *(27)*, the principal regulatory factor of the lipolytic pathways.

In obese males, administration of testosterone is followed by a reduction in lipoprotein lipase (LPL) activity (that regulates lipogenesis) and free fatty acid (FFA) uptake in abdominal but not in subcutaneous adipose tissue *(28)*. Therefore, in normal men, testosterone activates HSL in adipocytes thereby favoring a decrease in body fat mass. By contrast, this does not occur in obese males, who are characterized by a progressively reduced total and free testosterone with increasing body weight *(25)*. This is exactly what happens in hypogonadal men, where low testosterone levels impair lipolysis in adipocytes and favor fat gain, particularly visceral fat *(29)*.

In normal-weight women, in the presence of normal insulin sensitivity, adipocytes release limited amounts of FFA and regular amounts of LPL *(29)*, and normal testosterone supports insulin in suppressing FFA release from adipocytes. Obese women, by contrast, are characterized by increased production of FFA and inhibition of LPL secretion because of the presence of high insulin due to the insulin-resistant state *(29)*. Increased androgens then aggravate the detrimental effects of insulin resistance on FFA release from adipocytes. Therefore, testosterone would be expected to diminish visceral fat depots in women *(25)*. It is currently thought that this does not occur because of the protective effect of estrogens. In fact, the androgen receptors in female adipose tissue seem to have the same characteristics as those found in male adipose tissue *(29)*, but estrogens down-regulate the density of these receptors *(30)*. It has been clearly demonstrated that testosterone increases visceral fat in women. Female-to-male transsexuals treated with testosterone do in fact have an increase in visceral fat only when oophorectomized *(31)*. In addition, administration of androgens in postmenopausal women has been documented to increase visceral fat while reducing subcutaneous fat *(32)*. This indicates that testosterone causes accumulation of visceral adipose tissue, consistent with the important role of testosterone in determining the high prevalence of abdominal fat distribution pattern in hyperandrogenized women with PCOS.

6. THE INFLUENCE OF OBESITY ON THE PHENOTYPE OF PCOS

Obesity has profound effects on the clinical, hormonal, and metabolic features of PCOS, which largely depend on the degree of excess body fat and on the pattern of fat distribution. The recognition of the impact of obesity on PCOS may have some relevance in the pathophysiology of the disorder. In addition, obesity intuitively represents a target for therapeutic strategies, as weight loss produces several benefits on major complaints of women with PCOS, including hormonal and metabolic abnormalities, menses and ovulation, and therefore, fertility (*see* subsequent paragraph).

6.1. Clinical Hyperandrogenism and Androgen Blood Levels

Various studies have evaluated the impact of obesity on the hyperandrogenic state in women with PCOS. They have uniformly demonstrated that obese PCOS women are characterized by significantly lower sex hormone-binding globulin (SHBG) plasma levels and worsened hyperandrogemia (particularly total and free testosterone and androstenedione) in comparison with their normal-weight counterparts *(3)*. In addition, a negative correlation has been reported between body fat mass and circulating androgens *(3)*. A higher proportion of obese PCOS women complain of hirsutism and other androgen-dependent disorders, such as acne and androgenic alopecia, in comparison with normal-weight women *(3)*. The androgen profile can be further negatively affected in PCOS women by the presence of the abdominal body fat distribution with respect to those with the peripheral phenotype, regardless of BMI values *(3)*.

6.2. Menses Abnormalities and Infertility

PCOS is one of the most common causes of anovulation and endocrine infertility in women. Several studies have clearly demonstrated that menstrual abnormalities are more frequent in obese than in normal-weight PCOS women *(3)*. Moreover, there is evidence of a reduced incidence of pregnancy and blunted responsiveness to pharmacological treatments to induce ovulation in obese PCOS women *(33,34)*. In a prospective study carried out in 158 anovulatory women, the dose of clomiphene required to achieve ovulation was in fact positively correlated, whereas ovulatory outcome negatively correlated with body weight *(35)*. In addition, it has also been reported that, compared with normal-weight women, obese PCOS may have lower ovulatory responses to pulsatile gonadotropin-releasing hormone (GnRH) analog administration *(36)*. Accordingly, the pregnancy rate after a low-dose human menopausal gonadotropin (hMG) or pure follicle-stimulating hormone (FSH) administration has been found to be significantly lower in obese PCOS women than in normal-weight counterpart *(37)*. Finally, in recent studies performed in PCOS women conceiving after in vitro fertilization or intracytoplasmatic sperm injection, it was observed that those with obesity had higher gonadotropin requirements during stimulation, fewer oocytes, a higher abortion rate, and a lower live-birth rate than their non-obese counterpart *(38)*. In conclusion, a decreased efficiency of the different treatments for anovulation and infertility may be expected in obese PCOS women. These findings additionally support the negative impact of obesity on fertility in women with PCOS.

6.3. Metabolic Abnormalities: Insulin Resistance and Hyperinsulinemia

Reports on the prevalence of insulin resistance in women with PCOS are not homogeneous, depending on the sensitivity and specificity of the test employed, nor are cross-sectional or epidemiological studies available as yet. However, insulin resistance in women with PCOS appears more common than in the general population *(1,23)*. In one study examining the characteristics of more than 1,000 consecutive women with androgen excess, Azziz and co-workers *(39)* found that 716 of them had PCOS and were characterized, as a group, by hyperinsulinemia and insulin resistance. Interestingly, 60% of them were obese, which implies that obesity is significantly related to the insulin-resistant state. Many other studies have in fact reported that insulin resistance is very common in the presence of obesity, particularly the abdominal phenotype *(3,40,41)*, although it may be present even in those with normal weight *(3,40,41)*. It is commonly accepted that obesity and PCOS have an additional deleterious effect on insulin sensitivity, by mechanisms that have still not been adequately defined and could be different among obese and non-obese PCOS *(40–42)*.

Both fasting and glucose-stimulated insulin concentrations are usually significantly higher in PCOS than in non-PCOS controls *(3,40,41)*. Accordingly, studies examining insulin sensitivity by different methods, such as the euglycemic–hyperinsulinemic clamp technique, the frequent-sampling intravenous glucose tolerance test (FSIVGTT) or the insulin tolerance test (ITT) have demonstrated that PCOS women had significantly lower insulin sensitivity compared to age- and weight-matched controls (reviewed in refs *3,40,41*). This appears to be largely dependent on the presence of obesity. More recent studies have however confirmed this metabolic abnormality in obese PCOS women but not in those with normal weight *(43,44)*. At variance, another study performed in European PCOS women showed that, although insulin sensitivity and β-cell function, measured by the FSIVGTT technique, were preserved, glucose effectiveness (which is the insulin-independent glucose uptake) was decreased in normal-weight PCOS women *(45)*.

Intriguingly, additional studies have found that when insulin secretion is most appropriately expressed in relation to the magnitude of ambient insulin resistance and their product is quantified (the so-called disposition index), there is a subset of PCOS women exhibiting a significant impairment of β-cell function. Interestingly, all the women examined in these studies were obese and the β-cell dysfunction was particularly present in those who had a first-degree relative with T2DM *(46,47)*. On the contrary, similar findings were not confirmed by other studies performed in Europe *(48,49)*, although Holte and co-workers *(50)* reported that some differences in the insulin sensitivity index (ISI), defined as the ratio of the glucose disposal rate to the insulin concentrations at the end of a euglycemic–hyperinsulinemic clamp, were present only in subjects with high BMI values. Because a heritable component to β-cell dysfunction in families of women with PCOS has been suggested *(51)*, it could be speculated that differences among ethnicities could be related to some genetic trait. However, the influence of environmental factors (such as dietary factors, etc.) *(52)*, and the pattern of fat distribution, which is in fact very common in both obese and non-obese women, should be considered.

6.4. Metabolic Abnormalities: Glucose Intolerance and T2DM

Undoubtedly, worsening insulin resistance in the long term may represent an important factor in the development of glucose intolerance states (including impaired glucose tolerance and T2DM) in PCOS *(53,54)*. Clinical studies have in fact shown that impaired glucose intolerance is present, at the first clinical examination, in as many as 30–40% of obese PCOS women in the USA *(40)* and, probably, to a lesser extent in those living in Europe *(49)*, whilst it is uncommon in their normal-weight counterparts *(40,49)*. Different studies in American *(53,55)*, Asian *(56)*, and Italian *(49)* cohorts have shown that women with PCOS have a tendency to early development of T2DM and that its prevalence was higher when compared with the general population, regardless of ethnicity and geographical area. Interestingly, in all these studies, it was also found that this occurred almost always in those women who were obese and very rarely in their non-obese counterparts. Therefore, obesity seems to represent a condition for the development of T2DM in PCOS women.

Insulin resistance has a fundamental role for the development of glucose intolerance states in PCOS subjects. In fact, long-term prospective studies performed in PCOS women, most of whom were overweight or obese, found that insulin resistance tended to worsen over time in the majority of affected women, together with a deterioration of fasting or stimulated glucose values after oral glucose challenge in many cases *(49,57)*. Despite this, the presence of insulin resistance does not however imply a concomitant alteration of glucose tolerance, as most obese insulin-resistant PCOS women still maintain a normal glucose tolerance state. Factors influencing individual susceptibility toward T2DM in obese women with PCOS therefore remain to be elucidated. In this context, an early defect in insulin secretion may be necessary for the development of T2DM, as briefly discussed above (in the Section 6.3.).

6.5. Metabolic Abnormalities: Lipid Abnormalities

Although PCOS per se may be associated with alterations of both lipid and lipoprotein metabolisms, the coexistence of obesity usually leads to a more atherogenetic lipoprotein pattern. A greater reduction of high-density lipoproteins (HDLs), together with a higher increase of both triglycerides and total cholesterol levels, has in fact been observed in obese PCOS women with respect to those in normal weight *(3)*.

6.6. The Metabolic Syndrome

We are faced with a great debate on the definition of the metabolic syndrome, which includes more relevant risk factors for CVD definable on a clinical basis *(58–60)*.

Whatever the criteria proposed, there is no doubt that the abdominal obesity phenotype is a fundamental factor in the definition, being otherwise present even in a subset of subjects with normal BMI (<25). Some recent studies used the NCEP/ATPIII criteria to assess the prevalence of the metabolic syndrome in PCOS women. Collectively, the available studies *(61–63)* found a prevalence rate of approximately 40–50%, which is nearly twofold higher than that reported in the general population, according to different geographical areas and ethnicities.

As reported above, there are several conceptual reasons to indicate that insulin resistance and the metabolic syndrome should be considered as separate entities *(64)*. Therefore, the attempt to define the metabolic syndrome because of a simple unifying pathophysiological process is problematic. Very few studies describing the relationship between reliable measurements of insulin resistance and all of the components of each cluster used to define the metabolic syndrome have been reported. In a large group of healthy volunteers, Cheal et al. *(65)* recently found that, although insulin resistance and the presence of the metabolic syndrome were significantly associated ($p < 0.001$), the sensitivity and positive predictive values equalled 46 and 76%, the presence of overweight with high triglycerides, low HDL-cholesterol, or elevated blood pressure being the most common factors included in the diagnosis of the metabolic syndrome itself. In a recent study *(66)* performed in a cohort of 289 PCOS women with a wide range of BMI and an age-matched normal-weight healthy control group, we investigated the prevalence of insulin resistance (measured by simple mathematical tests and insulin concentrations) and how many PCOS women with the metabolic syndrome, according to the NCEP/ATP III criteria, were insulin resistant in comparison with PCOS women without the metabolic syndrome. We found that 55% of PCOS women had fasting hyperinsulinemia, 37% had higher HOMA values, and 49.5% had a higher ISI (applied to the oral glucose tolerance test) *(67)*, which indicates that approximately 40–50% of PCOS subjects were insulin-resistant, based on these measurements. Moreover, when PCOS subjects were classified as having or not having the metabolic syndrome, we found that in those with the metabolic syndrome, fasting hyperinsulinemia was present in 87.3%, higher HOMA in 74.6%, and higher ISI in 79.4%, compared with 54.7% ($p < 0.001$), 32.8% ($p < 0.001$), and 56.7% ($p < 0.001$) in those without the metabolic syndrome. Notably, BMI was very significantly higher in the former than in the latter. It therefore appears that insulin resistance is present in at least 70–85% of women with PCOS and that obesity plays a major role in distinguishing those with and without the metabolic syndrome.

6.7. Other Cardiovascular Risk Factors

There is a great debate as to whether women with PCOS are susceptible to a significant risk for CVDs *(68)*. In the last few years, a growing amount of data have been published showing that states of insulin resistance such as T2DM, obesity (particularly the abdominal phenotype), and PCOS are characterized, among other well-defined factors, including hormonal and metabolic alterations, by impaired coagulation and fibrinolysis, both anatomical and functional endothelial injury and vascular dysfunctions, and a state of subclinical inflammation, which overall represent independent risk factors for CVDs *(69–71)*. Although obese PCOS women have been found to be characterized by a worsened state in all these pro-atheroscleric alterations as a function of their BMI, it nonetheless remains controversial whether they are prevalently related to obesity and the insulin-resistant state rather than to PCOS per se.

7. PATHOPHYSIOLOGICAL ROLE OF OBESITY ON PCOS

The pathophysiology of the relationship between obesity and PCOS and mechanisms involved in determining hyperandrogenism and associated infertility has been extensively reviewed in recent publications to which the reader can refer for more information *(3,16,24)*. Here, we will briefly summarize the main factors responsible, including insulin, androgens, estrogens, gonadotropins, the growth hormone (GH)–insulin-like growth factor (IGF)-1 axis, the hypothalamic pituitary axis, leptin, and others.

7.1. Insulin

In female physiology, insulin acts as a true gonadotropic hormone *(40,41)*. At ovarian level, by acting through its own receptors and the IGF-I, insulin synergizes LH action and stimulates ovarian steroidogenesis both in granulosa and in thecal cells. In addition, insulin appears to increase pituitary sensitivity to GnRH action *(41)*. Notably, a huge number of PCOS women show a condition of insulin resistance and compensatory hyperinsulinemia and, in this way, ovarian androgen production can be overstimulated. This is particularly evident in the presence of obesity, although it may occur even in non-obese PCOS women, and obesity probably acts as an amplifier of insulin resistance and hyperinsulinemia *(40,41)*. This can explain why hyperandrogenism and related clinical features, particularly menstrual disorders and anovulation are worsened in obese PCOS women. Both insulin resistance and hyperinsulinemia, which parallel the increase of body fat, may be responsible for the alteration of both spontaneous and induced ovulation observed in the obese PCOS women *(16,24)*. The abdominal phenotype of obesity amplifies this disorder.

7.2. Androgens and SHBG

In a previous paragraph (Section 5), we described how the abdominal obesity phenotype may be the consequence of androgen excess, which characterizes PCOS. However, abdominal obesity per se is also a condition of sex hormone imbalance. The marked reduction of SHBG levels may favor a greater free androgen fraction to be delivered to target tissues. In addition, women with central obesity have higher testosterone and dihydrotestosterone production rates than those with peripheral obesity, which may exceed their metabolic clearance rates *(72)*. An increased production rate occurs even for androgens not bound to SHBG, such as dehydroepiandrosterone (DHEA) and androstenedione *(73)*. Therefore, the abdominal phenotype of obesity can be defined as a condition of a relative functional hyperandrogenic state. The role of adipose tissue is also crucial in controlling the balance of sex hormone availability in the target non-fat tissues. In fact, adipose tissue is able to store various lipid soluble steroids, including androgens. Most sex hormones appear to be preferentially concentrated within the adipose tissue rather than in the blood. As a consequence, because the amount of fat tissue is greater than the intravascular space in obesity, and the steroid tissue concentration is much higher than in plasma, the steroid pool in obese subjects is greater than that found in normal-weight individuals *(74)*. In addition, fat represents a site of intensive sex hormone metabolism and inter-conversion, because of the presence of several steroidogenetic enzymes, such as 3β-hydroxysteroid deydrogenase, 17β-hydroxysteroid deydrogenase and the aromatase system *(3,74)*. Obesity, particularly the abdominal phenotype, may thus add further specific mechanisms in the development of androgen excess in women with PCOS *(74)*.

7.3. Estrogens

The influence of obesity on hyperandrogenism can also be indirectly mediated by estrogens, whose increased production rates in the adipose tissue render obesity a hyperestrogenic state *(25)*. Excess estrogens may exert positive feedback regulation on gonadotropin release, triggering in turn a rise in ovarian androgen production, according to a still valid theory proposed many years ago by Yen *(75)*.

7.4. Gonadotropins

Gonadotropin secretion is affected by the presence of obesity in PCOS. An increase in circulating LH levels is inconsistently found in PCOS women, because of a GnRH-mediated increase in the amplitude and frequency of pulsatile LH secretory pattern *(76)*. The occurrence of spontaneous ovulation is associated with a normalization of LH secretion in PCOS women *(76)*. The concentrations of LH are however inversely related to body weight in PCOS women, depending on the effect of obesity in decreasing LH pulse amplitude and LH response to GnRH *(3)*. By contrast, increased LH concentrations are commonly found in normal-weight women with PCOS. Obese PCOS women are therefore characterized by significantly lower LH concentrations than their normal-weight counterpart, which can resemble the normal range in massively obese PCOS women *(3)*. This implies that obesity attenuates the responsibility of altered gonadotropin secretion in the pathogenesis of hyperandrogenism in PCOS women.

7.5. The Growth Hormone–IGF-1 Axis

Another factor involved in the pathophysiological impact of obesity on PCOS is the growth hormone (GH)/IGF-1 system, which may play a role in favoring altered ovarian androgen secretion and granulosa cell function in PCOS *(41)*. IGF-1 bioavailability appears to be reduced in obese PCOS women in comparison with their normal-weight counterpart, because of the combined low GH and high insulin levels, which depends on obesity per se *(77,78)*. By contrast, IGF-1 bioavailability seems to be increased in normal-weight PCOS women, probably because of the insulin-induced suppression of hepatic and ovarian IGF-binding protein-1 (IGFBP1) and the GH-induced hepatic IGF-1 stimulation *(77,78)*. Given the close interaction between insulin and IGF-1 in stimulating ovarian steroidogenesis *(41)*, a primary abnormality of the IGF-IGFBP1 system appears to be important in normal-weight PCOS women, whereas obesity appears to be associated with reduced IGF-1 bioavailability. Because insulin may interact with IGF-1 receptors in the ovarian tissues, it is reasonable to believe that insulin excess, rather than IGF-1, has a major responsibility in stimulating androgen production in obese PCOS women.

7.6. The Hypothalamic–Pituitary–Adrenal Axis

Obesity, particularly the abdominal phenotype, is characterized by a hyperactivity of the hypothalamic–pituitary–adrenal (HPA) axis *(79)*. Two distinct alterations are present. The first, which appears to be central in origin, is characterized by altered adrenocorticotropin (ACTH) pulsatile secretory dynamics, hyperresponsiveness of the HPA axis to different neuropeptides and acute stress events, dysregulation of the noradrenergic control of the corticotropin releasing hormone (CRH)–ACTH system, and, possibly, distinct dietary factors. The other appears to be located in the periphery, namely the visceral adipose tissue, which is characterized by elevated cortisol traffic, increased cortisol clearance, because of the influence of several distinct factors, including alterations of the enzymes involved in cortisol metabolism *(80)*.

In physiological conditions, it is well known that a functional cross-talk exists between the HPA axis and sex hormones *(81)*. In normal subjects, the response of the HPA axis to physiological stress is higher in females than in males, which suggests a regulatory role of androgens (and estrogens) *(82)*. We have shown that this occurs even in the presence of obesity *(83)*. ACTH and cortisol response in women with abdominal obesity is exaggerated with respect to their peripheral counterparts and normal-weight controls *(81)*. An increased response of adrenal androgens and ACTH and cortisol to CRH administration may also occur in PCOS women *(84)*. Overall, these findings suggest that these women may present a hyper-responsiveness of the neuroendocrine centers regulating the HPA axis to external environmental stress factors, as previously suggested *(80)*. In addition, we have suggested that a hyperresponsive HPA axis could be responsible, at least in part, for the condition of relative hyperandrogenism in women with simple abdominal obesity. Conditions of hypercortisolism such as Cushing's syndrome are good examples of how the HPA axis may differently regulate gonadal function according to sex. In men, in fact, Cushing's syndrome is associated with reduced gonadotropin levels and low testosterone concentrations regardless of the extent of hypercortisolism *(85)*. On the contrary, women with Cushing's syndrome and mild hypercortisolism may present a condition of androgen excess of both adrenal and ovarian origin and polycystic ovaries, whereas when severe hypercortisolism is present, the gonadal axis may be inhibited, sharing a similar condition to Cushing's syndrome in men *(85)*. We recently reported that, compared with obese men in whom a negative relationship exists, a significant positive one is conversely present between the activity of the HPA axis and the free testosterone levels in obese females, which suggests a partial responsibility of increased HPA axis activity in determining testosterone levels *(83)*. These findings are in line with studies performed by Rodin and co-workers *(86)* who reported increased urinary excretion of cortisol metabolites and C19 steroid sulfates and an increased ratio of the 11-oxo metabolites of cortisol and corticosterone to their 11-hydroxy metabolites in obese women with and without PCOS, which is consistent with enhanced oxidation by the 11βHSD1 enzyme system. If this is true, increased activation of the HPA axis to compensate for the peripheral cortisol defect might therefore be responsible in turn for increased adrenal androgen production.

7.7. The Opioid System

PCOS women are characterized by increased levels of plasma immunoreactive β-endorphin (reviewed in ref. *3*). In humans, β-endorphin administration increases insulin secretion from β cells *(3)*. An inhibition of the opioid tone may induce a decreased hyperinsulinemia in PCOS women because of reduced insulin secretion and improved hepatic clearance. In addition, β-endorphin administration reduces LH release in normal women but not in PCOS women, suggesting a condition of β-endorphin resistance in PCOS. Obesity by itself is characterized by an increased opioid system activity *(3)*. Moreover, infusion of physiological doses of β-endorphin has been found to induce a significant increase in insulin concentration in obese but not in normal-weight subjects, suggesting β-cell hypersensitivity to opioids in the obese state *(64)*. In addition, both acute and chronic administration of opioid antagonists, such as naloxone and naltrexone, are able to suppress both basal and glucose-stimulated insulin blood concentrations in obese women, particularly in those with the abdominal phenotype *(3)*, but not in normal-weight controls. An increased β-endorphin response to acute CRH administration has also been found in women with abdominal obesity *(3)*. However, there are no studies investigating the net contribution of obesity to the opioid tone and its ability to regulate insulin in PCOS women.

7.8. Leptin

Several cytokines have also been suggested as being involved in female reproduction, and available data are particularly relevant for leptin. Leptin, a product of the *OB* gene, is not only an adipose-derived messenger of the amount of energy stores to the brain, one of the most important orexigenic hormones acting at the central neuroendocrine nuclei to control food intake and energy balance *(87)*, but also a crucial hormone for gonadal function and reproduction *(88)*. Obesity is characterized by increased leptin concentrations, and hyperleptinemia is thought to be indicative of leptin resistance at central levels, thereby explaining the lack of reduced feeding in the presence of excess leptin concentrations. There is evidence that leptin participates in the regulation of the gonadal axis at both central and peripheral levels *(88)*. Leptin, in fact, regulates GnRH and gonadotropin secretion, leptin receptors being highly expressed in the hypothalamus *(88)*. In addition, high leptin concentrations in the ovary may participate in the regulation of theca cell function and interfere with the development of dominant follicles and oocyte maturation *(88)*, In addition, leptin appears to directly stimulate ovarian 17α-hydroxylase activity, which is involved in both ovarian and adrenal steroidogenesis *(88)*. Convincing studies on the effect of excess leptin on gonadotropin or ovarian sex hormone release in obese women, whether normally cycling or with ovulation impairment (such as in PCOS), are still lacking however. To date, contradictory results have been reported on leptin levels in women with PCOS, and higher levels than those expected for their BMI or normal concentrations have been detected *(89)*. This topic therefore requires much more detailed studies.

7.9. Other Potential Factors

Other potential factors include diet *(82)*, ghrelin *(82)*, and the endocannabinoid system *(90)*. There are several recent review articles to which the reader can refer for more in-depth information. The major factors involved in the pathophysiology of obesity in PCOS and their interrelationships is shown in Fig. 1.

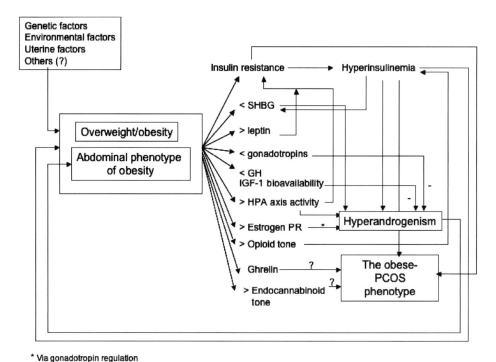

Fig. 1. The major factors involved in pathophysiology of obesity on polycystic ovary syndrome (PCOS).

8. BENEFITS INDUCED BY LIFESTYLE INTERVENTION EMPHASIZE THE PATHOPHYSIOLOGICAL ROLE OF OBESITY IN PCOS

Treatment of PCOS is influenced by the presence of obesity, but whether this implies differential therapeutic strategies with respect to patients with different patterns of obesity has not been adequately investigated. On the contrary, there is no doubt that, because of the importance of obesity in the pathogenesis of PCOS and the implications that metabolic alterations associated with the obesity state affect long-term health, weight loss should be pursued in all obese women with PCOS. This may help, in fact, to improve the hyperandrogenic state and even fertility, because of the negative effect of obesity per se on factors regulating ovulatory function and uterine performance *(15,16)*. Although obese women with PCOS may report some difficulty in losing weight and maintaining weight loss, the resting metabolic rate and postprandial thermogenesis, when studied, do not however differ in obese women with PCOS and weight-matched control subjects, suggesting that the same need for caloric restriction relative to energy expenditure is necessary for weight loss in both groups *(91)*. Moreover, no differences in hormonal responses to physical exercises were found between PCOS and weight-matched control women *(92)*.

The best therapeutic strategy for favoring weight loss in obese PCOS women has not yet been investigated. Lifestyle interventions, particularly a hypocaloric diet alone or in conjunction with increased physical activity, have proven efficacy *(93)*. Physical exercise could have an important impact on insulin resistance. In the context of overall glucose homeostasis, a single instance of exercise can markedly increase rates of whole body glucose disposal *(94)* and increase the sensitivity of skeletal muscle glucose uptake to insulin *(95)*. Regular physical activity is nevertheless required to have a lasting effect on insulin responsiveness *(96)*.

8.1. Metabolic and Hormonal Effects

Dietary-induced weight loss improves insulin-resistance and hyperinsulinemia *(3,16, 93)*. Insulin sensitivity before and after weight loss has been studied using several methodologies, including the euglycemic–hyperinsulinemic clamp technique. Both fasting and glucose-stimulated insulin levels tend to significantly decrease even after a weight decrease by approximately 5–10 percent baseline values. Using the euglycemic–hyperinsulinemic clamp technique, one study found that glucose disposal rate returned to baseline values after a few months of hypocaloric diet *(48)*. In a more recent randomized study performed to evaluate the efficacy of hypocaloric diet alone or associated with insulin sensitizers (metformin) or antiandrogens (flutamide) for a period of 6 months *(97)* in different groups of obese PCOS women, we found that although all groups improved fasting and glucose-stimulated insulin levels and insulin resistance, these effects could be mostly attributed to dietary weight loss rather than to specific drugs, which suggests a primary role of weight loss in improving alterations of the insulin–glucose system. Longer term studies performed by Hoeger *(98)* and our group *(99)* have confirmed these findings and additionally showed that metabolic effects were maintained in the long-term despite no change in weight loss in the last period of treatment. This is exactly what happens in much larger studies performed in simple obesity, using available antiobesity agents, such as sibutramine, orlistat *(100)*, or a new drug blocking the endocannabinoid receptor type 1, rimonabant, the phase III results of which have recently been published *(101)*. As a surrogate marker of the metabolic benefit, several studies documented a significant improvement of acanthosis nigricans, a cutaneous marker of insulin resistance *(3)*.

Weight loss also induces significant benefits on hyperandrogenism. Harlass and co-workers *(102)* first reported a decrease in total and free testosterone in a small group of obese anovulatory women after modest weight loss. In subsequent larger non-controlled studies *(3,16,93)*, a significant reduction of total and free testosterone levels after dietary-induced weight loss was confirmed. Additional controlled studies have obtained similar findings, although others did not report any effect. Weight loss can be followed by a significant increase of SHBG concentrations *(3,93)*, which is consistent with a reduction of the bioavailable free androgens. Reports on the beneficial effects of dietary-induced weight loss over a 12-month period on hirsutism and total testosterone concentrations in obese PCOS women have also been reported *(98,99)*. Jakubowicz and Nestler *(103)* performed a leuprolide test before and after a 6-month hypocaloric diet and found the 17α-hydroxyprogesterone response returned to baseline values, suggesting a decrease in the activity of P450c17α, a key enzyme involved in ovarian androgen production.

Whether diet composition may have a different impact on androgen and metabolism has been investigated in two studies *(104,105)*. They were performed in small groups of obese women with PCOS, randomly prescribed a high-protein (30%), low-carbohydrate (40%) versus a low-protein (15%), high-carbohydrate (55%) hypocaloric diet for a short time (1–3 months, respectively). In both studies, the final results were consistent with a significant effect of weight loss on total testosterone and fasting or glucose-stimulated insulin levels, without any significant effect of diet composition, suggesting that caloric restriction, rather than diet composition, is responsible for the beneficial effect of weight loss on hormones and metabolism. This may have a practical relevance from the clinical point of view, although there may be difficulties in achieving patient compliance, particularly in the long term, as clearly documented by the growing epidemic of obesity worldwide. Interestingly, there are studies demonstrating that pharmacological treatment may improve not only weight loss but also therapeutic compliance in responder obese patients, therefore favoring weight loss maintenance over time. Unfortunately, there are still very few studies available on this potentially interesting therapeutic approach to PCOS *(106,107)*.

8.2. Effects on Menses, Ovulation, and Fertility

Chronic anovulation is a common feature of PCOS patients, and the restoration of normal menstrual cycles and of ovulatory function represents the primary goal to be achieved for many women with PCOS complaining of oligo-amenorrhea and/or infertility. Evidence exists that dietary-induced weight loss may improve both menstrual abnormalities and spontaneous ovulation in the majority of PCOS women (reviewed in refs *3,16,24*). On the contrary, it should be noted that available data on the consequences of weight loss on menses and ovulatory abnormalities among obese women with PCOS have often been obtained in uncontrolled open studies, in studies including a control group who failed to complete the study program, and even with minimal (5% of baseline) weight loss during therapy *(108–112)*. Mechanisms responsible for the beneficial effect of weight loss on menses alterations and fertility probably depend on the coexistent reduction of both hyperinsulinemia and hyperandrogenemia. This is further confirmed by studies using insulin sensitizers, such as metformin and thiazolidinediones, in PCOS women with insulin resistance, demonstrating that by improving insulin resistance and associated hyperinsulinemia, androgen levels may decline, menses abnormalities may improve, and ovulation may be restored in most women, often regardless of weight loss and even after just a few weeks of pharmacological treatment *(34,113–115)*. However, two recent meta-analyses on the effects of metformin on ovulation *(116,117)* clearly demonstrated that where metformin was used as a sole agent, ovulation was achieved in 46% of recipients compared with 24% in the placebo group and that where metformin and clomifene were used in combination, 76% of recipients ovulated versus 42% of those receiving placebo. The conclusion is that equal or better ovulation rates have been achieved by a lifestyle intervention to achieve weight loss compared with metformin use.

Long-term lifestyle intervention may be needed to achieve weight loss and improve fertility. In another study performed by Hoeger and co-workers *(98)*, a group of 38 overweight or obese PCOS women were treated with metformin or placebo plus lifestyle intervention (including a 500–1000 kcal deficit per day, weekly behavioral education program, and exercise), or metformin alone. In the 23 women completing the trial, the authors found an overall weight loss of 7–10%; hirsutism did not significantly change, although total and free testosterone decreased by approximately 20% in the combined treatment group, whereas fasting and glucose-stimulated insulin decreased by approximately 25%. Most importantly, all treatments significantly improved ovulation rate, with a greater efficacy in those who lost weight compared with those who did not. Interestingly, however, prediction of three or more ovulations per 24 weeks by a logistic regression analysis indicated that weight loss (odds ratio: 8.97; $p = 0.030$), rather than metformin treatment (odds ratio: 1.14; $p = 0.891$), was responsible for this effect. This is in agreement with our own data obtained in a large cohort of women treated for 12 months with a low-calorie diet alone or combined with metformin and/or a pure antiandrogen, flutamide *(99)*. These findings further support the beneficial effect of weight loss on ovulation in obese PCOS women also in the long term and suggest that weight loss should be encouraged in these women, despite difficulties in achieving and maintaining adequate compliance on an individual basis. Ultimately, the goal represented by an increased probability of ovulating and, hopefully, becoming pregnant may have a great impact on improving compliance. This has been demonstrated in one study where obese PCOS women with patent Fallopian tubes and chronic anovulation were invited to follow a hypocaloric diet to achieve a 5% weight loss in a 6-month period, after which they were forced to achieve further weight loss in the presence of a poor ovulatory response. Overall, after 8–10 months, approximately 80% achieved regular menses, 60% had ovulatory cycles, and 40% became pregnant *(118)*.

9. SUMMARY AND PERSPECTIVES

Obesity is a costly and increasingly prevalent condition in western societies. Among other comorbidities, it is frequently associated with reduced fertility and signs and symptoms of androgen excess. In women with PCOS obesity is very common, although its prevalence in this disorder has not been estimated on an epidemiological basis. Intriguingly, obesity has an important pathophysiological impact on PCOS, and obese PCOS women are characterized by worsened endocrine and metabolic profiles and poorer fertility. Although it is believed that obesity simply emphasizes most common alterations such as hyperandrogenism and the insulin-resistant state, it is nonetheless likely that the obesity–PCOS phenotype represents a heterogeneous group of women with different pathophysiological events. In our opinion, this represents an exciting area for future research.

Whatever the mechanisms (Fig. 2), treatment with lifestyle intervention programs has clearly demonstrated its efficacy in obese PCOS women. Unfortunately, this approach is probably underestimated by many physicians. This is probably because of the well-known and considerable difficulties in the management of obesity and related disorders. The recognition that many benefits can be achieved even in the short term may however improve patient compliance. In fact, in many patients, a small amount of weight loss will improve menses, ovulation, and therefore fertility. There is however the need for lifestyle intervention programs targeted to women affected by PCOS. Preliminary data from an Australian Infertility Centre are encouraging *(119)*. On the contrary, there are still many unanswered question on this important topic. Should dietary management focus only on weight loss in the presence of obesity or on increasing insulin sensitivity regardless of weight loss. Available data do not support a greater efficacy of different dietary composition, either restricted in carbohydrates or in lipids in the short term, and therefore much longer trials are needed. In addition, whether low-saturated fat and high fibre diet with predominant low glycemic index carbohydrate foods are more helpful

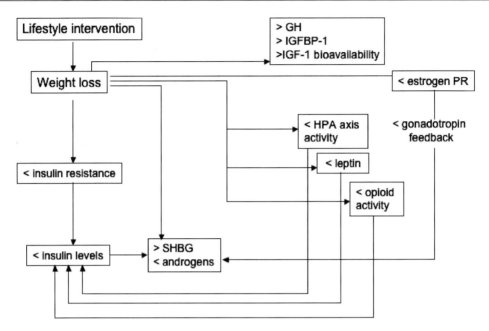

Fig. 2. Mechanisms by which weight loss may improve hormonal and metabolic derangements and ovulatory dysfunction in obese polycystic ovary syndrome (PCOS) women.

has not yet been adequately investigated. The long story of metformin in PCOS seems to demonstrate that by reducing insulin a great benefit can be achieved regardless of minor changes in body weight. These and other related treatment areas represent excellent opportunities for future research in the field of PCOS.

REFERENCES

1. Ehrmann DA. Polycystic ovary syndrome. *N Engl J Med* 2005; 352: 1223–1236.
2. Pasquali R, Gambineri A. PCOS: a multifaceted disease from adolescence to adult age. *Ann NY Acad Sci* 2006; 1092: 158–174.
3. Gambineri A, Pelusi C, Vicennati V, Pagotto, U, Pasquali R. Obesity and the polycystic ovary syndrome. *Int J Obes Relat Metab Dis* 2002; 26: 883–896.
4. Knochenhauer ES, Key TJ, Kahsar-Miller M, Waggoner W, Boots LR, Azziz R. Prevalence of the polycystic ovary syndrome in unselected black and white women of the southeastern United States: a prospective study. *J Clin Endocrinol Metab* 1998; 83: 3078–3082.
5. Michelmore KF, Balen HA, Dunger DB, Vessey MP. Polycystic ovaries and associated clinical and biochemical features in young women. *Clin Endocrinol (Oxf)* 1999; 51: 779–786.
6. Diamanti-Kandarakis E, Kouli CR, Bergiele AT, Filandra FA, Tsianateli TC, Spina GG, Zapanti ED, Bartzis MI. A survey of the prevalence of the polycystic ovary syndrome in the Greek island of Lesbos: hormonal and metabolic profiles. *J Clin Endorinol Metab* 1999; 84: 4006–4011.
7. Asuncion M, Calvo RM, San Millan JL, Sancho J, Avila S, Escobar-Morreale HF. A prospective study of the prevalence of the polycystic ovary syndrome in unselected Caucasian women from Spain. *J Clin Endorinol Metab* 2000; 85: 2434–2438.
8. Azziz R, Keslie S, Reyna R, Key TJ, Knochenhauer ES, Yildiz B. The prevalence and features of the polycystic ovary syndrome in an unselected population. *J Clin Endorinol Metab* 2004; 89: 2745–2749.

9. Wu FC, Von Eckardstein A. Androgens and coronary artery disease. *Endocr Rev* 2003; 24: 183–217.

10. Kousta E, Cela E, Lawrence N, Penny A, Millauer B, White D, Wilson H, Robinson S, Johnston D, McCarthy M, Franks S. The prevalence of polycystic ovaries in women with a history of gestational diabetes. *Clin Endocrinol (Oxf)* 2000; 53:501–507.

11. Haslan DW, James WPT. Obesity. *Lancet* 2005; 366:1197–1209.

12. James WPT, Rigby N, Leach R. The obesity epidemic, metabolic syndrome and future preventive strategies. *Eur J Cardiovasc Prev Rehabil* 2004; 11:3–8.

13. Hippocrates. The influence of climate, water supply and situation on health. *Essay to Scynthians* 4th century B.C.

14. Ford ES. Prevalence of the metabolic syndrome in US population. *Endocr Metab Clin N Am* 2004; 33: 333–350.

15. Linnè Y. Effects of obesity on women's reproduction and complications during pregnancy. *Obes Rev* 2004; 5: 137–143.

16. Pasquali R, Pelusi C, Genghini S, Cacciari M, Gambineri A. Obesity and reproductive disorders in women. *Hum Reprod Up* 2003; 9: 359–372.

17. Stein IF, Leventhal ML. Amenorrhea associated with bilateral polycystic ovaries. *Am J Obstet Gynecol* 1935; 29: 181–191.

18. Rogers J, Mitchell GW. The relation of obesity to menstrual disturbances. *N Engl J Med* 1952; 247: 53–56.

19. Hartz AJ, Barboriak PN, Wong A, Katayama KP, Rimm AA. The association of obesity with infertility and related menstrual abnormalities in women. *Int J Obes Relat Metab Dis* 1979; 3: 57–77.

20. Pelusi C, and Pasquali R. Polycystic ovary syndrome in adolescents. Pathophysiology and treatment implication. *Treat Endocrinol* 2003; 2: 215–230.

21. Lake JK, Power C, and Cole TJ. Women's reproductive health: the role of body mass index in early and adult life. *Int J Obes Relat Metab Dis* 1997; 21: 432–438.

22. Zawadzki JK, Dunaif A. Diagnostic criteria for polycystic ovary syndrome. In *Polycystic Ovary Syndrome* Dunaif A, Givens JR, Haseltine FP, Merriam GR, eds. Boston: Blackwell 1992; 377–384.

23. The Rotterdam ESHRE/ASRM-Sponsored PCOS consensus workshop group. Revised 2003 consensus on diagnostic criteria and long-term health risks related to polycystic ovary syndrome (PCOS). *Hum Reprod* 2004; 19: 41–47.

24. Pasquali R, Gambineri A, Pagotto U. The impact of obesity on reproduction in women with polycystic ovary syndrome. *Br J Obstet Gynecol* 2006; 113: 1148–1159.

25. Pasquali R. Vicennati V, Pagotto U. Endocrine determinants of fat distribution. In *Handbook of obesity* Bray GA, Bouchard C, eds. M. Dekker, Inc. New York 2003; 671–692.

26. De Pergola G, Xu XF, Yang SM, Giorgino R, Bjorntorp P. Up-regulation of androgen receptor binding in male rat fat pad adipose precursor cells exposed to testosterone: study in a whole cell assay system. *J Steroid Biochem Mol Biol* 1990; 37: 553–558.

27. Dicker A, Ryden M, Naslund E, Muchlen IE, Wiren M, Lafontan M, Arner P. Effect of testosterone on lipolysis in human pre-adipocytes from different fat depots. *Diabetologia* 2004; 47: 420–428.

28. Marin P, Oden B, Bjorntorp P. Assimilation and mobilization of triglycerides in subcutaneous abdominal and femoral adipose tissue in vivo in men: effects of androgens. *J Clin Endocrinol Metab* 1995; 80: 239–243.

29. Bjorntorp P. The regulation of adipose tissue distribution in humans. *Int J Obes* 1996; 20: 291–302.

30. Bjorntorp P. Centralization of body fat. *International Textbook of obesity* Chichester, UK: John Wiley & Sons, 2001; 213–224.

31. Elbers JMH, Asscheman H, Seidel JC, Megens JA, Gooren LJG. Long-term testosterone administration increases visceral fat in female to male transsexuals. *J Clin Endocrinol Metab* 1997; 79: 265–271.

32. Lovejoy JC, Bray GA, Bourgeois MO, Macchiavelli R, Rood JC, Greeson C, et al. Exogenous androgens influence body composition and regional body fat distribution in obese postmenopausal women - A clinical research center study. *J Clin Endocrinol Metab* 1996; 81: 2198–2203.

33. Lobo RA, Gysler M, March CM, Goebelman U, Mischell DR Jr. Clinical and laboratory predictors of clomiphene response. *Fertil Steril* 1982; 37: 168–174.

34. Nestler JE, Jakubowicz DJ, Evans WS and Pasquali R. Effects of metformin on spontaneous and clomiphene-induced ovulation in the polycystic ovary syndrome. *N Engl J Med* 1998; 25: 1876–1880.

35. De Leo V, la Marca A, Petraglia F. Insulin-lowering agents in the management of polycystic ovary syndrome. *Endocr Rev* 2003; 24: 633–637.

36. Filicori M, Flamigni C, Dellai P. Treatment of anovulation with pulsatile gonadotropin-releasing hormone: prognostic factors and clinical results in 600 cycles. *J Clin Endocrinol Metab* 1994; 79: 1215–1220.

37. White DM, Polson DW, Kiddy D, Sagle P, Watson H, Gilling-Smith C, Hamilton-Fairley D, Franks S. Induction of ovulation with low-dose gonadotropins in polycystic ovary syndrome: an analysis of 109 pregnancies in 225 women. *J Clin Endocrinol Metab* 1996; 81: 3821–3824.

38. Fedorcsák P, Dale PO, Storeng R, Tanbo T, Abyholm T. The impact of obesity and insulin resistance on the outcome of IVF or ICSI in women with polycystic ovarian syndrome. *Hum Reprod* 2001; 16: 1086–1091.

39. Azziz JR, Sanchez LA, Knochenhauer ES, Moran C, Lazenby J, Stephens KC, Taylor A, Boots LR. Androgen excess in women: experience with over 1000 consecutive patients. *J Clin Endocrinol Metab* 2004; 89: 453–462.

40. Dunaif A. Insulin resistance and the polycystic ovary syndrome: mechanisms and implications for pathogenesis. *Endocr Rev* 1997, 18: 774–800.

41. Poretsky L, Cataldo NA, Rosenwaks Z, Giudice LC. The insulin-related ovarian regulatory system in health and disease. *Endocr Rev* 1999; 20: 535–582.

42. Cibula D. Is insulin resistance an essential component of PCOS? *Hum Reprod* 2004; 19: 757–759.

43. Morin Papunen LC, Vahkonen I, Koivunen RM, Ruokonen A, Tapanainen JS. Insulin sensitivity, insulin secretion and metabolic and hormonal parameters in healthy women and women with polycystic ovary syndrome. *Hum Reprod* 2004; 15: 1266–1274.

44. Vrbikova J, Cibula D, Dvorakova K, Stanicka S, Sindelka G, Hill M, Fanta M, Vondra K, Skrha J. Insulin sensitivity in women with polycystic ovary syndrome. *J Clin Endocrinol Metab* 2004; 89: 2942–2945, 2004.

45. Gennarelli G, Roveri RNovi F, Holte J, Bongiovanni F, Revelli A, Pacini A, Cavallo-Perin P, Massobrio P. Preserved insulin sensitivity and β-cell activity, but decreased glucose effectiveness in normal weight women with polycystic ovary syndrome. *J Clin Endocrinol Metab* 2005; 90: 3381–3386.

46. Dunaif A, Finegood DT. β-cell dysfunction independent of obesity and glucose intolerance in the polycystic ovary syndrome. *J Clin Endocrinol Metab* 1996; 81: 942–947.

47. Ehrmann DA, Sturis J, Byrne MM, Karrison T, Rosenfield RL, Polonsky KS. Insulin secretory defects in polycystic ovary syndrome. Relationship to insulin sensitivity and family history of non-insulin-dependent diabetes mellitus. *J Clin Invest* 1995; 96: 520–527.

48. Holte J, Bergh T, Berne C, Wide L, Lithell H. Restored insulin sensitivity but persistently increased early insulin secretion after weight loss in obese women with polycystic ovary syndrome. *J Clin Endocrinol Metab* 1995, 80: 2586–2593.

49. Gambineri A, Pelusi C, Manicardi E, Vicennati V, Cacciari M, Morselli-Labate AM, Pagotto U, Pasquali R. Glucose intolerance in a large cohort of Mediterranean women with polycystic ovary syndrome: phenotype and associated factors. *Diabetes* 2004; 53: 2353–2358.

50. Holte J, Bergh Ch, Berglund L, Litthell H. Enhanced early phase insulin response to glucose in relation to insulin resistance in women with polycystic ovary syndrome. *J Clin Endocrinol Metab* 1994; 78: 1052–1058.

51. Colilla S, Cox NJ, Ehrmann DA. Heritability of insulin secretion and insulin action in women with polycystic ovary syndrome and their first-degree relatives. *J Clin Endocrinol Metab* 2001; 86: 2027–2031.

52. Wijeyartne CN, Balen AH, Barth JH, and Belchetz PE. Clinical manifestation and insulin resistance (IR) in polycystic ovary syndrome (PCOS) among South Asians and Caucasians: Is there a difference? *Clin Endocrinol (Oxf)* 2002; 57: 343–350.

53. Pasquali R, Gambineri A, Anconetani B, Vicennati V, Colitta D, Caramelli E, Casimirri F, Morselli-Labate AM. The natural history of the metabolic syndrome in young women with the polycystic ovary syndrome and the long-term effect of oestrogen-progestagen treatment. *Clin Endocrinol (Oxf)* 1999; 50: 517–527.

54. Ehrmann DA, Barnes RB, Rosenfield RL, Cavaghan MK, Imperial J. Prevalence of impaired glucose tolerance and diabetes in women with polycystic ovary syndrome. *Diabetes Care* 1999; 22: 141–146.

55. Legro RS, Kunselman AR, Dodson WC, Dunaif A. Prevalence and predictors of risk for type 2 diabetes mellitus and impaired glucose tolerance in polycystic ovary syndrome: a prospective, controlled study in 254 affected women. *J Clin Endocrinol Metab* 1999; 84: 165–169.

56. Weerakiet S, Srisombut C, Bunnag P, Sangtong S, Chuangsoongnoen N, Rojanasakul A. Prevalence of type 2 diabetes mellitus and impaired glucose tolerance in Asian women with polycystic ovary syndrome. *Int J Gynaecol Obstet* 2001; 75: 177–184.

57. Legro RS, Gnatuk CL, Kunselman AR, Dunaif A. Changes in glucose tolerance over time in women with polycystic ovary syndrome: a controlled study. *J Clin Endocrinol Metab* 2005; 90: 3236–3242.

58. Executive Summary of the Third Report of The National Cholesterol Education Program (NCEP) Expert Panel on Detection, Evaluation, and Treatment of High Blood Cholesterol In Adults (Adult Treatment Panel III). *JAMA* 2001; 285: 2486–2497.

59. World Heath Organization. Definition, diagnosis and classification of diabetes mellitus and its complications. Part 1: diagnosis and classification of diabetes mellitus. Geneva (Switzerland): Department of Noncommunicable Disease Surveillance; 1999.

60. Eckel RH, Grundy SM, Zimmet PZ. The metabolic syndrome. *Lancet* 2005; 365: 1415–1428.

61. Glueck CJ, Papanna R, Wang P, Goldemberg N, Sieve-Smith L. Incidence and treatment of metabolic syndrome in newly referred women with confirmed polycystic ovarian syndrome. *Metabolism* 2003, 52: 908–915.

62. Apridonidze T, Essah P, Iourno MJ, and Nestler JE. Prevalence and characteristics of the metabolic syndrome in women with PCOS. *J Clin Endocrinol Metab* 2005, 90: 1929–1935.

63. Kohronen S, Hippelainen M, Vanhala M, Heinonen S, Niskanen L. The androgenic sex hormone profile is an essential feature of metabolic syndrome in premenopausal women: a controlled community-based study. *Fertil Steril* 2003, 79:1327–1334.

64. Kahn R, Ferrannini E, Buse J, Stern M. The metabolic syndrome: time for a critical reappraisal. Joint statement from the American Diabetes Association and the European Association for the study of Diabetes. *Diabetes Care* 2005; 28: 2289–2304.

65. Cheal KL, Abbasi F, Lamendola C, McLaughlin T, Reaven GM, Ford ES. Relationship to insulin resistance of the Adult Treatment Panel III Diagnostic Criteria for Identification of the Metabolic Syndrome. *Diabetes* 2004; 53: 1195–1200.

66. Pasquali R, Gambineri A. Insulin resistance: definition and epidemiology in normal women and PCOS women. In *Insulin Resistance and Polycystic Ovarian Syndrome: Pathogenesis, Evaluation, and Treatment* Diamanti-Kandarakis E, Nestler JE, Pasquali R, Panidis D, eds. Totowa, NJ: The Humana Press (in press).

67. Matusda M, De Fronzo RA. Insulin sensitivity indices obtained from oral glucose tolerance testing. *Diabetes Care* 1999; 22: 1462–1470.

68. Legro RS. Polycystic ovary syndrome and cardiovascular disease: a premature association? *Endocr Rev* 2003; 24:302–312.

69. Kishore J, Harjai MBBS. Potential new cardiovascular risk factors: left ventricular hypertrophy, homocysteine, lipoprotein (a), triglycerides, oxidative stress, and fibrinogen. *Ann Int Med* 1999; 131: 376–386.

70. Bloomgarden ZT. Inflammation and insulin resistance. *Diabetes Care* 2003; 26: 1922–1926.

71. Diamanti-Kandarakis E, Paterakis T, Alexandraki K, Piperi C, Aessopos A, Katsikis I, Katsilambros N, Kreatsas G, Panidis D. Indices of low-grade chronic inflammation in polycystic ovary syndrome and the beneficial effect of metformin. *Hum Reprod* 2006 [Epub ahead of print].

72. Kirschner MA, Samojlik E, Drejka M, Szmal E, Schneider G, Ertel N. Androgenestrogen metabolism in women with upper body versus lower body obesity. *J Clin Endocrinol Metab* 1990; 70: 473–479.

73. Kurtz BR, Givens JR, Koinindir S, Stevens MD, Karas JG, Bitte JB, Judge D, Kitabchi AE. Maintenance of normal circulating levels of Δ4androstenedione and dehydroepiandrosterone in simple obesity despite increased metabolic clearance rate: evidence for a servo-control mechanism. *J Clin Endocrinol Metab* 1987; 64: 1261–1267.

74. Azziz, R. Reproductive endocrinologic alterations in female asymptomatic obesity. *Fertil Steril* 1989; 52: 703–725.

75. Yen SSC. The polycystic ovary syndrome. *Clin Endocrinol (Oxf)* 1980; 12: 177–208.

76. Taylor AE, McCourt B, Martin KA, Anderson EJ, Adams JM, Schoenfeld D, et al. Determinants of abnormal gonadotropin secretion in clinically defined women with polycystic ovary syndrome. *J Clin Endocrinol Metab* 1997; 82: 2248–2256.

77. Morales AJ, Laughlin GA, Butzow T, Maheshwari H, Baumann G, Yen SS. Insulin, somatotropic, and luteinizing hormone axes in lean and obese women with polycystic ovary syndrome: common and distinct features. *J Clin Endocrinol Metab* 1996; 81: 2854–2864.

78. Van Dam EW, Roelfsema F, Helmerhorst FH, Frolich M, Meinders AE, Veldhuis JD, Pijl H. Low amplitude and disorderly spontaneous growth hormone release in obese women with or without polycystic ovary syndrome. *J Clin Endocrinol Metab* 2002; 87: 4225–4230.

79. Wajchenberg BL. Subcutaneous and visceral adipose tissue: their relation to the metabolic syndrome. *Endocr Rev* 2000; 21: 697–738.

80. Pasquali R, Vicennati V. The abdominal obesity phenotype and insulin resistance are associated with abnormalities of the hypothalamic-pituitary-adrenal axis in humans. *Horm Metab Res* 2000; 32: 521–525.

81. Tilbrook AJ, Turner AI, Clarke IJ. Effects of stress on reproduction in non-rodent mammals: the role of glucocorticoids and sex differences. *Rev Reprod* 2000; 5: 105–113.

82. Pasquali R. Obesity and androgens: fact and perspectives. *Fertil Steril* 2006; 85: 1319–1340.

83. Vicennati V, Ceroni L, Genghini S, Patton L, Pagotto U, Pasquali R. Sex difference in the relationship between the hypothalamic-pituitary-adrenal (HPA) axis and sex hormones in obesity. *Obes Res* 2006; 14: 235–243.

84. Pasquali R, Vicennati V. Obesity and hormonal abnormalities. In *International Textbook of obesity* Bjorntorp P, ed. Chichester, UK: John Wiley & Sons, 2001; 225–239.

85. Lado-Abeal J, Rodriguez-Arnao J, Newell-Price JD, Perry LA, Grossman AB, Besser GM, et al. Menstrual abnormalities in women with Cushing's disease are correlated with hypercortisolemia rather than raised circulating androgen levels. *J Clin Endocrinol Metab* 1998; 83: 3083–3088.

86. Rodin A, Thakkar H, Taylor N, Clayton R. Hyperandrogenism in polycystic ovary syndrome. Evidence of dysregulation of 11 beta-hydroxysteroid dehydrogenase. *N Engl J Med* 1994; 330: 460–465.

87. O'Rahilly S. Life without leptin. *Nature* 1998; 392: 330–331.

88. Moschos S, Chan JL, Mantzoros CS. Leptin and reproduction: a review. *Fertil Steril* 2002; 77: 433–444.

89. Mitchell M, Armstrong DT, Robker RL, Norman DJ. Adipokines: implications for female fertility and obesity. *Reproduction* 2005; 130: 583–597.

90. Pagotto U, Marsicano G, Cota D, Lutz B, Pasquali R. The emerging role of the endocannabinoid system in endocrine regulation and energy balance. *Endocr Rev* 2006; 27:73–100.

91. Segal KR, Dunaif A. Resting metabolic rate and postprandial thermogenesis in polycystic ovary syndrome. *Int J Obes Relat Metab Dis* 1990; 14: 559–567.

92. Jaatinen T-A, Anttila L, Erkkola R, Koskinen P, Laippala P, Ruutiainen K, Scheinin M, Irjala K. Hormonal responses to physical exercise in patients with polycystic ovarian syndrome. *Fertil Steril* 1993; 60: 262–267.

93. Pasquali R, Gambineri A. Treatment of the polycystic ovary syndrome with lifestyle intervention. *Curr Opin Endocrinol Metab* 2002; 9: 459–468.

94. Richter EA, Mikines KJ, Galbo H, Kiens B. Effect of exercise on insulin action in human skeletal muscle. *J Appl Physiol* 1989; 66: E876–885.

95. Mikines KJ, Sonne B, Farrell PA, Tronier B, Gelbo H. Effect of physical exercise on sensitivity and responsiveness to insulin in humans. *Am J Physiol* 2001, 254: E248–259.

96. Marshall K. Polycystic ovary syndrome: clinical considerations. *Altern Med Rev* 2001; 6: 272–292.

97. Gambineri A, Pelusi C, Genghini S, Morselli-Labate AM, Cacciari M, Pagotto U, Pasquali R. Effect of flutamide and metformin administered alone or in combination in dieting obese women with polycystic ovary syndrome. *Clin Endocrinol (Oxf)* 2004; 60: 241–249.

98. Hoeger KM, Kochman L, Wixom N, Craig K, Miller RK, Guzick DS. A randomized, 48-week, placebo-controlled trial of intensive lifestyle modification and/or metformin therapy in overweight women with polycystic ovary syndrome: a pilot study. *Fertil Steril* 2004; 82: 421–429.

99. Gambineri A, Patton L, Vaccina A, Pagotto U, Pasquali R. Effect of flutamide and metformin administered alone or in combination in dieting obese women with polycystic ovary syndrome (PCOS): a randomized, 12-months, placebo-controlled study. Androgen Excess Society 3[rth] Meeting, San Diego, USA, 2005.

100. Li Z, Maglione M, Tu W, Mojica W, Arterburn D, Shugarman LR, Hilton L, Suttorp M, Solomon V, Shekelle PG, Morton SC. Meta-analysis: pharmacologic treatment of obesity. *Ann Intern Med* 2005; 142: 532–546.

101. Van Gaal LF, Rissanen AM, Scheen AJ, Ziegler O, Rossner S, for the RIO-Europe Study Group. Effects of the cannabinoid-1 receptor blocker rimonabant on weight reduction and cardiovascular risk factors in overweight patients: 1-year experience from the RIO-Europe study. *Lancet* 2005; 365: 1389–1397.

102. Harlass FE, Plymate SR, Fariss BL, Belts RP. Weight loss is associated with correction of gonadotropin and sex steroid abnormalities in the obese anovulatory female. *Fertil Steril* 1984, 42: 649–652.

103. Jakubowicz DA, Nestler JE. 17?*a*-Hydroxyprogesterone responses to leuprolide and serum androgens in obese women with and without polycystic ovary syndrome after weight loss. *J Clin Endocrinol Metab* 1997, 82: 556–560.

104. Stamets K, Taylor DS, Kunselman A, Demers LM, Pelkman CL, Legro RS. A randomized trial of the effects of two types of short-term hypocaloric diets on weight loss in women with polycystic ovary syndrome. *Fertil Steril* 2004; 81:630–637.

105. Moran LJ, Noakes M, Clifton PM, Tomlinson L, Galletly C, Norman RJ. Dietary composition in restoring reproductive and metabolic physiology in overweight women with polycystic ovary syndrome. *J Clin Endocrinol Metab* 2003; 88: 812–819.

106. Sabuncu T, Harma M, Harma M, Nazligul Y, Kilic F. Sibutramine has a positive effect on clinical and metabolic parameters in obese patients with polycystic ovary syndrome. *Fertil Steril* 2003; 80: 1199–1204.

107. Jayagopal V, Kilpatrick ES, Holding S, Jennings PE, Atkin SL. Orlistat is as beneficial as metformin in the treatment of polycystic ovarian syndrome. *J Clin Endocrinol Metab* 2005; 90: 729–733.

108. Pasquali R, Antenucci D, Casimirri F, Venturoli S, Paradisi R, Fabbri R, Balestra V, Melchionda N, Barbara L. Clinical and hormonal characteristics of obese amenorrheic hyperandrogenic women before and after weight loss. *J Clin Endocrinol Metab* 1989; 68: 173–179.

109. Guzick DS, Wing R, Smith D, Barga SL, Winters SJ. Endocrine consequences of weight loss in obese, hyperandrogenic anovulatory women. *Fertil Steril* 1994; 61: 598–604.

110. Hollmann M, Runnebaum B, Gerhard. Effects of weight loss on the hormonal profile in obese, infertile women. *Hum Reprod* 1996; 11: 1884–1891.

111. Clark AM, Ledger W, Galletly C, Tomlinson L, Blaney F, Wang X, Norman RJ. Weight loss results in significant improvement in pregnancy and ovulation rates in anovulatory obese women. *Hum Reprod* 1995; 10: 2705–2712.

112. Kiddy DS, Hamilton-Fairley D, Bush A, Short F, Anyaoku V, Reed MJ, Franks S. Improvement in endocrine and ovarian function during dietary treatment of obese women with polycystic ovary syndrome. *Clin Endocrinol (Oxf)* 1992; 36: 105–111.

113. Dunaif A, Scott D, Finegood D, Quintana B, Whitcomb R. The insulin-sensitizing agent troglitazone improves metabolic and reproductive abnormalities in the polycystic ovary syndrome. *J Clin Endocrinol Metab* 1996; 81: 3299–3306.

114. Ehrmann DA. Insulin-lowering therapeutic modalities for polycystic ovary syndrome. *Endocrinol Metab Clin North Am* 1999; 28: 423–438.

115. Kim LH, Taylor AE, Barbieri RL. Insulin sensitizers and polycystic ovary syndrome: Can a diabetes medication treat infertility? *Fertil Steril* 2000; 73: 1097–1098.

116. Lord JM, Flight IH, Norman RJ. Metformin in polycystic ovary syndrome: systematic review and meta-analysis. *BMJ* 2003; 327: 951–953.

117. Kashyap S, Wells GA, Rosenwaks Z. Insulin-sensitizing agents as primary therapy for patients with polycystic ovarian syndrome. *Hum Reprod* 2004; 19: 2474–2483.

118. Crosignani PG, Colombo M, Vegetti W, Somigliana E, Gessati A, Ragni G. Overweight and obese anovulatory patients with polycystic ovaries: parallel improvements in anthropometric indices, ovarian physiology and fertility rate induced by diet. *Hum Reprod* 2003; 18: 1928–1932.

119. Norman RJ, and Moran LJ. Diet and lifestyle factors in the aetiology and management of polycystic ovary syndrome. In *Insulin Resistance and Polycystic Ovarian Syndrome: Pathogenesis, Evaluation, and Treatment*. Diamanti-Kandarakis E, Nestler JE, Pasquali R, Panidis D, eds. Totowa, NJ: The Humana Press (in press).

15 Metabolic and Endocrine Effects of Statins in Polycystic Ovary Syndrome

Pinar H. Kodaman, MD, PhD,
and Antoni J. Duleba, MD

CONTENTS

Summary

Polycystic ovary syndrome (PCOS), a common endocrinopathy affecting women of reproductive age, is characterized by oligo-ovulation and androgen excess. The hyperandrogenemia is secondary to ovarian theca-interstitial hyperplasia and excessive androgen production induced by various factors, including elevated gonadotropins, hyperinsulinemia, and increased oxidative stress. In addition to hyperinsulinemia and systemic inflammation, PCOS is often associated with other cardiovascular risk factors including dyslipidemia and endothelial dysfunction. Statins block HMG CoA reductase, the rate-limiting enzyme in cholesterol biosynthesis, and thereby reduce cardiovascular morbidity and mortality. Blockade of this enzyme and the downstream mevalonate pathway may also lead to decreased maturation of insulin receptors, inhibition of steroidogenesis, and alteration of signal transduction pathways that mediate cellular proliferation. Furthermore, statins have intrinsic antioxidant properties. Given the pleiotropic actions of statins, they are likely to exert beneficial metabolic and endocrine effects in addition to improving the lipid profile in women with PCOS.

Key Words: Polycystic ovary syndrome; theca; statins; oxidative stress; testosterone.

From: *Contemporary Endocrinology: Polycystic Ovary Syndrome*
Edited by: A. Dunaif, R. J. Chang, S. Franks, and R. S. Legro © Humana Press, Totowa, NJ

1. INTRODUCTION

Women with polycystic ovary syndrome (PCOS) suffer from menstrual dysfunction, infertility, and hirsutism. In addition, these women have increased cardiovascular risk factors, including dyslipidemia, which typically consists of elevated total cholesterol and low-density lipoprotein (LDL) *(1–4)*, hypertension, increased carotid intima-media thickness, and a greater prevalence of subclinical atherosclerosis *(3,5)*. In the long term, many, but not all studies, indicate that women with PCOS may have significant cardiovascular morbidity and mortality *(2,6–10)*.

Statins are selective inhibitors of 3-hydroxy-3-methylglutaryl-coenzyme A (HMG-CoA) reductase, the rate-limiting enzyme in the cholesterol biosynthetic pathway. Statins improve the lipid profile, primarily by decreasing total cholesterol and LDL levels *(11,12)* and, therefore, also decrease both cardiovascular morbidity and mortality *(11,13)*. Statins significantly reduce both fatal and non-fatal cardiovascular disease (CVD) events in primary and secondary prevention trials *(11,14,15)*. Statins appear to stabilize atherosclerotic plaques by decreasing levels of metalloproteases and reducing oxidized LDL levels *(16,17)*, thereby preventing plaque rupture, which is the direct cause of most acute coronary events. Other beneficial effects of statins include improvement of endothelial function, such as increased nitric oxide production and inhibition of endothelin *(18,19)*, enhanced cellular immunity, and antiproliferative *(20)* and anti-inflammatory actions *(16)*. More recently, it has become apparent that statins also possess potent antioxidant activities *(21)*.

The potential use of statins for PCOS is related not only to the dyslipidemia frequently associated with this endocrinopathy, but also the recent finding that the dysregulation of ovarian theca-interstitial growth and excessive steroidogenesis appear to be mediated by oxidative stress. PCOS is associated with increased oxidative stress, elevation of markers of systemic inflammation, such as C-reactive protein *(22,23)* and tumor necrosis factor (TNF)-α *(24,25)*, and decreased antioxidant reserve *(22)*. TNF-α and insulin stimulate theca-interstitial cell proliferation *(26–28)*, and several in vitro and in vivo studies have shown that insulin and TNF-α also induce oxidative stress *(29–31)*. It is well known that reactive oxygen species (ROS) induce proliferation of various cell types, including fibroblasts and aortic endothelial cells *(32)*, whereas antioxidants, such as α-tocopherol, inhibit proliferation of vascular smooth muscle, fibroblasts, and many cancer cell lines *(33–36)*.

This chapter will focus on the metabolic and endocrine disturbances associated with PCOS and the novel use of statins in the treatment of this disorder. This approach appears to have beneficial effects not only on the cardiovascular risk factors associated with PCOS, but it may also improve the thecal hyperplasia and hyperandrogenism of PCOS by various mechanisms.

2. HORMONAL DYSREGULATION IN PCOS

The ovaries of women with PCOS are usually enlarged with prominent hyperplasia of theca-interstitial cells that produce excessive amounts of androgens *(37–39)*. Most patients with PCOS have elevated plasma concentrations of luteinizing hormone (LH) and normal or relatively decreased levels of follicle-stimulating hormone (FSH) *(40)*. Increased LH promotes thecal steroidogenesis and thus contributes to the hyperandrogenism seen with the disorder.

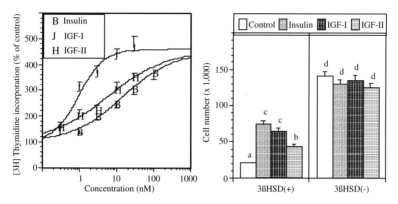

Fig. 1. Dose-dependent stimulation of theca-interstitial cell proliferation by insulin and IGFs. Right graph: effect of insulin and insulin-like growth factors (IGFs) on the number of steroidogenically active [3βHSD(+)] and steroidogenically inactive [3βHSD(–)] theca-interstitial cells. Means with no superscripts in common are significantly different ($p < 0.05$).

Insulin resistance with consequent compensatory hyperinsulinemia, which occurs in both obese and non-obese women with PCOS *(41–43)*, is likely a major contributor to hyperandrogenism, as insulin stimulates the production of androgens by thecal and stromal cells *(44,45)*. Furthermore, free, bioavailable insulin-like growth factor (IGF)-I levels are also elevated in women with PCOS *(46–49)*. Both insulin and IGF-I stimulate proliferation of rat and human theca-interstitial cells *(26,27,50,51)*, and insulin and IGF-I also protect these cells from apoptosis *(52)*. Insulin and IGF-I increase the growth of steroidogenically active ovarian cells, while having little effect on the non-steroidogenic cells *(26)*, demonstrating the relationship between hyperinsulinemia, thecal hyperplasia, and hyperandrogenism (Fig. 1). Furthermore, insulin and IGF-I appear to induce oxidative stress as demonstrated by an increase in LDL peroxidation *(31)*.

3. PCOS AND OXIDATIVE STRESS

Oxidants and antioxidants are involved in the regulation of gene expression under both physiological and pathological conditions. For example, although high concentrations of ROS induce oxidative damage and are cytotoxic, at moderate concentrations, ROS can play a role in signal transduction-mediating cell growth and differentiation and protection from apoptosis *(53–55)*. ROS appear to act as intra- and intercellular messengers capable of producing these cellular responses *(56–58)*.

This biphasic effect of ROS was demonstrated in rat theca-interstitial cell cultures *(59)*. Specifically, modest oxidative stress induced by hypoxanthine and xanthine oxidase stimulated a twofold increase in theca-interstitial cell proliferation, whereas greater oxidative stress profoundly inhibited proliferation (Fig. 2). On the contrary, antioxidants, such as vitamin E succinate, the glutathione peroxidase mimetic ebselen, and superoxide dismutase all inhibited the growth of ovarian theca-interstitial cells *(59)*. The inhibitory effects of antioxidants occurred under basal conditions, that is, in the absence of ROS induction, indicating that the source of ROS resides within

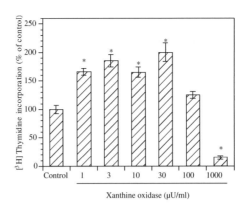

Fig. 2. Effect of hypoxanthine/xanthine oxidase on DNA synthesis of rat theca-interstitial cells. The cells were cultured for 48 h under serum-free conditions with hypoxanthine (1 mmol/l) with and without xanthine oxidase (1–1000 μM/ml). Cultures were carried out in 96-well plates (35,0000 cells/well). Each bar represents the mean +/– SEM of eight replicates. *$p < 0.01$ compared with control.

theca-interstitial cells. Both oxidants and antioxidants had comparable effects on steroidogenically active and inactive cells *(59)*.

These findings raise the possibility that the increased oxidative stress associated with PCOS may contribute to ovarian mesenchymal hyperplasia in addition to the cardiovascular risk factors associated with the syndrome. Furthermore, besides increasing the number of steroidogenically active cells, ROS induce the expression of steroidogenic enzymes, including cholesterol side-chain cleavage (P450scc), 17α-hydroxylase/17,20 lyase (P450c17), and 3-β-hydroxysteroid dehydrogenase (3βHSD) as well as the steroidogenic acute regulatory protein (StAR), which mediates the transport of cholesterol for steroid synthesis *(60)*. In this way, ROS may further exacerbate the hyperandrogenemia of PCOS. At present, the specific mechanisms involved in the generation of ROS in PCOS remain elusive; however, in intact cells, the major intracellular source of ROS is NADPH oxidase, a multisubunit enzyme.

4. STATINS AND THE MEVALONATE PATHWAY

To understand how statins produce their effects, it is essential to understand the mevalonate pathway (Fig. 3). This pathway consists of the reactions starting from acetyl-coenzyme A (acetyl-CoA) and leads to the formation of farnesyl pyrophosphate (FPP). This compound serves as the substrate for several biologically important agents, including cholesterol, isoprenylated proteins, coenzyme Q, and dolichol *(12,61)*. The rate-limiting step in the mevalonate pathway is conversion of HMG-CoA to mevalonate by HMG-CoA reductase. The resulting depletion of mevalonate leads to a decrease in downstream agents, including FPP and geranylgeranyl-pyrophosphate (GGPP). FPP and GGPP farnesylate and geranylgeranylate proteins, respectively, and these post-translational modifications, known collectively as isoprenylation, have important consequences *(62)*.

Isoprenylation is important to membrane attachment and subsequent function of several families of proteins, including Ras, Ras-related GTP-binding proteins, and

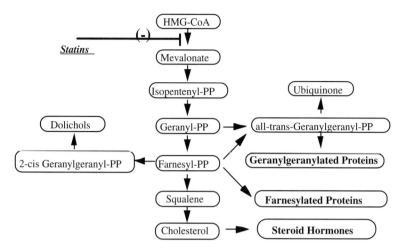

Fig. 3. The mevalonate pathway and its major products.

protein kinases *(62)*. Particularly relevant members of the Ras superfamily include Ras, Rho, Rac, and Cdc42. These small GTPases modulate proliferation, apoptosis, and other cellular functions. Major signal transduction pathways involved in the regulation of proliferation and apoptosis include mitogen-activated protein kinase (MAPK) pathways and the PI3 kinase (PI3K)/Akt and p70S6 kinase (p70S6K) pathways. MAPK pathways are particularly important with respect to cellular proliferation, and downstream effectors include Ras-Raf-extracellular signal-regulated kinase 1/2 (Erk 1/2), P38 kinase (p38K), and c-Jun N terminal protein kinase (JNK). Key steps required for activation of these pathways include farnesylation of Ras and geranylgeranylation of Rho, Rac, and Cdc42 (Fig. 4).

Isoprenylation also affects the generation of ROS by NADPH oxidase, as the assembly of this enzyme requires the presence of isoprenylated Rac at the plasma

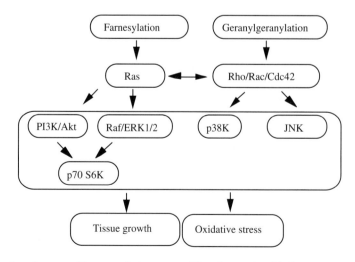

Fig. 4. Proposed pathways of isoprenylation on proliferation and oxidative stress.

ccll mcmbrane *(63)*. Two cytosolic components of NADPH oxidase: p47phox and p67phox complex with Rac1 to induce NADPH oxidase activity *(64)*. Thus, disruption of isoprenylation can lead to profound disturbances in cellular function, including decreased generation of intracellular ROS.

5. MECHANISM OF STATIN ACTION

Statins characterized to date include mevastatin, lovastatin (Mevacor), fluvastatin (Lescol), simvastatin (Zocor), pravastatin (Pravachol), atorvastatin (Lipitor), and rosuvastatin (Crestor). The competitive and reversible inhibition of HMG-CoA reductase by statins impairs hepatic cholesterol synthesis and induces a compensatory increase in the expression of LDL receptors in the liver *(16,65,66)*. This mechanism results in the binding and subsequent removal of LDL and very low-density lipoprotein (VLDL) particles from the circulation, leading to a reduction of total cholesterol, LDL, and triglycerides. Thus, by inhibiting HMG-CoA reductase, statins block the meval-onate biosynthetic pathway, which results in many downstream effects including not only decreased cholesterol synthesis but also a decrease in downstream agents involved in intracellular signaling. Specifically, the blockade of the conversion of HMG-CoA to mevalonate by statins, which is the rate-limiting step in the pathway, results in depletion of mevalonate and, subsequently, leads to decreased isoprenylation of proteins in the form of geranylgeranylation or farnesylation *(62)*.

Inhibition of HMG-CoA and a consequent decrease of isoprenylation of Ras and Rho may inactivate important signal transduction pathways regulating mitotic activity as shown by the recent study in mesangial cells in which statin-induced inhibition of proliferation was associated with suppression of Rho GTPase/p21 signaling *(67)*. Of note, this effect of statins was independent of the cholesterol-lowering actions. Statin-induced inhibition of proliferation is blocked by the addition of mevalonic acid and FPP, but not squalene, suggesting a central role of isoprenylation *(68)*. However, the antiproliferative actions of statins are not ubiquitous and depend on cell type. For example, statins induce proliferation in endothelial progenitor cells *(69)*.

The pleiotropic actions of statins also include their inhibitory effect on N-linked glycosylation *(70)*. Decreased N-linked glycosylation inhibits the maturation of insulin and Type I IGF-I receptors *(71)*. In addition, statins possess both indirect and direct antioxidant activity *(21)*. The antioxidant actions of statins include inhibition of NADPH oxidase activity, preservation of relative levels of vitamins C and E, as well as inhibition of the uptake and generation of oxidized LDL *(63,72)*. Statins have intrinsic antioxidant activity with both antihydroxyl and antiperoxyl radical activity *(21)*. In vitro, simvastatin is the most effective antihydroxyl radical antiox-idant, whereas fluvastatin is the most effective antiperoxyl radical antioxidant *(21)*. In vivo, statins reduce plasma levels of nitrotyrosine and chlorotyrosine *(73)*. Statins also exert anti-inflammatory effects by lowering C-reactive protein levels and suppressing pro-inflammatory agents, such as TNF-α *(74)*.

6. RATIONALE FOR THE USE OF STATINS IN PCOS

Given the pleiotropic nature of the mechanism of statin action, the effects of statins on ovarian function, specifically in women with PCOS, are likely to involve multiple pathways (Fig. 5). First, by directly inhibiting production of cholesterol, the substrate

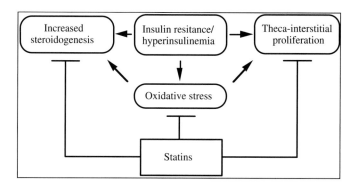

Fig. 5. Rationale for use of statins in polycystic ovary syndrome (PCOS).

for testosterone, statins can improve hyperandrogenemia. Second, the decreased isoprenylation of small GTPases, such as Ras, may also decrease steroidogenesis. This was demonstrated in adrenocortical cells, for example, where an activating K-Ras mutation increased mRNA levels of P450scc, P450c17, and 3βHSD and thereby stimulated steroidogenesis *(75)*, and statins abrogated this effect *(76)*.

By decreasing N-linked glycosylation and thus maturation of insulin and Type I IGF-I receptors, statins can block the actions of insulin and IGF-I on ovarian cells. Furthermore, the effects of the mevalonate pathway correlate with the sites of insulin action as insulin stimulates ovarian steroidogenesis, protein isoprenylation, and ovarian theca-interstitial cell proliferation *(50,77–80)*. Specifically, insulin stimulates the activity of both farnesyltransferase as well as geranylgeranyl transferases I and II *(77,78,81–83)*, thereby augmenting the activity of Ras and other small GTPases *(77–79,84)*. This leads to cellular proliferation by activation of the MAPK pathway, which is mediated by the small GTPases and their effectors, such as Erk1/2.

Although resistance to the effects of insulin on glucose transport is a prominent feature of PCOS, compensatory hyperinsulinemia and elevation of free IFG-I stimulates other aspects of ovarian function, such as proliferation. This suggests that insulin resistance is limited to glucose transport while the other effects of insulin are maintained. Two different signaling pathways mediate these effects: glucose transport is stimulated by insulin through the PI3-kinase pathway, whereas it appears that insulin-induced proliferation is mediated by p70S6K or MAPK pathways *(85,86)*. Thus, insulin resistance may be due to defects in some, but not all, signal transduction pathways. Furthermore, oxidative stress shares some signal transduction pathways with insulin and IGF-I, specifically the Erk 1/2 and p70s6K pathways *(87)*. A convergence of the actions of insulin/IGF-I and ROS at the Erk1/2 and p70s6 K pathways may explain the comparable effects of these agents on proliferation.

Thus, blockade of the mevalonate pathway by statins can lead to an abrogation of the effects of hyperinsulinemia. In addition, by decreasing isoprenylation of small GTPases, such as Ras and Rac, statins can directly inhibit cellular proliferation and ROS generation by NADPH oxidase. As alluded to above, the intrinsic antioxidant activities of statins can also block cellular proliferation and decrease the oxidative stress and inflammation associated with PCOS. The latter, along with the statin-mediated improvcmcnt in lipid profile, can have a beneficial effect on the potential cardiovascular morbidity and mortality associated with this syndrome.

7. EFFECTS OF STATINS ON OVARIAN FUNCTION

The statin mevastatin inhibits the proliferation of theca-interstitial cells in vitro *(88)*; Figure 6 demonstrates that mevastatin decreases DNA synthesis of theca-interstitial cells in a concentration-dependent fashion by 72–92% *(88)*. Furthermore, mevastatin inhibits LH-stimulated production of both progesterone and testosterone by these cells that is independent of its effect on cell number (Fig. 7) *(88)*. The inhibition of theca-interstitial cell proliferation by statins persists in the presence of 5% serum, indicating that the statin-induced inhibition of proliferation is independent of the supply of cholesterol *(89)*. The inhibitory effects of mevastatin on ovarian cell proliferation are consistent with previous reports regarding other mesenchymal cell types, including vascular smooth muscle *(90–92)*, cardiomyocytes *(93)*, and mesangial cells *(67)*.

The effects of statins on ovarian steroidogenesis may be due to several mechanisms. Besides impairing the availability of the substrate cholesterol, statins also decrease the expression of several key enzymes involved in testosterone production including P450scc, P450c17, and 3βHSD as demonstrated in adrenocortical cells *(94,95)*, and similar findings have been observed in ovarian cells *(96)*. It has been established previously that oxidative stress increases the expression of these same steroidogenic enzymes in the ovary *(60)*.

As described above in Section 3, NADPH oxidase is a major source of intracellular ROS. Mevastatin and simvastatin, in the presence of LH, inhibit the expression of p22phox, a membrane-bound subunit essential for function of NADPH oxidase in theca-interstitial cells *(97)*. The expression of another NADPH oxidase subunit p47phox, which requires isoprenylated Rac for its activity, is also decreased by these statins *(97)*. In addition, mevastatin blocks basal and insulin-dependent activation of the MAP kinase pathway in vitro as measured by phosphorylation of Erk1/2, a downstream kinase, which requires farnesylation of Ras *(89)*.

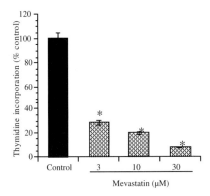

Fig. 6. Effect of mevastatin on DNA synthesis in theca-interstitial cell cultures. The cells were cultured for 48 h under serum-free conditions without (control) or with mevastatin (3–30 μM). Each bar represents the mean of eight replicates. *$p < 0.01$ significantly different from control.

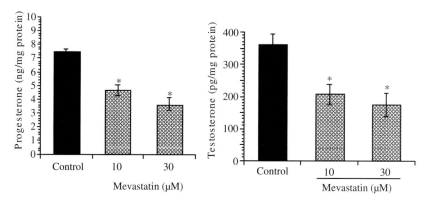

Fig. 7. Effect of mevastatin on progesterone and testosterone production by theca-interstitial cell cultures. The cells were cultured for 48 h under serum-free conditions in the presence of LH (100 ng/ml) without (control) or with mevastatin (3–30 M). Each bar represents the mean of four replicates. *$p < 0.01$ significantly different from control.

Thus, in summary, the in vitro studies on ovarian theca-interstitial cells demonstrate that statins decrease cell proliferation and testosterone production, inhibit the expression of steroidogenic enzymes, decrease expression of NADPH oxidase subunits, and block MAPK-dependent phosphorylation. Taken together, these finding raise the possibility that the use of statins in women with PCOS could decrease thecal hyperplasia, hyperandrogenism, and oxidative stress.

8. TREATMENT OF PCOS WITH STATINS

Recently, a randomized, prospective clinical trial investigated for the first time the effects of simvastatin on women with PCOS *(98)*. PCOS was defined according to the definition adopted at a recent international consensus workshop *(99)*. Specifically, all eligible patients had at least two of the three following criteria: *(1)* chronic anovulation; *(2)* hyperandrogism and/or hyperandrogenemia; and *(3)* polycystic ovaries. Forty-eight women with PCOS were randomized to one of two groups: *(1)* the Statin group [simvastatin, 20 mg daily plus oral contraceptive pill (OCP) containing 20 µg ethinyl estradiol and 150 µg desogestrel] or *(2)* the OCP group (OCP alone). Both groups consisted of OCPs as statins are designated pregnancy category X given their broad-ranging and potentially detrimental effects on cellular function and proliferation.

After 12 weeks of treatment, testosterone levels declined by an average of 41% ($p < 0.0001$) in the Statin group and by 14% ($p = 0.1$) in the OCP group, and the treatment effect between groups was significant ($p < 0.006$) (Fig. 8). Hirsutism slightly, but significantly, declined in the Statin group as measured by the Ferriman & Gallway scale and declined non-significantly in the OCP group. In contrast to the effects on testosterone, simvastatin had no effect on dehydroepiandrosterone sulfate (DHEAS) levels, suggesting that the actions of statins are selective and may not alter adrenal steroidogenesis.

However, simvastatin did affect the hypothalamo–pituitary axis, because between the groups, there were distinctly different responses noted with respect to gonadotropin levels. LH declined by 43% in the Statin group and only by 9% in the OCP group.

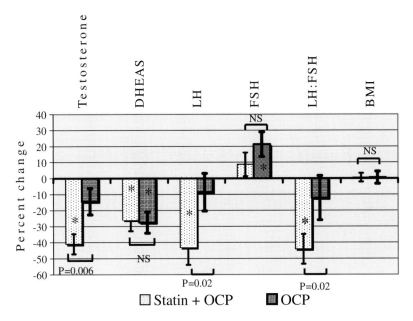

Fig. 8. Effect of statin (simvastatin 20 mg/day) and oral contraceptive pill (OCP) versus OCP alone on serum levels on androgens, gonadotropins, and body mass index (BMI) in women with polycystic ovary syndrome (PCOS) after 12 weeks of treatment. Asterisks denote significant effect of treatment versus baseline; *p*-values listed above or below brackets refer to significant differences between treatment groups. NS refers to non-significant differences.

As the FSH levels did not significantly change, the net effect was a reduction in the LH : FSH ratio by approximately 44% in the Statin group and a non-significant decrease by 12% in the OCP group. Neither of the treatments had a significant effect on body mass index (BMI). The improvements in testosterone and LH in the Statin group were not mediated by changes in insulin sensitivity, as determined by fasting and post-glucose challenge levels of insulin and glucose.

As expected, total cholesterol and LDL decreased in the Statin group by 10 and 24%, respectively, whereas there were small increases in these parameters in the OCP group (Fig. 9). There was a small, but significant, increase in HDL in both groups, and triglyceride levels were not affected by simvastatin treatment. The improvement of the lipid profile by simvastatin is of particular value in PCOS, a condition characterized by dyslipidemia and other cardiovascular risk factors. Use of statins in these patients is likely to offer significant protection from long-term cardiovascular morbidity.

This is the first study demonstrating the effects of a statin on endocrine and metabolic parameters in women with PCOS. Although the design of the above-described clinical trial did not allow for direct dissociation of the effects of statins on the ovary from those on the hypothalamus and pituitary, it is likely that the primary actions of statins are exerted at the ovarian level by decreasing testosterone, which in turn, may cause a decrease of LH. This is supported by in vitro studies that show direct effects of statins on testosterone production by theca-interstitial cells *(88)* and also by the finding that ovarian wedge resection or laparoscopic diathermy both decrease ovarian androgen production in parallel with a marked decline of LH and the LH : FSH ratio *(100,101)*.

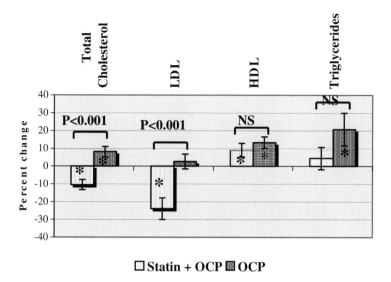

□ Statin + OCP ▨ OCP

Fig. 9. Effect of statin (simvastatin 20 mg/day) and oral contraceptive pill (OCP) versus OCP alone on lipid profile in women with polycystic ovary syndrome (PCOS) after 12 weeks of treatment. Asterisks denote significant effect of treatment versus baseline; *p*-values listed above brackets refer to significant differences between treatment groups. NS refers to non-significant differences.

The statin-induced decrease of testosterone levels in the above-described study is consistent with findings of two randomized trials in men *(95,102)*. However, the decline in testosterone levels in these men was modest, and several other studies evaluating men failed to demonstrate a significant effect of statins on testosterone production *(103–105)*. A possible explanation for this may be the ability of the testes to adapt to statins through compensatory mechanisms involving an increased capacity of Leydig cells to produce cholesterol as was demonstrated in the rat *(106)*. Much less is known about the effects of statins on steroidogenesis in women. The use of statins in postmenopausal women was associated with a small, but significant, decrease in progesterone levels *(107)*, whereas other studies showed no effect on steroidogenesis *(108)*. It remains to be seen what the long-term effects of statins are in women with PCOS. The above-described randomized controlled study has been extended in duration to 24 weeks, and the results are pending analysis.

9. CONCLUSION

Prominent features of PCOS include hyperinsulinemia, increased oxidative stress, and elevation of growth factors and cytokines, including IGF-I and TNF-α. These alterations may contribute to the increased size of the ovarian theca-interstitial compartment and to increased production of androgens. Furthermore, PCOS is associated with a broad range of cardiovascular risk factors, including dyslipidemia, endothelial dysfunction, and systemic inflammation.

Growing evidence points to statins as agents capable of not only correcting dyslipidemia but also improving systemic inflammation, endothelial function, and oxidative stress. In vitro studies have shown that statins inhibit both proliferation and steroidogenesis of ovarian theca-interstitial cells. The actions of statins may be, in part, related to reduction of oxidative stress and consequent reduction of steroidogenesis and cellular proliferation. The inhibition of N-glycosylation of insulin and IGF-I receptors along with the inhibition of the mevalonate pathway by statins can abrogate the actions of insulin, which otherwise would contribute to the thecal hyperplasia and hyperandrogenemia that occurs with PCOS. In the first clinical trial in women with PCOS, simvastatin decreased testosterone level, normalized gonadotropins, and improved lipid profile.

Taken together, the available evidence supports the hypothesis that the mevalonate pathway plays a prominent role in the function of theca-interstitial cells and that modulation of this pathway by agents such as statins may provide both systemic cardiovascular benefits and improved ovarian function in PCOS. Given the involvement of the mevalonate pathway in the post-translational modification of small GTPases included in many signaling pathways, care must be taken to avoid the use of statins in women who are trying to conceive or who may be at risk of conceiving.

REFERENCES

1. Wild RA, Painter PC, Coulson PB, Carruth KB, Ranney GB. Lipoprotein lipid concentrations and cardiovascular risk in women with polycystic ovary syndrome. *J. Clin. Endocrinol. Metab.* 1985;61:946–951.

2. Mahabeer S, Naidoo C, Norman RJ, Jialal I, Reddi K, Joubert SM. Metabolic profiles and lipoprotein lipid concentrations in non-obese and obese patients with polycystic ovarian disease. *Horm. Metab. Res.* 1990;22:537–540.

3. Guzick DS, Talbott EO, Sutton-Tyrrell K, Herzog HC, Kuller LH, Wolfson SKJ. Carotid atherosclerosis in women with polycystic ovary syndrome: initial results from a case-control study. *Am. J. Obstet. Gynecol.* 1996;174:1224–1229.

4. Talbott EO, Guzick DS, Clerici A, Berga S, Detre K, Weimer K, et al. Coronary heart disease risk factors in women with polycystic ovary syndrome. *Arterioscler. Thromb. Vasc. Biol.* 1995;15: 821–826.

5. Talbott EO, Guzick DS, Sutton-Tyrrell K, McHugh-Pemu KP, Zborowski JV, Rembsberg KE, et al. Evidence for association between polycystic ovary syndrome and premature carotid atherosclerosis in middle-aged women. *Arterioscler. Thromb. Vasc. Biol.* 2000;20:2414–2421.

6. Wild RA, Applebaum-Bowden D, Demers LM, Bartholomew M, Landis JR, Hazzard WR, et al. Lipoprotein lipids in women with androgen excess: independent associations with increased insulin and androgens. *Clin. Chem.* 1990;36:283–289.

7. Dahlgren E, Johansson S, Lindstedt G, Knutsson F, Oden A, Janson PO, et al. Women with polycystic ovary syndrome wedge resected in 1956 to 1965: a long-term follow-up focusing on natural history and circulating hormones. *Fertil. Steril.* 1992;57:505–513.

8. Dahlgren E, Janson PO, Johansson S, Lapidus L, Oden A. Polycystic ovary syndrome and risk for myocardial infarction. *Acta Obstet. Gynecol. Scand.* 1992;71:599–604.

9. Wild S, Pierpoint T, McKeigue P, Jacobs H. Cardiovascular disease in women with polycystic ovary syndrome at long-term follow-up: a retrospective cohort study. *Clin. Endocrinol.* 2000;52:595–600.

10. Wild RA, Pierpoint T, Jacobs H, McKeigue P. Long-term consequences of polycystic ovary syndrome: results of a 31 year follow-up study. *Hum Fertil* 2000;3(2):101–105.

11. Anonymous. Randomised trial of cholesterol lowering in 4444 patients with coronary heart disease: the Scandinavian Simvastatin Survival Study (4S). *Lancet* 1994;344:1383–1389.

12. Goldstein JL, Brown MS. Regulation of the mevalonate pathway. *Nature* 1990;343:425–430.

13. Sacks FM, Pfeffer MA, Moye LA, Rouleau JL, Rutherford JD, Cole TG, et al. The effect of pravastatin on coronary events after myocardial infarction in patients with average cholesterol levels. *N. Engl. J. Med.* 1996;335:1001–1009.

14. Shepard J, Cobbe SM, Ford I, Isles CG, Lorimer AR, MacFarlane PW, et al. Prevention of coronary heart disease with pravastatin in men with hypercholesterolemia. West of Scotland Coronary Prevention Study Group. *N. Engl. J. Med.* 1995;333:1301–1307.

15. Downs JR, Clearfield M, Weis S, Whitney E, Shapiro DR, Beere PA, et al. Primary prevention of acute coronary events with lovastatin in men and women with average cholesterol levels: results of AFCAPS/TexCAPS. Air Force/Texas Coronary Atherosclerosis Prevention Study. *JAMA* 1998;279:1615–1622.

16. McFarlane SI, Muniyappa R, Francisco R, Sowers JR. Clinical review 145: Pleiotropic effects of statins: lipid reduction and beyond. *J. Clin. Endocrinol. Metab.* 2002;87:1451–1458.

17. Crisby M, Nordin-Fredriksson G, Shah PK, Yano J, Zhu J, Nilsson J. Pravastatin treatment increases collagen content and decreases lipid content, inflammation, metalloproteinases, and cell death in human carotid plaques: implications for plaque stabilization. *Circulation* 2001;103:926–933.

18. Perticone F, Ceravolo R, Maio R, Cloro C, Candigliota M, Scozzatava A, et al. Effects of atorvastatin and vitamin C on endothelial function of hypercholesterolemic patients. *Atherosclerosis* 2000;152:512–518.

19. Alvarez DS, M., Herrera MD, Marhuenda E, Andriantsitohaina R. Characterization of endothelial factors involved in the vasodilatory effect of simvastatin in aorta and small mesenteric artery of the rat. *Br. J. Clin. Pharmacol.* 2000;131:1179–1187.

20. Porter KE, Naik J, Turner NA, Dickinson T, Thompson MM, London NJ. Simvastatin inhibits human saphenous vein neointima formation via inhibition of smooth muscle cell proliferation and migration. *J. Vasc. Surg.* 2002;36:150–157.

21. Franzoni F, Quinones-Galvan A, Regoli F, Ferrannini E, Galetta F. A comparative study of the in vitro antioxidant activity of statins. *Int. J. Cardiol.* 2003;90:317–321.

22. Sabuncu T, Vural H, Harma M. Oxidative stress in polycystic ovary syndrome and its contribution to the risk of cardiovascular disease. *Clin. Biochem.* 2001;34:407–413.

23. Kelly CC, Lyall H, Petrie JR, Gould GW, Connell JM, Sattar N. Low grade chronic inflammation in women with polycystic ovarian syndrome. *J. Clin. Endocrinol. Metab.* 2001;86:2453–2455.

24. Naz RK, Thurston D, Santoro N. Circulating tumor necrosis factor (TNF)-alpha in normally cycling women and patients with premature ovarian failure and polycystic ovaries. *Am. J. Reprod. Immunol.* 1995;34:170–175.

25. Gonzalez F, Thusu K, Abdel-Rahman E, Prabhala A, Tomani M, Dandona P. Elevated serum levels of tumor necrosis factor alpha in normal-weight women with polycystic ovary syndrome. Metabolism: *Clin. Experim.* 1999;48:437–441.

26. Duleba AJ, Spaczynski RZ, Olive DL, Behrman HR. Effects of insulin and insulin-like growth factors on proliferation of rat ovarian theca-interstitial cells. *Biol. Reprod.* 1997;56:891–897.

27. Duleba AJ, Spaczynski RZ, Arici A, Carbone R, Behrman HR. Proliferation and differentiation of rat theca-interstitial cells: comparison of effects induced by platelet-derived growth factor and insulin-like growth factor-I. *Biol. Reprod.* 1999;60:546–550.

28. Spaczynski RZ, Arici A, Duleba AJ. Tumor necrosis factor-alpha stimulates proliferation of rat ovarian theca-interstitial cells. *Biol. Reprod.* 1999;61:993–998.

29. Adamson GM, Billings RE. Tumor necrosis factor induced oxidative stress in isolated mouse hepatocytes. *Arch. Biochem. Biophys.* 1992;294:223–229.

30. Krieger-Brauer HI, Kather H. Human fat cells possess a plasma membrane-bound H_2O_2 generating system that is activated by insulin via a mechanism bypassing the receptor kinase. *J. Clin. Invest.* 1992;89:1006–1013.

31. Rifici VA, Schneider SII, Khachadurian AK. Stimulation of low-density lipoprotein oxidation by insulin and insulin like growth factor I. *Atherosclerosis* 1994;107:99–108.

32. Ruiz-Gines JA, Lopez-Ongil S, Gonzalez-Rubio M, Gonzalez-Santiago L, Rodriguez-Puyol M, Rodriguez-Puyol D. Reactive oxygen species induce proliferation of bovine aortic endothelial cells. *J. Cardiovasc. Pharmacol.* 2000;35:109–113.

33. Ivanov VO, Ivanova SV, Niedzwiecki A. Ascorbate affects proliferation of guinea pig vascular smooth muscle cells by direct and extracellular matrix-mediated effects. *J. Mol. Cell Cardiol.* 1997;29:3293–3303.

34. Azzi A, Aratri E, Boscoboinik D, Clement S, Ozer NK, Ricciarelli R, et al. Molecular basis of alpha-tocopherol control of smooth muscle cell proliferation. *Biofactors* 1998;7:3–14.

35. Nesaretnam K, Stephen R, Dils R, Darbre P. Tocotrienols inhibit the growth of human breast cancer cells irrespective of estrogen receptor status. *Lipids* 1998;33:461–469.

36. Onat D, Boscoboinik D, Azzi A, Basaga H. Effects of alpha-tocopherol and silibin dihemisuccinate on the proliferation of human skin fibroblasts. *Biotechnol. Appl. Biochem.* 1999;29:213–215.

37. Hughesdon PE. Morphology and morphogenesis of the Stein-Leventhal ovary and of so-called "hyperthecosis". *Obstet. Gynecol. Surv.* 1982;37:59–77.

38. Wickenheisser JK, Quinn PG, Nelson VL, Legro RS, Strauss JF 3rd, McAllister JM. Differential activity of the cytochrome P450 17 alpha hydroxylase and steroidogenic acute regulatory protein gene promoters in normal and polycystic ovary syndrome theca cells. *J. Clin. Endocrinol. Metab.* 2000;85:2304–2311.

39. Nelson VL, Legro RS, Strauss JF 3rd, McAllister JM. Augmented androgen production is a stable steroidogenic phenotype of propagated theca cells from polycystic ovaries. *Mol. Endocrinol.* 1999;13:946–957.

40. Yen SS, Vela P, Rankin J. Inappropriate secretion of follicle-stimulating hormone and luteinizing hormone in polycystic ovarian disease. *J. Clin. Endocrinol. Metab.* 1970;30:435–442.

41. Burghen GA, Givens JR, Kitabchi AE. Correlation of hyperandrogenism with hyperinsulinism in polycystic ovarian disease. *J. Clin. Endocrinol. Metab.* 1980;50:113–116.

42. Chang RJ, Nakamura RM, Judd HL, Kaplan SA. Insulin resistance in non-obese patients with polycystic ovarian disease. *J. Clin. Endocrinol. Metab.* 1983;57:356–359.

43. Dunaif A, Graf M, Mandell J, Laumas V, Dobrjansky A. Characterization of groups of hyperandrogenic women with acanthosis nigricans, impaired glucose tolerance, and/or hyperinsulinemia. *J. Clin. Endocrinol. Metab.* 1987;65:499–507.

44. Barbieri RL, Makris A, Ryan KJ. Insulin stimulates androgen accumulation in incubations of human ovarian stroma and theca. *Obstet. Gynecol.* 1984;64:74S–80S.

45. Barbieri RL, Makris A, Randall RW, Daniels G, Kistner RW, Ryan KJ. Insulin stimulates androgen accumulation in incubations of ovarian stroma obtained from women with hyperandrogenism. *J. Clin. Endocrinol. Metab.* 1986;62:904–910.

46. Iwashita M, Mimuro T, Watanabe M, Setoyama T, Matsuo A, Adachi T, et al. Plasma levels of insulin-like growth factor-I and its binding protein in polycystic ovary syndrome. *Horm. Res.* 1990;33:21–26.

47. Homburg R, Pariente C, Lunenfeld B, Jacobs HS. The role of insulin-like growth factor-I (IGF-I) and IGF binding protein in patients with polycystic ovarian disease. *Hum. Reprod.* 1992;7: 1379–1383.

48. Suikkari AM, Ruutiainen K, Erkkola R, Seppala M. Low levels of low molecular weight insulin like growth factor binding protein in patients with polycystic ovarian disease. *Hum. Reprod.* 1989;4: 136–139.

49. Thierry van Dessel HJ, Lee PD, Faessen G, Fauser BC, Giudice L. Elevated serum levels of free insulin-like growth factor I in polycystic ovary syndrome. *J. Clin. Endocrinol. Metab.* 1999;84: 3030–3035.

50. Duleba AJ, Spaczynski RZ, Olive DL. Insulin and insulin-like growth factor I stimulate the proliferation of human ovarian theca-interstitial cells. *Fertil. Steril.* 1998;69:335–340.

51. Duleba AJ, Spaczynski RZ, Olive DL, Behrman HR. Divergent mechanism regulate proliferation/survival and steroidogenesis of theca-interstitial cells. *Mol. Hum. Reprod.* 1999;5:193–198.

52. Duleba AJ, Spaczynski RZ, Tilly JL, Olive DL. Insulin and insulin-like growth factors protect ovarian theca-interstitial cells from apoptosis. 45th Annual Meeting of the Society for Gynecologic Investigation 1998; Atlanta, GA.

53. Clement MV, Pervaiz S. Reactive oxygen intermediates regulate cellular response to apoptotic stimuli: a hypothesis. *Free Radical Res.* 1999,30.247–252.

54. Kamata H, Hirata H. Redox regulation of cellular signalling. *Cell Signal* 1999;11:1–14.

55. Kunsch C, Medford RM. Oxidative stress as a regulator of gene expression in the vasculature. *Circulation Res.* 1999;85:753–766.

56. Burdon RH, Alliangana D, Gill V. Hydrogen peroxide and the proliferation of BHK-2 cells. *Free Radical Res.* 1995;23:471–486.

57. Burdon RH, Gill V, Alliangana D. Hydrogen peroxide in relation to proliferation and apoptosis in BHK-21 hamster fibroblasts. *Free Radical Res.* 1996;24:81–93.

58. delBello B, Paolicchi A, Comporti M, Pompella A, Maellaro E. Hydrogen peroxide produced during gamma-glutamyl transpeptidase activity is involved in prevention of apoptosis and maintenance of proliferation in U937 cells. *FASEB J.* 1999;13:69–79.

59. Duleba AJ, Foyouzi N, Karaca M, Pehlivan T, Kwintkiewicz J, Behrman HR. Proliferation of ovarian theca-interstitial cells is modulated by antioxidants and oxidative stress. *Hum. Reprod.* 2004;19:1519–1524.

60. Piotrowski P, Rzepczynska I, Kwintkiewicz J, Duleba AJ. Oxidative stress induces expression of CYP11A, CYP17, StAR and 3bHSD in rat theca-interstitial cells. 52nd Annual Meeting of the Society for Gynecologic Investigation 2005; Los Angeles, CA (March 23–26).

61. Turunen M, Olsson J, Dallner G. Metabolism and function of coenzyme Q. *Biochem. Biophys. Acta* 2004;1660:171–199.

62. Zhang FL, Casey PJ. Protein prenylation: molecular mechanism and functional consequences. *Annu. Rev. Biochem.* 1996;65:241–269.

63. Wassmann S, Laufs U, Muller K, Konkol C, Ahlbory K, Baumer AT, et al. Cellular antioxidant effects of atorvastatin in vitro and in vivo. *Arterioscler. Thromb. Vasc. Biol.* 2002;22:300–305.

64. Gregg D, Rauscher FM, Goldschmidt-Clermont PJ. Rac regulates cardiovascular superoxide through diverse molecular interactions: more than a binary GTP switch. *Am. J. Cell Physiol.* 2003;285: C723–734.

65. Clearfield M. Evolution of cholesterol management therapies exploiting potential for further improvement. *Am. J. Ther.* 2003;10:275–281.

66. Corsini A, Bellosta S, Baetta R, Fumagalli R, Paoletti R, Bernini F. New insights into the pharmacodynamic and pharmacokinetic properties of statins. *Pharmacol. Ther.* 1999;84:413–428.

67. Danesh FR, Sadeghi MM, Amro N, Philips C, Zeng L, Lin S, et al. 3-Hydroxy-3-methylglutaryl CoA reductase inhibitors prevent high glucose-induced proliferation of mesangial cells via modulation of Rho GTPase/p21 signaling pathway: implications for diabetic nephropathy. *Proc. Natl. Acad. Sci. USA* 2002;99:8301–8305.

68. Raiteri M, Arnaboldi L, McGeady P, Gelb MH, Verri D, Tagliabue C, et al. Pharmacological control of the mevalonate pathway: effect on arterial smooth muscle cell proliferation. *J. Pharmacol. Exp. Ther.* 1997;281:1144–1153.

69. Assmus B, Urbich C, Aicher A, Hofmann WK, Haendeler J, Rossig L, et al. HMG-CoA reductase inhibitors reduce senescence and increase proliferation of endothelial progenitor cells via regulation of cell cycle regulatory genes. *Circ. Res.* 2003;92:1049–1055.

70. Siddals KW, Marshman E, Westwood M, Gibson JM. Abrogation of insulin-like growth factor-I (IGF-I) and insulin action by mevalonic acid depletion; synergy between protein prenylation and receptor glycosylation pathways. *J. Biol. Chem.* 2004;279:38353–38359.

71. Carlberg M, Dricu A, Blegen H, Wang M, Hjertman M, Zickert P, et al. Mevalonic acid is limiting for N-linked glycosylation and translocation of the insulin-like growth factor-I receptor to the cell surface. Evidence for a new link between 3-hydroxy-3-methylglutaryl coenzyme A reductase and cell growth. *J. Biol. Chem.* 1996;271:17453–17462.

72. Avram M, Dankner G, Cogan U, Hochgraf E, Brook JGW. Lovastatin inhibits low-density lipoprotein oxidation and alters its fluidity and uptake by macrophages: in vitro and in vivo studies. *Metabolism* 1992;41:229–235.

73. Shishehbor MH, Brennan ML, Aviles RJ, Fu X, Sprecher DL, Hazen SL. Statins promote potent systemic antioxidant effects through specific inflammatory pathways. *Circulation* 2003;108: 426–431.

74. Ando H, Takamura T, Ota T, Nagai Y, Kobayashi K. Cerivastatin improves survival of mice with lipopolysaccharide-induced sepsis. *J. Pharmacol. Exp. Ther.* 2000;294:1043–1046.

75. Wu CH, Chen YF, Wang JY, Hsieh MC, Yeh CS, Lian ST, et al. Mutant K-ras oncogene regulates steroidogenesis of normal human adrenocortical cells by the RAF-MEK-MAPK pathway. *Br. J. Cancer* 2002;87:1000–1005.

76. Wu CH, Lee SC, Chiu HH, Yang YC, Lian ST, Shin JR, et al. Morphologic change and elevation of cortisol secretion in cultured human normal adrenocortical cells caused by mutant p21K-ras protein. *DNA Cell Biol.* 2002;21:21–29.

77. Goalstone ML, Leitner JW, Wall K, Dolgonos L, Rother KI, Accili D, et al. Effect of insulin on farnesyltransferase. Specificity of insulin action and potentiation of nuclear effects of insulin-like growth factor-1, epidermal growth factor, and platelet-derived growth factor. *J. Biol. Chem.* 1998;273:23892–23896.

78. Goalstone ML, Draznin B. Effect of insulin on farnesyltransferase activity in 3T3-L1 adipocytes. *J. Biol. Chem.* 1996;271:27585–27589.

79. Goalstone ML, Leitner JW, Golovchenko I, Stjernholm MR, Cormont M, LeMarchand-Brustel Y, et al. Insulin promotes phosphorylation and activation of geranylgeranyltransferase II. Studies with geranylgeranylation of rab-3 and rab-4. *J. Biol. Chem.* 1999;274:2880–2884.

80. Barbieri RL, Makris A, Ryan KJ. Effects of insulin on steroidogenesis in cultured porcine ovarian theca. *Fertil. Steril.* 1983;40:237–241.

81. McCarty MF. Insulin's stimulation of endothelial superoxide generation may reflect up-regulation of isoprenyl transferase activity that promotes rac translocation. *Med. Hypotheses* 2002;58: 472–475.

82. Draznin B, Miles P, Kruszynska Y, Olefsky J, Friedman J, Golovchenko I, et al. Effects of insulin on prenylation as a mechanism of potentially detrimental influence of hyperinsulinemia. *Endocrinology* 2000;141:1310–1316.

83. Goalstone ML, Draznin B. What does insulin do to Ras? *Cell Signal* 1998;10:297–301.

84. Solomon CS, Leitner JW, Goalstone ML. Dominant negative alpha-subunit of farnesyl- and geranylgeranyl-transferase I inhibits insulin-induced differentiation of 3T3-L1 pre-adipocytes. *Int. J. Obes. Relat. Metab. Disord.* 2003;27:40–47.

85. Taha C, Klip A. The insulin signaling pathway. *J. Membr. Biol.* 1999;169:1–12.

86. Avruch J. Insulin signal transduction through protein kinase cascades. *Mol. Cell. Biochem.* 1998;182:31–48.

87. Lee WC, Choi CH, Cha SH, Oh HL, Kim YK. Role of ERK in hydrogen peroxide-induced cell death of human glioma cells. *Neurochem. Res.* 2005;30:263–270.

88. Izquierdo D, Foyouzi N, Kwintkiewicz J, Duleba AJ. Mevastatin inhibits ovarian theca-interstitial cell proliferation and steroidogenesis. *Fertil. Steril.* 2004;82:1193–1197.

89. Kwintkiewicz J, Foyouzi N, Piotrowski P, Rzepczynska I, Duleba AJ. Mevastatin inhibits proliferation of rat ovarian theca-interstitial cells by blocking the mitogen activated protein kinase pathway. *Fertil. Steril.* 2006;86:1053–1058.

90. O'Driscoll G, Green D, Taylor RR. Simvastatin, an HMG coenzyme A reductase inhibitor, improves endothelial function within 1 month. *Circulation* 1997;95:1126–1131.

91. Axel DI, Riessen R, Runge H, Viebahn R, Karsch KR. Effects of cerivastatin on human arterial smooth muscle cell proliferation and migration in transfilter cocultures. *J. Cardiovasc. Pharmacol.* 2000;35:619–629.

92. Buemi M, Allegra A, Senatore M, Marino D, Mcdici MA, Aloisi C, et al. Pro-apoptotic effect of fluvastatin on human smooth muscle cells. *Eur. J. Pharmacol.* 1999;370:201–203.

93. El-Ani D, Zimlichman R. Simvastatin induces apoptosis of cultured rat cardiomyocytes. *J. Basic Clin. Physiol. Pharmacol.* 2001;12:325–338.

94. Wu CH, Lee SC, Chiu HH, Yang YC, Lian ST, Shin SJ, et al. Morphologic change and elevation of cortisol secretion in cultured human normal adrenocortical cells caused by mutant p21K-ras protein. *DNA Cell Biol.* 2002;21:21–29.

95. Dobs AS, Schrott H, Davidson MH, Bays H, Stein EA, Kush D, et al. Effects of high-dose simvastatin on adrenal and gonadal steroidogenesis in men with hypercholesterolemia. *Met. Clin. Exp.* 2000;49:1234–1238.

96. Rzepczynska I, Piotrowski P, Kwintkiewicz J, Duleba AJ. Effect of mevastatin on expression of CYP17, 3bHSD, CYP11A and StAR in rat theca-interstitial cells. 52nd Annual Meeting of the Society for Gynecologic Investigation 2005; Los Angeles, CA (March 23–26).

97. Piotrowski P, Kwintkiewicz J, Rzepczynska I, Duleba AJ. Simvastatin and mevastatin inhibit expression of NADPH oxidase subunits: p22phox and p47phox in rat theca-interstitial cells. 52nd Annual Meeting of the Society for Gynecologic Investigation 2005; Los Angeles, CA (March 23–26).

98. Duleba AJ, Banaszweska B, Spaczynski RZ, Pawelczyk L. Simvastatin improves biochemical parameters of polycystic ovary syndrome: results of a prospective randomized trial. *Fertil. Steril.* 2006;85:996–1001.

99. Rotterdam ESHRE/ASRM-Sponsored PCOS Consensus Workshop Group. Revised 2003 consensus on diagnostic criteria and long-term health risks related to polycystic ovary syndrome. *Fertil. Steril.* 2004;81:19–25.

100. Duleba AJ, Banaszewska B, Spaczynski RZ, Pawelczyk L. Success of laparoscopic ovarian wedge resection is related to obesity, lipid profile, and insulin levels. *Fertil. Steril.* 2003;79: 1008–1014.

101. Amer SA, Li TC, Cooke ID. A prospective dose-finding study of the amount of thermal energy required for laparoscopic ovarian diathermy. *Hum. Reprod.* 2003;18:1693–1698.

102. Hyypa MT, Kronholm E, Virtanen A, Leino A, Jula A. Does simvastatin affect mood and steroid hormone levels in hypercholesterolemic men? A randomized double-blind trial. *Psychoneuroendocrinology* 2003;38:181–194.

103. Jay RH, Sturley RH, Stirling C, McGarrigle HH, Katz M, Reckless JP, et al. Effects of pravastatin and cholestyramine on gonadal and adrenal steroid production in familial hypercholesterolemia. *Br. J. Clin. Pharmacol.* 1991;32:417–422.

104. Bernini GP, Argenio GF, Gasperi M, Vivaldi MS, Franchi F, Salvetti A. Effects of long-term simvastatin treatment on testicular and adrenal steroidogenesis in hypercholesterolemic patients. *J. Endocrinol. Invest.* 1994;17:227–233.

105. Travia D, Tosi F, Negri C, Faccini G, Moghetti P, Muggeo M. Sustained therapy with 3-hydroxy-3-methylglutaryl-coenzyme A reductase inhibitors does not impair steroidogenesis by adrenals and gonads. *J. Clin. Endocrinol. Metab.* 1995;80:836–840.

106. Andreis PG, Cavallini L, Mazzocchi G, Nussdorfer GG. Effects of prolonged administration of lovastatin, an inhibitor of cholesterol synthesis, on the morphology and function of rat Leydig cells. *Exp. Clin. Endocrinol.* 1990;96:15–24.

107. Bairey-Merz CN, Olson MB, Johnson BD, Bittner V, Hodgson TK, Berga SL. Cholesterol lowering medication, cholesterol level, and reproductive hormones in women: the Women's Ischemia Syndrome Evaluation (WISE). *Am. J. Med.* 2002;113:723–727.

108. Ide H, Fujiya S, Aanuma Y, Agishi Y. Effects of simvastatin, a HMG-CoA reductase inhibitor, on plasma lipids and steroid hormones. *Clin. Ther.* 1990;12:410–420.

16

Recommended Therapies for Metabolic Defects in Polycystic Ovary Syndrome

Robert J. Norman, MD, PhD,
Anneloes E. Ruifrok, Medical Student,
Lisa J. Moran, PhD,
and Rebecca L. Robker, PhD

CONTENTS

Summary

Polycystic ovary syndrome (PCOS) is not just a reproductive condition but has metabolic sequelae. The heterogeneity of the condition is reflected in different emphases in patients on expression of these abnormalities. These conditions include effects on lipids, glucose and insulin metabolism, cardiovascular system and weight control. The metabolic syndrome appears to be more common in PCOS. Treatment of metabolic sequelae can be directed to lifestyle interventions including diet and exercise, insulin-sensitizing drugs and management of hyperlipidaemia. The primary goal of treatment in PCOS is to restore reproductive function while improving metabolic sequelae. This is most readily achieved by reducing insulin resistance through a decrease in weight and abdominal fat. Weight loss and exercise reduce insulin resistance, plasma lipids and blood pressure. In summary, there are a range of diets that may be used in PCOS ranging from high protein to high carbohydrate as well as combinations of glycaemic index (GI) foods. The difference in weight between women from the USA with PCOS and Europe may relate to the extensive use of the Mediterranean-type diet in women from Southern Europe who, while suffering from PCOS, do not appear to get the same metabolic sequelae.

From: *Contemporary Endocrinology: Polycystic Ovary Syndrome*
Edited by: A. Dunaif, R. J. Chang, S. Franks, and R. S. Legro © Humana Press, Totowa, NJ

Key Words: Polycystic overy syndrome (PCOS); metabolic syndrome (MBS); lifestyle; insulin sensitizing agents; impaired glucose tolerance.

1. INTRODUCTION

Polycystic ovary syndrome (PCOS) is the consequence of an interaction between the reproductive, endocrine, and metabolic systems. The heterogeneity of the condition is reflected in different emphases in patients on expression of these abnormalities. For instance, significant hair growth, acne, and other cosmetic aspects result from excess testosterone while excessive obesity is reflected in hyperinsulinaemia and the potential for impaired glucose tolerance or diabetes mellitus.

2. THE METABOLIC BASIS FOR ABNORMALITIES IN PCOS

Although the pathogenesis of PCOS is complex and not fully understood, insulin resistance is proposed to be a key metabolic defect in its aetiology (1). Insulin resistance is defined as the inability of insulin to exert its physiological effect and is manifested peripherally or centrally through a reduction in the ability of insulin to lower plasma glucose. This can be observed as impaired insulin-stimulated glucose uptake and suppression of lipolysis of the muscles or adipose tissue, hepatic glucose over-production, and suppression of glycine synthesis. Mechanisms implicated in the aetiology of insulin resistance include elevated levels of (2,3):

1. plasma free fatty acids (FFA);
2. cytokines such as tumor necrosis factor (TNF)-α and interleukin 6 (IL6);
3. leptin;
4. resistin; and
5. peroxisome proliferator activated receptor (PPAR)-γ.

Insulin resistance is affected strongly by obesity, and abdominal obesity is common in overweight subjects with PCOS (4–6). Obesity is implicated in insulin resistance through the release of FFA's from adipocytes, particularly the abdominal adipocytes that impair insulin-mediated glucose uptake in skeletal muscle, adipocytes and the liver, and decrease hepatic insulin sensitivity while increasing hepatic glucose uptake (2,7,8). A synergistic interaction appears to exist with a degree of insulin resistance present in lean women with PCOS, which is augmented by obesity (9,10).

Insulin resistance and compensatory hyperinsulinaemia are consistently documented in lean and obese women with PCOS compared with weight-matched controls.

Potential mechanisms to explain this association include insulin resistance in both muscle and adipose tissue through decreased activity of the insulin receptor, reduced beta-cell function, increased insulin secretion and response to dietary stimuli, and decreased hepatic clearance of insulin.

Hyperandrogenism correlates positively with insulin resistance in obese and lean women with PCOS (11). In PCOS, inhibition of follicular maturation and clinical hyperandrogenaemia occur because of increased ovarian androgen production and luteinizing hormone (LH) hypersecretion (12,13). The liver and ovarian tissue do not appear to display insulin resistance, unlike skeletal muscle and adipose tissue. Insulin synergistically increases the action of LH (14) by stimulating androgen production (15) in the theca and decreasing hepatic production of sex hormone binding globulin

(SHBG) *(16)*, resulting in increased concentrations of total and free androgens. Insulin may additionally stimulate the activity of cytochrome P450-C17α, a key enzyme in ovarian and adrenal androgen biosynthesis, as shown by the reduction of cytochrome P450-C17α activity by insulin-sensitizing agents *(17)* and also by weight loss *(18)*. A role for regulation of leptin and the family of insulin-like growth factors (IGF) and their binding proteins (IGFBP) might also exist *(19)*. A complex interaction thus exists between total body obesity, abdominal obesity and insulin resistance in the aetiology and pathogenesis of PCOS. Not all women with PCOS exhibit hyperinsulinaemia and insulin resistance *(20,21)*. The heterogeneity and complex aetiology of the syndrome might contribute to this discrepancy.

Diagnosis of PCOS is controversial and not all agree with the NIH or Rotterdam diagnostic criteria. The characterization of insulin resistance is additionally unclear. Although assessment methods of insulin sensitivity such as euglycaemic hyperinsulinaemia clamping and the intravenous glucose tolerance test are used for research purposes, the clinical measures of a fasting glucose insulin in response to oral glucose tolerance or the ratio between glucose and insulin as expressed by a homeostatic model assessment (HOMA) or quantitative insulin sensitivity check index (QUICKI) *(22,23)* ratio remain uncertain. The location of adipose tissue additionally influences insulin resistance in PCOS *(24)*. Alteration of obesity and adipose tissue location is fundamentally important to the management of the metabolic problems in PCOS.

3. METABOLIC SYNDROME DEFINITIONS AND PREVALENCE

In 1988, Reaven et al. *(25)* described the metabolic syndrome as a link between insulin resistance, hypertension, dyslipidaemia, type 2 diabetes and other metabolic abnormalities associated with an increased risk of atherosclerotic cardiovascular disease in adults. It is clear that many of these features are common in PCOS, and recent studies have emphasized the commoner occurrence of metabolic syndrome in PCOS. There are a number of definitions of metabolic syndrome in current use, and these are summarized in Table 1. They include the WHO criteria, the ATPIII definition and the more recent one from the International Study for Diabetes *(26)*. Most publications in PCOS use the ATPIII definition. Studies that described metabolic syndrome in PCOS are described in Table 2. Korhonen et al. *(27)* studied 204 women who had metabolic syndrome and compared them with 62 overweight women without central obesity or the metabolic syndrome and 53 healthy lean women. They observed that subjects with metabolic syndrome were more likely to have oligomenorrhea, especially in those with the most severe symptoms (46%, compared with obese 25% and lean 15% control subjects). Glueck et al. *(28)* in 2003, found the metabolic syndrome in 46% of women with PCOS, which was higher than a control group of women in a three-year National Health and Nutrition Examination Survey (NHANES) three year women. Apridonidze and colleagues *(29)* in 2005 did a chart study of women in the clinic of Dr John Nestler. The prevalence of metabolic syndrome was 43%, which was twice that of age-matched controls. Other studies have however not shown any significant difference in metabolic syndrome, particularly among thin women *(30)*. Most studies from the

Table 1
Definition of the Metabolic Syndrome

	NCEP ATPIII	WHO	IDF
Definition (26)	3 or more of the following	Diabetes or impaired fasting glucose, or impaired glucose tolerance or insulin resistance plus to or more of the following	Central obesity with specific cut-points for different ethnic groups plus two or more of the following
Waist circumference, cm	>102 (M); >88 (F)	–	≥94 (M); ≥80 (F)[a]
Waist hip ratio (WHR)	–	>0.9 (M); >0.85(F)	–
Body mass index, kg/m³	–	≥30	–
Serum triglycerides, mg/dl (and mmol/l)	≥150 (1.7)	≥150	≥150 or specific treatment
HDL cholesterol, mg/dl (and mmol/l)	≤40 (1.03) (M); ≤50 (1.29) (F)	<35 (0.9) (M); <39 (1.0) (F)	≤40 (1.03) (M) or specific treatment; ≤50 (1.29) (F) or specific treatment
Blood pressure, mmHg	≥130/85	≥140/90	≥130/85 or specific treatment
Fasting blood glucose, mg/dl (and mmol/l)	≥110 (6.1)	b	≥100 (5.6) or previously diagnosed diabetes
Microalbuminuria, μg/min	–	>20	–
Albumin : creatinine ratio, mg/g	–	≥30	–

M=male; F=female; HDL, high-density lipoprotein.

ATP3: any three of the traits in the same individual meet the criteria for the metabolic syndrome.

[a]For Europeans.

[b]WHO: High insulin levels, an elevated fasting blood glucose or an elevated post-meal glucose alone with at least two of the main criteria (bold) stated above.

IDF: Central obesity plus any two of the criteria stated above.

Table 2

Studies that Described Metabolic Syndrome in Polycystic Ovary Syndrome (PCOS)

Name study	Number of participants	% MBS	Study group	Definition used	Population
Apridonidze T (29)	106	43	PCOS	ATP3	USA
Carmina E (96)	282	8.2	PCOS	ATP3	European
		16	PCOS	WHO	
		2.4	Control		
Coviello AD (119)	49	37	PCOS	ATP3 and WHO	USA
	165	6	NHANES	Combination of ATP3 and IDF	USA
Ehrmann DA (48)	394	33.4	PCOS and control	ATP3	USA
Faloia E (30)	27	37	PCOS	ATP3	European (Italy)
	20	33.3	Control		
Glueck CJ (28)	138	46.4	PCOS	ATP3	USA
	1887	22.2	NHANES		
Korhonen S (27)	543	19.5	Female residents of Pieksamaki[a]	WHO	European (Finland)
Rabelo Acevedo M (120)	39	44	PCOS	NS	Puerto Rico
Sam S (121)	51	56.9	PCOS	ATP3	USA
	38	44.7	HA		
	143	59.4	Unaffected		
	153		Unknown phenotypes		
Vrbikova J (122)	64	1.6	PCOS	ATP3	European (Czech)
	73	0	Control		
Vural B (123)	43	11.6	PCOS	WHO	Turkey
	43	0	Control		

NS=not stated; NHANES=national health and nutrition examination survey.
[a]Born in 1942, 1947, 1952, 1957, 1962.

USA have shown an increase in the prevalence of metabolic syndrome whereas those from Europe have shown very much lower values. It remains to be seen whether all the changes can be explained by obesity alone as opposed to PCOS.

4. METABOLIC RISK FACTORS IN PCOS

4.1. Hypertension

In patients with PCOS, there is some evidence that there is an enhanced renin-angiotensin system function *(31)*. This was confirmed by several other studies. Li et al. *(32)* found elevated values of plasma renin activity (PRA) and plasma angiotensin II, and Morris et al. *(33)* and Jaatinen et al. *(34)* showed the PRA was elevated. Although Hacihanefioglu et al. *(35)* concluded that in PCOS women the plasma total renin level is higher than in healthy women, these PCOS women appeared to be normotensive.

4.2. Dyslipidaemia

This is extremely common in PCOS and may involve 60–70% of all women particularly those with obesity. However, a large number of women with PCOS may have completely normal lipid profiles. Wild et al. *(36)* initially evaluated women with PCOS and normal women by comparing lipoprotein, lipid, and androgen profiles. They showed that women with PCOS had higher triglycerides and very-low-density lipoprotein (VLDL) cholesterol with lower high-density lipoprotein 2 (HDL2) cholesterol and apolipoprotein A1:A2 ratios. Slowinska-Srzednicka et al. *(37)* compared lean and obese PCOS with control subjects. They also found lower levels of HDL2 cholesterol and higher levels of apolipoprotein B in PCOS. Obese women had lower levels of HDL cholesterol and apo-A1 with higher triglycerides and VLDL cholesterol. Overall, most investigators agree that women with PCOS have at least twice the level of serum triglyceride and 25% lower concentration of HDL. There is less agreement with thinner women where HDL2 cholesterol has been alleged lower by some investigators but not others. Obesity appears to be an important contributory factor to the elevated serum triglycerides, cholesterol and phospholipid concentrations. Elevated insulin appears to be a significant explanatory variable for abnormal triglycerides and apo-A1 levels *(38,39)*. Lipid abnormalities appear to be endogenous to the hyperinsulinaemia of PCOS rather than the hyperandrogenaemia as evidenced by lack of change following gonadotropin-releasing hormone (GnRH) agonist treatment.

4.3. Hyperandrogenism

There appears to be a relatively weak connection between hyperandrogenaemia and cardiovascular disease in women. Some studies have shown that circulating androgen levels do not correlate at all with cardiovascular events in women. Overall, this endocrine disturbance is not readily recognized as a cause for increased atherogenic events *(36,40)*.

4.4. Insulin Resistance

Following the initial identification of fasting hyperinsulinaemia and subsequent identification of this being associated with insulin resistance, there is now a strong literature regarding insulin and insulin resistance in PCOS. Obesity and PCOS have synergistic effects on the amount of insulin resistance and subsequent hyperinsulinaemia. The majority of obese PCOS patients have insulin resistance, whereas a small minority of leaner patients may also have it *(41)*. There is clearly an increased risk of type 2 diabetes (Section 4.5) and impaired glucose tolerance. Diabetes in a woman predisposes to cardiovascular disease *(42)* and certainly removes any gender advantage that she might have. There also appears to be a relationship between cardiovascular disease and insulin and glucose levels in non-diabetic subjects making hyperinsulinaemia important in cardiovascular disease as well as dyslipidaemia and glucose intolerance.

4.5. Disorders of Glucose Metabolism

There is a greater prevalence of impaired glucose tolerance and frank diabetes mellitus in patients with PCOS *(43–46)*. Although much of this is obesity-related, there is still an increased risk in non-obese patients with PCOS. A number of studies have followed cohorts of patients with PCOS longitudinally *(44,47–50)* and showed deteriorating glucose tolerance over time at a rate greater than that expected in controlled subjects. Subjects with impaired glucose tolerance also convert to diabetes at a greater rate given the relationship of diabetes with cardiovascular disease and microvascular problems. This is clearly an important issue in the metabolism of PCOS. Almost all the diabetes is type-2-related and is because of insulin resistance, although failure to secrete adequate insulin is also an issue.

4.6. Inflammatory Markers

There is an increasing recognition that PCOS has elements of an inflammatory disease. High-sensitivity C-reactive protein (hsCRP) is raised in many patients with PCOS and may be a precipitant of vascular disease *(51,52)* as well as a marker of inflammation generally *(53,54)*. IL6 is also raised in a number of patients and TNF-α is known to be produced by fat and tends to promote insulin resistance *(52,53,55–57)*. All these markers are raised in obesity together with leptin, which is related specifically to body mass index rather than PCOS itself *(58)*.

4.7. Coagulation Markers

Some studies have suggested that fibrinogen, Von Willebrand factor antigen, factor VII procoagulant activity, factor VII antigen, and plasminogen activator inhibitor levels are abnormal in PCOS *(59,60)*. There is some doubt as to whether these are due to PCOS per se or to obesity *(61)*.

4.8. The Effects of Therapy

There has been ongoing controversy about whether the oral contraceptive pill by aggravating insulin resistance has a marked impact on the metabolic factors in PCOS. In a recent review, it was concluded that the evidence was inconclusive and some studies showing an increased change in metabolic risk factors and other studies showing no change *(62)*. These are summarized in Table 3.

Table 3
Effect of Combined Oral Contraceptives on Polycystic Ovary Syndrome (PCOS)/Insulin Resistance

Study	BMI (kg/m³)	Design	Intervention/subgroups	Insulin sensitivity	Total cholesterol	HDL cholesterol	Triglycerides
Korytkowski (124)	28	CT	PCOS	↓	NS	NS	↑
			Control	↓	NS	NS	↑
Dahlgren (125)	<28	CT	COC	↓	NS	ND	↑
			GnRH analogues	↑	NS	ND	NS
Armstrong (126)	<28	Observational	PCOS	NS	ND	ND	ND
Cibula (62)	<30	CT	PCOS	NS	ND	ND	ND
			Control	NS	ND	ND	ND
Vrbikova (127)	<30	RCT	COC	↓	↑	↑	↑
			TTS-E/CPA	NS	NS	NS	NS
Guido (128)	<25	Observational	DRSP	NS	↑	↑	↑

NS = no significant change; ↓/↑ = significant change (p < 0.05); ND = not done; HDL = high-density lipoprotein; R/CT = randomized/controlled trial; PCOS = polycystic ovary syndrome; TTS-E = transdermal estrogens; CPA = cyproterone acetate; DRSP = drospirenone; IR = insulin resistance; COC = combined oral contraceptives. Table used from Vrbikova J, *Hum Rep Update*, 2005; 11(3):277.

5. CLINICAL DISEASE RELATED TO METABOLIC RISK FACTORS IN PCOS

5.1. Hypertension

Hypertension is common in older women with PCOS who are obese, but generally blood pressure is within the normal range for control subjects in young women. Twenty-four hour ambulatory systolic blood pressure measurements suggest that PCOS women may have higher nocturnal levels compared with controls and maybe an early expression of the risk of further development of sustained hypertension *(63,64)*. Some studies have suggested that treatment for hypertension is required more in women with PCOS.

5.2. Obesity

Obesity is common in PCOS with the percentage prevalence varying between countries. It is alleged that over 50% of women with PCOS are overweight or obese in the USA, reflecting the higher prevalence of weight disorders in that country. In some parts of Europe the levels of obesity are quite low, and in countries such as China and other East Asian countries obesity is not commonly seen. Obesity contributes to the insulin resistance and is predictive of many other reproductive disorders including menstrual abnormalities, infertility, miscarriage, hypertension and pregnancy, congenital abnormalities, disorders of labour and gestational diabetes *(65,66)*.

5.3. Vascular Lesions

A number of studies have suggested that atherosclerosis in the carotid artery as assessed by using ultrasonography or intimal medial thickness is accelerated and is related to blood cardiovascular risk profiles, particularly those of lipids *(67)*. There is a suggestion that the lipid alterations contribute to detectable abnormalities in younger women with PCOS *(68,69)*. Abnormal function of endothelium has also been implicated through abnormal dynamic tests of endothelial function in PCOS patients. There is also marked resistance to the vasodilatory aspects of insulin, suggesting that insulin resistance is contributory to the endothelial problem. Diamanti-Kandarakis et al. *(70,71)* have shown that endothelin-1 is elevated in women with PCOS and is positively correlated with testosterone.

5.4. Ischaemic Heart Disease

There is little clinical evidence at present to implicate an increased clinical incidence of ischaemic heart disease occurring in women with PCOS, despite the numerous risk factors (Section 4). A large retrospective study conducted in the United Kingdom *(72)* on women who had wedge resections of the ovary did not reveal an increased death rate from myocardial infarction. The Nurses' Health Study, which looked at the relationship of menstrual cycle links to coronary artery disease, did suggest an increased death rate in women with oligoamenorrhea *(73)*. This surrogate of PCOS may be the only clinical feature that we have at the moment to show increased death rates. Coronary heart disease as detected by angiography appears to be more common in women with hirsutism and acne, and PCOS is more common in young postmenopausal women who have cardiac events. There is some evidence that coronary artery segments of greater than 50% stenosis are found in some women with PCOS compared with normal women *(74)*. Coronary calcification is also more common in PCOS compared with that in controls *(75–77)*.

6. INTERVENTIONS

6.1. Lifestyle Change including Diet and Exercise

6.1.1. DIET TYPES

The primary goal of treatment in PCOS is to restore reproductive function while improving metabolic sequelae. This is most readily achieved by reducing insulin resistance through a decrease in weight and abdominal fat. Weight loss and exercise reduce insulin resistance, plasma lipids and blood pressure. Many authors have vigorously recommended weight management for women with PCOS and interventions over as little as 4 weeks with weight losses of 5–10% of initial body weight can reduce hyperandrogenism and circulating insulin levels *(65,78–80)*. In PCOS, caloric restriction improves insulin sensitivity measured through euglycaemic hyperinsulinaemic clamps, fasting glucose insulin ratios, HOMA, Oral glucose tolerance test (OGTT)-stimulated insulin and fasting insulin. Weight loss also decreases hyperandrogenism as measured by decreases in the free androgen index, free or total testosterone and increases in SHBG. It improves menstrual function, ovulation and fertility and hirsutism *(81)*. Other advantages of diet and weight loss are

1. Decrease in hyperlipidaemia;
2. Decrease in plasminogen activator inhibitor activity;
3. Decrease in FFA activity;
4. Decrease in ovarian cytokine P450 c17α activity;
5. Reduction in basal adipocyte lipolysis;
6. Enhancement of responses to anovulation induction drugs;
7. Improvement in physiological outcomes.

The location of adipose tissue reduction is also important in restoring metabolic and reproduction function. Holte *(82)* demonstrated that weight loss in PCOS women resulted primarily in reduction of truncal abdominal fat, and the endocrine and metabolic improvements between intervention and control groups were removed after adjusting for truncal abdominal fat. This was confirmed by Huber-Buchholz and colleagues *(83)*. The return of reproductive function occurs with modest weight loss even though the end of study BMI's are often greater than 30 kg/m^3 *(84)*. We found fertility and menstrual improvements after 3–5 months of weight loss *(85)*, whereas Andersen et al. *(86)* noted that improvements occurred within 4–6 weeks of a very-low-calorie diet. Reduction of fasting insulin and HOMA was observed after weight loss in patients with PCOS who developed normal cyclicity as opposed to those who did not *(81)*. Endocrine improvements occur maximally during energy restriction that correlates with a maximum change in insulin sensitivity and is consistent with short-term energy restriction studies in PCOS that report decreases in fasting insulin, increases in SHBG and decreases in testosterone after as early as 4 weeks of energy reduction.

There have been reports that women with PCOS have difficulty in achieving and maintaining weight loss, but this has not been specifically confirmed. It has also been suggested that women with PCOS may possibly exhibit abnormalities in energy expenditure as shown by post-prandial thermogenesis *(87)*. There are also possibilities of discrepancies in appetite regulation, possibly related to ghrelin. This is a stomach-derived hormone that increases sharply before feeding onset and decreases after a meal. In obesity, fasting levels of ghrelin are decreased and the post-prandial decrease might be impaired potentially compromising meal intervention. We have observed an improved post-prandial decrease in ghrelin after 16 weeks of weight loss. This indicates that ghrelin is down-regulated in obesity and that weight loss might restore normal ghrelin homeostasis *(88)*.

Weight loss is a desirable outcome in overweight women with PCOS for short- and long-term improvements in reproductive and metabolic health. Precise dietary evidence-based guidelines are needed for the treatment of this group, both in the amelioration of short-term reproductive and metabolic dysfunction and for minimizing long-term cardiovascular and diabetic mortality and morbidity. The most appropriate dietary intervention remains unclear. The traditional aid to weight loss under official guidelines has been a low-fat moderate protein and high-carbohydrate intake diet combined with regular exercise *(89)*. Whereas short-term weight loss is relatively easy, long-term maintenance of this loss is extremely difficult. There is some evidence to indicate that weight loss is maintained more effectively and compliance is increased when an ad libitum low-fat, high-carbohydrate dietary pattern (approximately 30% of daily energy is fat and 55% is carbohydrate) is followed over longer periods of time compared with fixed energy diets. Subjects who successfully maintain weight report continued consumption of a low-energy and low-fat diet. There has been a lot of interest in high-protein diets, and it is being proposed that a moderate increase in dietary protein at the expense of dietary carbohydrate might increase weight loss and improves insulin sensitivity *(90,91)*. For the purpose of the discussion, the term 'high protein diet' will refer to a moderate-protein, moderate-carbohydrate diet (approximately 30% protein, 40% carbohydrate, 30% fat). The term 'low-protein diet' refers to a low-fat, high-carbohydrate and low-protein diet (15% protein, 55% carbohydrate, 30% fat). While a greater decrease in weight has been observed with a high-protein than a low-protein isocaloric diet in non-PCOS patients, at least two studies have shown no significant difference in PCOS *(81)*.

Indeed, in non-PCOS patients, there has been concern about high-protein diets being related to cardiovascular mortality and morbidity through a deleterious affect on the lipid profile. There is very little evidence from the Nurses' Health Study to support this hypothesis. Although intravenous protein stimulates insulin release, there is little evidence clinically of a difference in fasting insulin levels, post-prandial insulin or insulin sensitivity as assessed by using HOMA. The evidence for increased dietary protein on metabolic parameters is inconclusive. There is also a paucity of data examining the relationship between dietary factors and reproductive hormones. There is concern about high-protein diets and the potential detrimental effects on bone metabolism with increased renal calcium excretion and bone resorption in acute studies. However, no difference in markers of bone turnover and calcium excretion has been observed in long-term dietary intervention studies *(92)*. There has also been concern that increase in dietary protein may impair kidney function by promoting renal hyper-filtration, but again, the evidence for this is marginal *(93)*. In summary, there is inconclusive evidence for the value of increasing dietary protein in PCOS or indeed or any detrimental effect of high protein in PCOS. Ultimately, weight loss will result from a decrease in energy intake with an increase in energy expenditure.

The potentially detrimental effects of a high-carbohydrate diet might also be minimized by modifying the source of dietary carbohydrate, achieved practically through changing the glycaemic index of a carbohydrate. The glycaemic index is a classification index of carbohydrate foods based on the effects on post-prandial blood glucose response *(94)*. It is proposed that a low glycaemic index diet would improve dislipidaemia, improve endothelial function, decrease insulin demand and adiposity and decrease post-prandial glucose *(95)*. This should lead to a decreased risk of cardiovascular disease and of diabetes. Epidemiologically, a low-GI diet is associated with reduced weight, reduced waist/hip ratio and reduced waist circumference in male type 1 diabetics and waist circumference in female type 1 diabetics. In acute intervention studies, high-GI meals decrease satiety and increase hunger and subsequently food intake compared with low-GI test meals. Conversely, high-GI foods appear to promote satiety in the short term, whereas low-GI foods are associated with increased satiety 2–6 h post-meal. The effect of altering dietary GI on reproductive parameters has not been studied extensively. The diet and androgens randomized trial studied the effect of an ad libitum, low in animal fat and high in low GI foods, monounsaturated and N-3 polyunsaturated fatty acids and phyto-oestrogens compared with normal eating patterns in 104 women with high levels of testosterone. The intervention diet reduced serum testosterone, fasting glucose, OGTT-stimulated insulin and increased SHBG. However, with this study design, it was not possible to identify which dietary component produced the beneficial endocrine effect, although weight loss occurred only in the treatment group.

In summary, there are a range of diets that may be used in PCOS ranging from high protein to high carbohydrate as well as combinations of GI foods. The difference in weight between women from the USA with PCOS and Europe may relate to the extensive use of the Mediterranean-type diet in women from Southern Europe who, while suffering from PCOS, do not appear to get the same metabolic sequelae *(96,97)*.

6.1.2. EXERCISE

All national guidelines for weight loss strategies emphasize exercise as it increases caloric burning. There have been few randomized controlled trials on the effect of exercise in PCOS, and most of these are relatively small in size. It remains uncertain as to whether aerobic or non-aerobic (resistance) exercise is best for patients with PCOS, but it is clearly known to everybody that an obese patient with PCOS is not enthusiastic to be seen in a tightly fitting uniform in a gymnasium or indeed to be seen jogging down the street. Exercise needs to be planned suitable for the overweight person, and some of the best are walking, aqua-aerobics and resistance exercises. Considerably more research needs to go into this area, as it is a critically important component of keeping weight under control and reducing insulin resistance. A combination of diet and exercise is the key to the prevention of further weight gain and inducing improvements in metabolic outcomes.

6.1.3. PSYCHOLOGICAL

Although metabolic therapies are physical and measurable, psychological disturbances in PCOS are common and less easily determined. There are a number of quality-of-life assessments for PCOS that have been validated and shown to be suitable for women with this condition *(98)*. It is recommended that they be used in collaboration with any medical or drug intervention in PCOS. We have documented a great improvement in psychological outcome when women join a group where they are given advice about diet and exercise, avoidance of smoking, alcohol and caffeine *(99)*. It goes without saying that addition of extra stresses to the metabolic environment including smoking, alcohol and caffeine are inadvisable and that the medical practitioner and paramedical staff should make every attempt to persuade patients to reduce their use of these addictive substances. A whole package of lifestyle modification should include advice in this area in addition to the other medical issues.

6.1.4. METFORMIN

Metformin has had wide spread use in treating anovulation and insulin resistance in PCOS *(100)*. Evidence-based guidelines indicate that it is efficacious on its own or in combination with lifestyle modification *(78,101)*. Experience from the diabetes prevention program in men with impaired glucose tolerance suggests that lifestyle modification is fundamental but that metformin adds an additional element *(102)*. There is not a lot of evidence that the use of metformin leads to further weight loss despite its well-known side effects of nausea, vomiting and diarrhoea *(78,103,104)*. However, a randomized controlled study of women who are overweight and had PCOS indicated the extra benefit of using metformin with a low caloric and lifestyle change. The adjunct use of such a drug with diet and exercise needs investigation. The data from Pasquali et al. *(105)* and colleagues are summarized in Tables 4 and 5 showing the differential effects of metformin on obesity and on PCOS versus non-PCOS.

6.1.5. OTHER INSULIN SENSITIZERS

Other drugs such as troglitazone (now discontinued) *(106)*, rosiglitazone *(107–109)* and pioglitazone *(110,111)* have dramatic effects on insulin sensitivity improvement

Table 4
Added Benefit of Metformin to Diet (Pasquali et al. 2000) – Metformin versus Placebo

	Metformin = Placebo	*Metformin > Placebo*
Weight		Yes
Waist circumference		Yes
Visceral fat		Yes
Fasting glucose	Yes	
Fasting insulin	Yes	
Testosterone		Yes
SHBG	Yes	

Table 5
Added Benefit of Metformin to Diet (Pasquali et al. 2000) – PCOS versus
Non-PCOS

	PCOS responds the same as obese only	PCOS responds better than obese
Weight	Yes	
Waist circumference	Yes	
Visceral fat		Yes
Fasting glucose	Yes	
Fasting insulin	Yes	
Testosterone		Yes
SHBG		Obese responds more

and improvement in reproductive outcomes such as ovulation and pregnancy. There are however marginal effects on weight and indeed in some of these drugs weight increase continues. It is generally recommended that these agents should only be used where there is diabetes mellitus that cannot be controlled by diet and lifestyle. The potential dangers of these drugs in early pregnancy has been emphasized, but as yet, there is very little evidence of their harm. It is generally recommended that they should be avoided in women seeking to achieve a pregnancy.

6.1.6. LIPID-LOWERING DRUGS

Cholesterol is increased in many patients with PCOS as is triglyceride. HDL is often low. There have been recent attempts to use statins to alter cholesterol metabolism, and this has led to changes in other aspects of PCOS including improved ovarian function (112).

6.2. Management of Hirsutism

6.2.1. HYPERANDROGENISM

The oral contraceptive pill is commonly used in trying to control cosmetic and hyperandrogenaemia issues because of PCOS. There is little doubt that testosterone is reduced and SHBG is increased thereby lowering the free testosterone index or free testosterone measured by equilibrium dialysis (113,114). There is no overwhelming evidence that one oral contraceptive pill is better than another, but the use of progestins such as cyproterone acetate and drosperidone may have additional effects on the hair follicle in terms of blocking androgen action. However, the doses in the contraceptive pill are probably too low for this amount, and as a result, cyproterone acetate 50–100 mg/day has been added into the pill or to ethnylestradiol to substantially change hair growth. Other drugs used have been finasteride, spironolactone and flutamide (115,116). There is little evidence of the difference between these drugs, but great caution needs to be exercised when pregnancy is desired.

6.2.2. CALCIUM AND VITAMIN D

There is some literature around the use of calcium and vitamin D in PCOS indicating an improvement in outcome. According to Thys-Jacobs et al. (117), vitamin D repletion with calcium therapy can result in normalized menstrual cycles within 2 months; however, only thirteen women were included in this study. Pasquali et al. *(118)* tested whether calcium channel blockers may play a role in the treatment of hyperandrogenism and hyperinsulinaemia in obese women with PCOS. In the seven women who were tested no significant results were found.

6.2.3. FERTILITY MANAGEMENT

Although not a topic to be covered in this chapter, reproductive and metabolic consequences have an impact on fertility. Many of the treatments above will restore fertility or are pertinent for fertility induction.

REFERENCES

1. Dunaif A. Insulin action in the polycystic ovary syndrome. *Endocrinol Metab Clin North Am* 1999; 28:341–59.
2. Boden G. Role of fatty acids in the pathogenesis of insulin resistance and NIDDM. *Diabetes* 1997; 46:3–10.
3. Kahn BB, Flier JS. Obesity and insulin resistance. *J Clin Invest* 2000; 106:473–81.
4. Pasquali R, Casimirri F, Venturoli S, et al. Body fat distribution has weight-independent effects on clinical, hormonal, and metabolic features of women with polycystic ovary syndrome. *Metabolism* 1994; 43:706–13.
5. Bringer J, Lefebvre P, Boulet F, et al. Body composition and regional fat distribution in polycystic ovarian syndrome. Relationship to hormonal and metabolic profiles. *Ann N Y Acad Sci* 1993; 687:115–23.
6. Holte J, Bergh T, Berne C, Wide L, Lithell H. Restored insulin sensitivity but persistently increased early insulin secretion after weight loss in obese women with polycystic ovary syndrome. *J Clin Endocrinol Metab* 1995; 80:2586–93.
7. Roden M, Price TB, Perseghin G, et al. Mechanism of free fatty acid-induced insulin resistance in humans. *J Clin Invest* 1996; 97:2859–65.
8. Randle PJ, Garland PB, Hales CN, Newsholme EA. The glucose fatty-acid cycle. Its role in insulin sensitivity and the metabolic disturbances of diabetes mellitus. *Lancet* 1963; 1:785–9.
9. Morales AJ, Laughlin GA, Butzow T, Maheshwari H, Baumann G, Yen SS. Insulin, somatotropic, and luteinizing hormone axes in lean and obese women with polycystic ovary syndrome: common and distinct features. *J Clin Endocrinol Metab* 1996; 81:2854–64.
10. Moran L, Norman RJ. Understanding and managing disturbances in insulin metabolism and body weight in women with polycystic ovary syndrome. *Best Pract Res Clin Obstet Gynaecol* 2004; 18:719–36.
11. Pasquali R, Antenucci D, Casimirri F, et al. Clinical and hormonal characteristics of obese amenorrheic hyperandrogenic women before and after weight loss. *J Clin Endocrinol Metab* 1989; 68:173–9.
12. Franks S, Mason H, Willis D. Follicular dynamics in the polycystic ovary syndrome. *Mol Cell Endocrinol* 2000; 163:49–52.
13. Nelson VL, Legro RS, Strauss JF 3rd, McAllister JM. Augmented androgen production is a stable steroidogenic phenotype of propagated theca cells from polycystic ovaries. *Mol Endocrinol* 1999; 13:946–57.
14. Barbieri RL, Makris A, Randall RW, Daniels G, Kistner RW, Ryan KJ. Insulin stimulates androgen accumulation in incubations of ovarian stroma obtained from women with hyperandrogenism. *J Clin Endocrinol Metab* 1986; 62:904–10.
15. Poretsky L, Kalin MF. The gonadotropic function of insulin. *Endocr Rev* 1987; 8:132–41.

16. Nestler JE, Powers LP, Matt DW, et al. A direct effect of hyperinsulinemia on serum sex hormone-binding globulin levels in obese women with the polycystic ovary syndrome. *J Clin Endocrinol Metab* 1991; 72:83–9.

17. Nestler JE, Jakubowicz DJ. Decreases in ovarian cytochrome P450c17 alpha activity and serum free testosterone after reduction of insulin secretion in polycystic ovary syndrome. *N Engl J Med* 1996; 335:617–23.

18. Jakubowicz DJ, Nestler JE. 17 alpha-Hydroxyprogesterone responses to leuprolide and serum androgens in obese women with and without polycystic ovary syndrome offer dietary weight loss. *J Clin Endocrinol Metab* 1997; 82:556–60.

19. Poretsky L, Cataldo NA, Rosenwaks Z, Giudice LC. The insulin-related ovarian regulatory system in health and disease. *Endocr Rev* 1999; 20:535–82.

20. Dale PO, Tanbo T, Vaaler S, Abyholm T. Body weight, hyperinsulinemia, and gonadotropin levels in the polycystic ovarian syndrome: evidence of two distinct populations. *Fertil Steril* 1992; 58:487–91.

21. Ovesen P, Moller J, Ingerslev HJ, et al. Normal basal and insulin-stimulated fuel metabolism in lean women with the polycystic ovary syndrome. *J Clin Endocrinol Metab* 1993; 77:1636–40.

22. Chen H, Sullivan G, Quon MJ. Assessing the predictive accuracy of QUICKI as a surrogate index for insulin sensitivity using a calibration model. *Diabetes* 2005; 54:1914–25.

23. Carnevale Schianca GP, Sainaghi PP, Castello L, Rapetti R, Limoncini AM, Bartoli E. Comparison between HOMA-IR and ISI-gly in detecting subjects with the metabolic syndrome. *Diabetes Metab Res Rev* 2006; 22:111–7.

24. Holte J, Bergh T, Berne C, Berglund L, Lithell H. Enhanced early insulin response to glucose in relation to insulin resistance in women with polycystic ovary syndrome and normal glucose tolerance. *J Clin Endocrinol Metab* 1994; 78:1052–8.

25. Reaven GM. Banting lecture 1988. Role of insulin resistance in human disease. *Diabetes* 1988; 37:1595–607.

26. Reisin E, Alpert MA. Definition of the metabolic syndrome: current proposals and controversies. *Am J Med Sci* 2005; 330:269–72.

27. Korhonen S, Hippelainen M, Niskanen L, Vanhala M, Saarikoski S. Relationship of the metabolic syndrome and obesity to polycystic ovary syndrome: a controlled, population-based study. *Am J Obstet Gynecol* 2001; 184:289–96.

28. Glueck CJ, Papanna R, Wang P, Goldenberg N, Sieve-Smith L. Incidence and treatment of metabolic syndrome in newly referred women with confirmed polycystic ovarian syndrome. *Metabolism* 2003; 52:908–15.

29. Apridonidze T, Essah PA, Iuorno MJ, Nestler JE. Prevalence and characteristics of the metabolic syndrome in women with polycystic ovary syndrome. *J Clin Endocrinol Metab* 2005; 90: 1929–35.

30. Faloia E, Canibus P, Gatti C, et al. Body composition, fat distribution and metabolic characteristics in lean and obese women with polycystic ovary syndrome. *J Endocrinol Invest* 2004; 27:424–9.

31. Wu X, Lu K, Su Y. [Renin-angiotensin system: involvement in polycystic ovarian syndrome]. *Zhonghua Fu Chan Ke Za Zhi* 1997; 32:428–31.

32. Li X, Shen H, Ge X. [Changes of plasma renin activity and angiotensin II levels in women with polycystic ovary syndrome]. *Zhonghua Fu Chan Ke Za Zhi* 2000; 35:586–7.

33. Morris RS, Wong IL, Hatch IE, Gentschein E, Paulson RJ, Lobo RA. Prorenin is elevated in polycystic ovary syndrome and may reflect hyperandrogenism. *Fertil Steril* 1995; 64:1099–103.

34. Jaatinen TA, Matinlauri I, Anttila L, Koskinen P, Erkkola R, Irjala K. Serum total renin is elevated in women with polycystic ovarian syndrome. *Fertil Steril* 1995; 63:1000–4.

35. Hacihanefioglu B, Seyisoglu H, Karsidag K, et al. Influence of insulin resistance on total renin level in normotensive women with polycystic ovary syndrome. *Fertil Steril* 2000; 73:261–5.

36. Wild RA, Painter PC, Coulson PB, Carruth KB, Ranney GB. Lipoprotein lipid concentrations and cardiovascular risk in women with polycystic ovary syndrome. *J Clin Endocrinol Metab* 1985; 61:946–51.

37. Slowinska-Srzednicka J, Zgliczynski S, Wierzbicki M, et al. The role of hyperinsulinemia in the development of lipid disturbances in nonobese and obese women with the polycystic ovary syndrome. *J Endocrinol Invest* 1991; 14:569–75.

38. Maitra A, Pingle RR, Menon PS, Naik V, Gokral JS, Meherji PK. Dyslipidemia with particular regard to apolipoprotein profile in association with polycystic ovary syndrome: a study among Indian women. *Int J Fertil Womens Med* 2001; 46:271–7.

39. Rajkhowa M, Neary RH, Kumpatla P, et al. Altered composition of high density lipoproteins in women with the polycystic ovary syndrome. *J Clin Endocrinol Metab* 1997; 82:3389–94.

40. Dunaif A. Hyperandrogenemia is necessary but not sufficient for polycystic ovary syndrome. *Fertil Steril* 2003; 80:262–3.

41. Dunaif A, Segal KR, Futterweit W, Dobrjansky A. Profound peripheral insulin resistance, independent of obesity, in polycystic ovary syndrome. *Diabetes* 1989; 38:1165–74.

42. Grimaldi A, Heurtier A. [Epidemiology of cardio-vascular complications of diabetes]. *Diabetes Metab* 1999; 25 Suppl 3:12–20.

43. Legro RS. Diabetes prevalence and risk factors in polycystic ovary syndrome. *Obstet Gynecol Clin North Am* 2001; 28:99–109.

44. Ehrmann DA, Barnes RB, Rosenfield RL, Cavaghan MK, Imperial J. Prevalence of impaired glucose tolerance and diabetes in women with polycystic ovary syndrome. *Diabetes Care* 1999; 22:141–6.

45. Pelusi B, Gambineri A, Pasquali R. Type 2 diabetes and the polycystic ovary syndrome. *Minerva Ginecol* 2004; 56:41–51.

46. Weerakiet S, Srisombut C, Bunnag P, Sangtong S, Chuangsoongnoen N, Rojanasakul A. Prevalence of type 2 diabetes mellitus and impaired glucose tolerance in Asian women with polycystic ovary syndrome. *Int J Gynaecol Obstet* 2001; 75:177–84.

47. Norman RJ, Masters L, Milner CR, Wang JX, Davies MJ. Relative risk of conversion from normo-glycaemia to impaired glucose tolerance or non-insulin dependent diabetes mellitus in polycystic ovarian syndrome. *Hum Reprod* 2001; 16:1995–8.

48. Ehrmann DA, Liljenquist DR, Kasza K, Azziz R, Legro RS, Ghazzi MN. Prevalence and predictors of the metabolic syndrome in women with polycystic ovary syndrome. *J Clin Endocrinol Metab* 2006; 91:48–53.

49. Legro RS, Gnatuk CL, Kunselman AR, Dunaif A. Changes in glucose tolerance over time in women with polycystic ovary syndrome: a controlled study. *J Clin Endocrinol Metab* 2005; 90:3236–42.

50. Legro RS, Kunselman AR, Dodson WC, Dunaif A. Prevalence and predictors of risk for type 2 diabetes mellitus and impaired glucose tolerance in polycystic ovary syndrome: a prospective, controlled study in 254 affected women. *J Clin Endocrinol Metab* 1999; 84:165–9.

51. Talbott EO, Zborowski JV, Boudreaux MY, McHugh-Pemu KP, Sutton-Tyrrell K, Guzick DS. The relationship between C-reactive protein and carotid intima-media wall thickness in middle-aged women with polycystic ovary syndrome. *J Clin Endocrinol Metab* 2004; 89:6061–7.

52. Boulman N, Levy Y, Leiba R, et al. Increased C-reactive protein levels in the polycystic ovary syndrome: a marker of cardiovascular disease. *J Clin Endocrinol Metab* 2004; 89:2160–5.

53. Kelly CC, Lyall H, Petrie JR, Gould GW, Connell JM, Sattar N. Low grade chronic inflammation in women with polycystic ovarian syndrome. *J Clin Endocrinol Metab* 2001; 86:2453–5.

54. Tarkun I, Arslan BC, Canturk Z, Turemen E, Sahin T, Duman C. Endothelial dysfunction in young women with polycystic ovary syndrome: relationship with insulin resistance and low-grade chronic inflammation. *J Clin Endocrinol Metab* 2004; 89:5592–6.

55. Diamanti-Kandarakis E, Paterakis T, Alexandraki K, et al. Indices of low-grade chronic inflammation in polycystic ovary syndrome and the beneficial effect of metformin. *Hum Reprod* 2006; 21:1426–31.

56. Fenkci V, Fenkci S, Yilmazer M, Serteser M. Decreased total antioxidant status and increased oxidative stress in women with polycystic ovary syndrome may contribute to the risk of cardiovascular disease. *Fertil Steril* 2003; 80:123–7.

57. Taponen S, Martikainen H, Jarvelin MR, et al. Hormonal profile of women with self-reported symptoms of oligomenorrhea and/or hirsutism: Northern Finland birth cohort 1966 study. *J Clin Endocrinol Metab* 2003; 88:141–7.

58. Mohlig M, Spranger J, Osterhoff M, et al. The polycystic ovary syndrome per se is not associated with increased chronic inflammation. *Eur J Endocrinol* 2004; 150:525–32.

59. Sampson M, Kong C, Patel A, Unwin R, Jacobs HS. Ambulatory blood pressure profiles and plasminogen activator inhibitor (PAI-1) activity in lean women with and without the polycystic ovary syndrome. *Clin Endocrinol (Oxf)* 1996; 45:623–9.

60. Atiomo WU, Bates SA, Condon JE, Shaw S, West JH, Prentice AG. The plasminogen activator system in women with polycystic ovary syndrome. *Fertil Steril* 1998; 69:236–41.

61. Landin K, Stigendal L, Eriksson E, et al. Abdominal obesity is associated with an impaired fibrinolytic activity and elevated plasminogen activator inhibitor-1. *Metabolism* 1990; 39:1044–8.

62. Cibula D, Sindelka G, Hill M, Fanta M, Skrha J, Zivny J. Insulin sensitivity in non-obese women with polycystic ovary syndrome during treatment with oral contraceptives containing low-androgenic progestin. *Hum Reprod* 2002; 17:76–82.

63. Orbetzova MM, Shigarminova RG, Genchev GG, et al. Role of 24-hour monitoring in assessing blood pressure changes in polycystic ovary syndrome. *Folia Med (Plovdiv)* 2003; 45:21–5.

64. Vrbikova J, Cifkova R, Jirkovska A, et al. Cardiovascular risk factors in young Czech females with polycystic ovary syndrome. *Hum Reprod* 2003; 18:980–4.

65. Norman RJ, Noakes M, Wu R, Davies MJ, Moran L, Wang JX. Improving reproductive performance in overweight/obese women with effective weight management. *Hum Reprod Update* 2004; 10: 267–80.

66. Norman RJ, Clark AM. Obesity and reproductive disorders: a review. *Reprod Fertil Dev* 1998; 10:55–63.

67. Legro RS. Polycystic ovary syndrome and cardiovascular disease: A premature association? *Endocr Rev* 2003; 24:302–12.

68. Lakhani K, Leonard A, Seifalian AM, Hardiman P. Microvascular dysfunction in women with polycystic ovary syndrome. *Hum Reprod* 2005; 20:3219–24.

69. Kravariti M, Naka KK, Kalantaridou SN, et al. Predictors of endothelial dysfunction in young women with polycystic ovary syndrome. *J Clin Endocrinol Metab* 2005; 90:5088–95.

70. Diamanti-Kandarakis E, Spina G, Kouli C, Migdalis I. Increased endothelin-1 levels in women with polycystic ovary syndrome and the beneficial effect of metformin therapy. *J Clin Endocrinol Metab* 2001; 86:4666–73.

71. Diamanti-Kandarakis E, Alexandraki K, Protogerou A, et al. Metformin administration improves endothelial function in women with polycystic ovary syndrome. *Eur J Endocrinol* 2005; 152:749–56.

72. Pierpoint T, McKeigue PM, Isaacs AJ, Wild SH, Jacobs HS. Mortality of women with polycystic ovary syndrome at long-term follow-up. *J Clin Epidemiol* 1998; 51:581–6.

73. Solomon CG, Hu FB, Dunaif A, et al. Long or highly irregular menstrual cycles as a marker for risk of type 2 diabetes mellitus. *JAMA* 2001; 286:2421–6.

74. Birdsall MA, Farquhar CM, White HD. Association between polycystic ovaries and extent of coronary artery disease in women having cardiac catheterization. *Ann Intern Med* 1997; 126:32–5.

75. Talbott EO, Zborowski JV, Rager JR, Boudreaux MY, Edmundowicz DA, Guzick DS. Evidence for an association between metabolic cardiovascular syndrome and coronary and aortic calcification among women with polycystic ovary syndrome. *J Clin Endocrinol Metab* 2004; 89:5454–61.

76. Talbott EO, Zborowski JV, Sutton-Tyrrell K, McHugh-Pemu KP, Guzick DS. Cardiovascular risk in women with polycystic ovary syndrome. *Obstet Gynecol Clin North Am* 2001; 28:111–33, vii.

77. Christian RC, Dumesic DA, Behrenbeck T, Oberg AL, Sheedy PF 2nd, Fitzpatrick LA. Prevalence and predictors of coronary artery calcification in women with polycystic ovary syndrome. *J Clin Endocrinol Metab* 2003; 88:2562–8.

78. Lord JM, Flight IH, Norman RJ. Metformin in polycystic ovary syndrome: systematic review and meta-analysis. *BMJ* 2003; 327:951–3.

79. Norman RJ, Davies MJ, Lord J, Moran LJ. The role of lifestyle modification in polycystic ovary syndrome. *Trends Endocrinol Metab* 2002; 13:251–7.

80. Pasquali R, Gambineri A. Role of changes in dietary habits in polycystic ovary syndrome. *Reprod Biomed Online* 2004; 8:431–9.

81. Moran LJ, Noakes M, Clifton PM, Tomlinson L, Galletly C, Norman RJ. Dietary composition in restoring reproductive and metabolic physiology in overweight women with polycystic ovary syndrome. *J Clin Endocrinol Metab* 2003; 88:812–9.

82. Holte J. Disturbances in insulin secretion and sensitivity in women with the polycystic ovary syndrome. *Baillieres Clin Endocrinol Metab* 1996; 10:221–47.

83. Huber-Buchholz MM, Carey DG, Norman RJ. Restoration of reproductive potential by lifestyle modification in obese polycystic ovary syndrome: role of insulin sensitivity and luteinizing hormone. *J Clin Endocrinol Metab* 1999; 84:1470–4.

84. Clark AM, Thornley B, Tomlinson L, Galletley C, Norman RJ. Weight loss in obese infertile women results in improvement in reproductive outcome for all forms of fertility treatment. *Hum Reprod* 1998; 13:1502–5.

85. Clark AM, Ledger W, Galletly C, et al. Weight loss results in significant improvement in pregnancy and ovulation rates in anovulatory obese women. *Hum Reprod* 1995; 10:2705–12.

86. Andersen P, Seljeflot I, Abdelnoor M, et al. Increased insulin sensitivity and fibrinolytic capacity after dietary intervention in obese women with polycystic ovary syndrome. *Metabolism* 1995; 44: 611–6.

87. Franks S, Robinson S, Willis DS. Nutrition, insulin and polycystic ovary syndrome. *Rev Reprod* 1996; 1:47–53.

88. Moran LJ, Noakes M, Clifton PM, et al. Ghrelin and measures of satiety are altered in polycystic ovary syndrome but not differentially affected by diet composition. *J Clin Endocrinol Metab* 2004; 89:3337–44.

89. NIH. National Institutes of Health. Clinical guidelines on the identification, evaluation and treatment of overweight and obesity in adults: Executive Summary. *Am J Clin Nutr* 68(4): 899–917.

90. Brinkworth GD, Noakes M, Keogh JB, Luscombe ND, Wittert GA, Clifton PM. Long-term effects of a high-protein, low-carbohydrate diet on weight control and cardiovascular risk markers in obese hyperinsulinemic subjects. *Int J Obes Relat Metab Disord* 2004; 28:661–70.

91. Howard BV, Manson JE, Stefanick ML, et al. Low-fat dietary pattern and weight change over 7 years: the Women's Health Initiative Dietary Modification Trial. *JAMA* 2006; 295:39–49.

92. Barzel US, Massey LK. Excess dietary protein can adversely affect bone. *J Nutr* 1998; 128:1051–3.

93. Calvo MS, Bell RR, Forbes RM. Effect of protein-induced calciuria on calcium metabolism and bone status in adult rats. *J Nutr* 1982; 112:1401–13.

94. Monro J. Redefining the glycemic index for dietary management of postprandial glycemia. *J Nutr* 2003; 133:4256–8.

95. Brand-Miller JC. Glycemic load and chronic disease. *Nutr Rev* 2003; 61:S49–55.

96. Carmina E, Napoli N, Longo RA, Rini GB, Lobo RA. Metabolic syndrome in polycystic ovary syndrome (PCOS): lower prevalence in southern Italy than in the USA and the influence of criteria for the diagnosis of PCOS. *Eur J Endocrinol* 2006; 154:141–5.

97. Carmina E, Legro RS, Stamets K, Lowell J, Lobo RA. Difference in body weight between American and Italian women with polycystic ovary syndrome: influence of the diet. *Hum Reprod* 2003; 18:2289–93.

98. Cronin L, Guyatt G, Griffith L, et al. Development of a health-related quality-of-life questionnaire (PCOSQ) for women with polycystic ovary syndrome (PCOS). *J Clin Endocrinol Metab* 1998; 83:1976–87.

99. Galletly C, Clark A, Tomlinson L, Blaney F. A group program for obese, infertile women: weight loss and improved psychological health. *J Psychosom Obstet Gynaecol* 1996; 17:125–8.

100. Nestler JE. Should patients with polycystic ovarian syndrome be treated with metformin? an enthusiastic endorsement. *Hum Reprod* 2002; 17:1950–3.

101. Lord JM, Flight IH, Norman RJ. Insulin-sensitising drugs (metformin, troglitazone, rosiglitazone, pioglitazone, D-chiro-inositol) for polycystic ovary syndrome. *Cochrane Database Syst Rev* 2003:CD003053.

102. Kitabchi AE, Temprosa M, Knowler WC, et al. Role of insulin secretion and sensitivity in the evolution of type 2 diabetes in the diabetes prevention program: effects of lifestyle intervention and metformin. *Diabetes* 2005; 54:2404–14.

103. Norman RJ, Wu R, Stankiewicz MT. 4: Polycystic ovary syndrome. *Med J Aust* 2004; 180:132–7.

104. Nestler JE. Metformin and the polycystic ovary syndrome. *J Clin Endocrinol Metab* 2001; 86:1430.

105. Pasquali R, Gambineri A, Biscotti D, et al. Effect of long-term treatment with metformin added to hypocaloric diet on body composition, fat distribution, and androgen and insulin levels in abdominally obese women with and without the polycystic ovary syndrome. *J Clin Endocrinol Metab* 2000; 85:2767–74.

106. Azziz R, Ehrmann D, Legro RS, et al. Troglitazone improves ovulation and hirsutism in the polycystic ovary syndrome: a multicenter, double blind, placebo-controlled trial. *J Clin Endocrinol Metab* 2001; 86:1626–32.

107. Yilmaz M, Biri A, Karakoc A, et al. The effects of rosiglitazone and metformin on insulin resistance and serum androgen levels in obese and lean patients with polycystic ovary syndrome. *J Endocrinol Invest* 2005; 28:1003–8.

108. Rautio K, Tapanainen JS, Ruokonen A, Morin-Papunen LC. Endocrine and metabolic effects of rosiglitazone in overweight women with PCOS: a randomized placebo-controlled study. *Hum Reprod* 2006; 21:1400–7.

109. Yilmaz M, Karakoc A, Toruner FB, et al. The effects of rosiglitazone and metformin on menstrual cyclicity and hirsutism in polycystic ovary syndrome. *Gynecol Endocrinol* 2005; 21:154–60.

110. Ortega-Gonzalez C, Luna S, Hernandez L, et al. Responses of serum androgen and insulin resistance to metformin and pioglitazone in obese, insulin-resistant women with polycystic ovary syndrome. *J Clin Endocrinol Metab* 2005; 90:1360–5.

111. Brettenthaler N, De Geyter C, Huber PR, Keller U. Effect of the insulin sensitizer pioglitazone on insulin resistance, hyperandrogenism, and ovulatory dysfunction in women with polycystic ovary syndrome. *J Clin Endocrinol Metab* 2004; 89:3835–40.

112. Izquierdo D, Foyouzi N, Kwintkiewicz J, Duleba AJ. Mevastatin inhibits ovarian theca-interstitial cell proliferation and steroidogenesis. *Fertil Steril* 2004; 82 Suppl 3:1193–7.

113. Van der Spuy ZM, le Roux PA. Cyproterone acetate for hirsutism. *Cochrane Database Syst Rev* 2003:CD001125.

114. Cibula D, Fanta M, Vrbikova J, et al. The effect of combination therapy with metformin and combined oral contraceptives (COC) versus COC alone on insulin sensitivity, hyperandrogenaemia, SHBG and lipids in PCOS patients. *Hum Reprod* 2005; 20:180–4.

115. Venturoli S, Marescalchi O, Colombo FM, et al. A prospective randomized trial comparing low dose flutamide, finasteride, ketoconazole, and cyproterone acetate-estrogen regimens in the treatment of hirsutism. *J Clin Endocrinol Metab* 1999; 84:1304–10.

116. O'Brien RC, Cooper ME, Murray RM, Seeman E, Thomas AK, Jerums G. Comparison of sequential cyproterone acetate/estrogen versus spironolactone/oral contraceptive in the treatment of hirsutism. *J Clin Endocrinol Metab* 1991; 72:1008–13.

117. Thys-Jacobs S, Donovan D, Papadopoulos A, Sarrel P, Bilezikian JP. Vitamin D and calcium dysregulation in the polycystic ovarian syndrome. *Steroids* 1999; 64:430–5.
118. Pasquali R, Cantobelli S, Vicennati V, et al. Nitrendipine treatment in women with polycystic ovarian syndrome: evidence for a lack of effects of calcium channel blockers on insulin, androgens, and sex hormone-binding globulin. *J Clin Endocrinol Metab* 1995; 80:3346–50.
119. Coviello AD, Legro RS, Dunaif A. Adolescent girls with polycystic ovary syndrome have an increased risk of the metabolic syndrome associated with increasing androgen levels independent of obesity and insulin resistance. *J Clin Endocrinol Metab* 2006; 91:492–7.
120. Rabelo Acevedo M, Vick MR. Association between the polycystic ovary syndrome and the metabolic syndrome in Puerto Rico. *P R Health Sci J* 2005; 24:203–6.
121. Sam S, Legro RS, Bentley-Lewis R, Dunaif A. Dyslipidemia and metabolic syndrome in the sisters of women with polycystic ovary syndrome. *J Clin Endocrinol Metab* 2005; 90:4797–802.
122. Vrbikova J, Vondra K, Cibula D, Dvorakova K, Stanicka S, Sramkova D, Sindelka G, Hill M, Bendlova B, Skrha J. Metabolic syndrome in young Czech women with polycystic ovary syndrome. *Hum Reprod* 2005; 20:3328–32.
123. Vural B, Caliskan E, Turkoz E, Kilic T, Demirci A. Evaluation of metabolic syndrome frequency and premature carotid atherosclerosis in young women with polycystic ovary syndrome. *Hum Reprod* 2005; 20:2409–13.
124. Korytkowski MT, Mokan M, Horwitz MJ, Berga SL. Metabolic effects of oral contraceptives in women with polycystic ovary syndrome. *J Clin Endocrin Metab* 1995; 80:3327–34.
125. Dahlgren E, Landin K, Krotkiewski M, Holm G, Janson PO. Effects of two antiandrogen treatments on hirsutism and insulin sensitivity in women with polycystic ovary syndrome. *Hum Reprod* 1998; 13:2706–11.
126. Armstrong VL, Wiggam MI, Ennis CN, Sheridan B, Traub AI, Atkinson AB, Bell PM. Insulin action and insulin secretion in polycystic ovary syndrome treated with ethinyl oestradiol/cyproterone acetate. *Q J Med* 2001; 94:31–7.
127. Vrbikova J, Stanicka S, Dvorakova K, Hill M, Vondra K, Bendlova B, Starka L. Metabolic and endocrine effects of treatment with peroral or transdermal oestrogens in conjunction with peroral cyproterone acetate in women with polycystic ovary syndrome. *Eur J Endocrinol* 2004; 150:215–23.
128. Guido M, Romualdi D, Guilliani M, Suriano R, Salvaggi L, Apa R, Lanzone A. Drospirenone for the treatment of hirsute women with polycystic ovary syndrome: a clinical, endocrinological, metabolic pilot study. *J Clin Endocrinol Metab* 2004; 89:2817–23.
129. Vrbikova J, Cibula D. Combined oral contraceptives in the treatment of polycysticovary syndrome. *Hum Reprod Update* 2005; 11:277–91.

17 Pathogenesis of Hyperandrogenism in Polycystic Ovary Syndrome

Wendy Y. Chang, MD, and Ricardo Azziz, MD, MPH

CONTENTS

Summary

Androgen excess (AE) is an important, even essential feature of the polycystic ovary syndrome (PCOS), and arises primarily from ovarian AE, although a hyperactivity of adrenocortical function and adrenal androgen (AA) excess are present in a significant number of patients. Increased ovarian theca cell function, and possibly number, and augmented expression of steroidogenic enzymes have been demonstrated in PCOS. Increased LH stimulation of thecal androgen biosynthesis also appears to be an important, early event in PCOS. Abnormalities in other intrinsic ovarian factors such as inhibin, activin, and follistatin appear to modulate ovarian LH response. Granulosa cell dysfunction may also contribute, with PCOS women demonstrating arrested granulose development and increased 5α-reductase expression. Adrenal AE, possibly arising from generalized adrenocortical hyper-responsivity, is a relatively common feature of PCOS. Finally, the metabolic consequences of obesity and insulin resistance appear to potentiate excess androgen production in adolescent and adult PCOS patients. In short, the hyperandrogenism of PCOS appears to be aptly multifactorial, consistent with the complex nature of the syndrome itself.

Key Words: Adrenal, androgens, polycystic ovary syndrome, hirsutism, luteinizing hormone, insulin.

1. INTRODUCTION

Polycystic ovary syndrome (PCOS) is a heterogeneous disorder characterized by hyperandrogenism, ovulatory dysfunction, and polycystic ovarian morphology. A complex disease entity, PCOS consists of a spectrum of clinical findings, likely arising from

From: *Contemporary Endocrinology: Polycystic Ovary Syndrome*
Edited by: A. Dunaif, R. J. Chang, S. Franks, and R. S. Legro © Humana Press, Totowa, NJ

multiple possible etiologies. Two sets of diagnostic criteria have been proposed for the disorder. The first arose from the proceedings of an expert conference sponsored in part by the National Institute of Child Health and Human Disease (NICHD) of the United States National Institutes of Health (NIH) in 1990. The summary of conference participants' survey concluded that the major criteria for PCOS should include (in order of importance): *(1)* hyperandrogenism and/or hyperandrogenemia; *(2)* oligo-ovulation, and *(3)* the exclusion of other known disorders *(1)*. In 2003, an expert conference was convened in Rotterdam, The Netherlands. Jointly sponsored by the European Society for Human Reproduction and Embryology and the American Society for Reproductive Medicine, the meeting proceedings recommended that PCOS be defined when at least two of the following three features were present: *(1)* oligo- and/or anovulation, *(2)* clinical and/or biochemical signs of hyperandrogenism, and *(3)* polycystic ovaries *(2)*. The revised Rotterdam criteria have essentially included two additional groups that were previously excluded under the NIH criteria: *(1)* patients with hyperandrogenism and polycystic ovaries who demonstrate no ovulatory dysfunction; and *(2)* patients with ovulatory dysfunction and polycystic ovaries who demonstrate no evidence of hyperandrogenism.

The inclusion of women demonstrating no evidence of hyperandrogenism in PCOS diagnosis remains controversial *(3)*. Androgen excess (AE) is the most common, underlying biochemical defect in PCOS *(4,5)*. PCOS is the most common cause of hyperandrogenism in women *(6)*. Evidence supporting the central role of AE includes the reversible development of polycystic ovaries in female-to-male transsexuals treated with high-dose testosterone *(7)*.

In the established non-human primate PCOS model, adult female rhesus monkeys exposed to testosterone in utero demonstrated many clinical and biochemical features

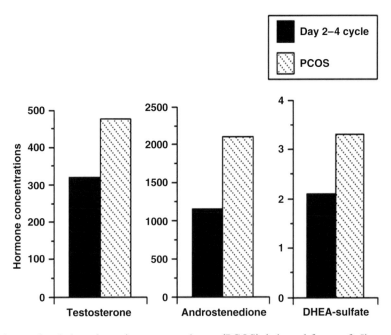

Fig. 1. Androgen levels in polycystic ovary syndrome (PCOS) (adapted from ref. *9*).

of PCOS, including hyperandrogenism, oligomenorrhea, luteinizing hormone (LH) hypersecretion, and impaired insulin response *(8)*.

As a whole, women with PCOS demonstrate significantly increased serum levels of the androgens androstenedione (A4), testosterone (T), and dehydroepiandrosterone (DHEA) and the DHEA metabolite, DHEAS sulfate (DHEAS), compared with non-PCOS women (Fig. 1) *(1,9)*. The pathogenesis of hyperandrogenism in PCOS may be as varied as the disorder itself, and central roles have been ascribed to *(1)* abnormal hypothalamic/pituitary function; *(2)* abnormal ovarian steroidogenesis and granulosa/theca function; *(3)* enhanced peripheral and hepatic 5α-reductase (5α-RA) activity; *(4)* increased adrenal hyperandrogenism; *(5)* disordered insulin metabolism and insulin resistance; *(6)* intrinsic ovarian factors; and *(7)* extrinsic factors. Following we will review the role of each of these mechanisms in determining the hyperandrogenism of PCOS.

2. ABNORMAL HYPOTHALAMIC PITUITARY FUNCTION AND HYPERANDROGENISM

Ovarian androgen production in the theca cell is stimulated by LH (Fig. 2) *(10)*. Excessive pituitary LH secretion was among the first laboratory abnormalities identified in PCOS. Both adult PCOS patients and hyperandrogenic adolescent girls demonstrate greater LH pulse frequency ascribed to increased gonadotropin-releasing hormone (GnRH) pulse frequency and overall elevated LH levels. In hyperandrogenic pubertal girls, LH pulse frequency was increased in both sleep and waking hours compared with controls; LH pulse amplitude was increased only during waking hours *(11)*. In

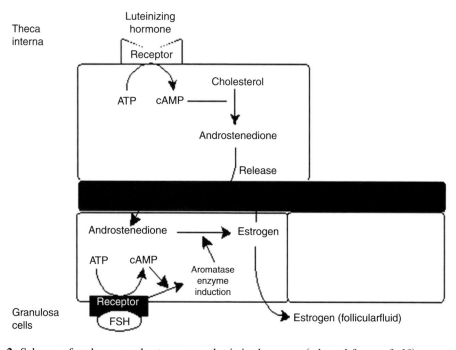

Fig. 2. Scheme of androgen and estrogen synthesis in the ovary (adapted from ref. *10*).

adults, this disordered GnRH pulse generator and LH secretion may result in part from abnormal sex steroid feedback.

The GnRH pulse generator in PCOS patients appears to demonstrate reduced sensitivity to and inhibition by estradiol and progesterone *(12)*. A study using flutamide indicated that GnRH pulse generator sensitivity to estradiol and progesterone feedback inhibition could be restored with anti-androgen therapy *(13)*. This finding accentuates the central role of hyperandrogenism in the disorder and suggests that the hyperandrogenism may precede disordered GnRH pulsatility. In addition, an immunologically anomalous form of LH, arising from two point mutations in the *LH-beta* gene, has been identified (termed vLH). The presence of vLH is frequently detected in healthy obese and non-obese women; vLH levels are low in obese women with PCOS. Overall, while the significance of vLH is unclear, it is thought that vLH may confer some degree of protection from PCOS symptoms *(14)*.

3. OVARIAN HYPERANDROGENISM

Androgen excess (AE) in PCOS is thought to result primarily from dysregulated ovarian androgen secretion. Ovarian steroidogenesis follows the two-cell model in which LH stimulates theca cells to produce androstenedione de novo (Fig. 2). The theca cells of non-PCOS women express little 17α-hydroxysteroid dehydrogenase (17α-HSD) and, therefore, produce low levels of testosterone. In the granulosa cell, androstenedione is then converted to estrone and subsequently estradiol. Approximately 80% of PCOS patients demonstrate a generalized ovarian steroidogenic hyperresponsiveness to gonadotropin stimulation *(15)*. Both in vivo and in vitro stimulation with LH or hCG result in marked elevations in testosterone and 17α-hydroxyprogesterone (17-OHP), a marker of ovarian androgen response *(16,17)*. These elevations persist despite adrenocortical suppression with dexamethasone. The suppression of circulating androgens in PCOS with selective GnRH-agonists supports the important role of the ovary as the source of AE in PCOS *(18)*. Two principal mechanisms of ovarian AE include excessive theca cell proliferation and increased theca steroidogenic capacity.

3.1. Excessive Theca Cell Proliferation and Androgen Production in PCOS

Clinical and in vitro studies implicate an intrinsic abnormality in theca cell steroidogenesis in PCOS. Women with PCOS and isolated polycystic ovaries demonstrate a higher 17-OHP production in response to hCG challenge than do control women *(19)*. Theca cells culture studies similarly demonstrate increased basal and LH-stimulated androstenedione secretion in PCOS compared with controls *(20)*. The PCOS ovary is characterized by an increased number of small, 3- to 7-mm antral follicles compared with non-PCOS ovaries. Many of the PCOS follicles demonstrate hypertrophy of the theca interna, resulting in many more layers of differentiated steroidogenic cells than the 3–5 layers normally seen in the theca interna of non-PCOS ovaries *(21)*. As a result, the PCOS ovary contains a greater number of steroidogenic cells in the theca interna, consistent with excessive androgen production. Much of the data on theca cell proliferation and regulation comes from animal studies showing that chronic exposure to LH or hCG results in increased theca cell number.

In addition to increased theca proliferation, PCOS ovaries also demonstrate overexpression of steroidogenic enzymes. Compared with ovulatory women, theca cells from

PCOS patients demonstrate greater mRNA content of LH receptor, steroidogenesis acute regulatory protein (StAR), CYP11A, and CYP17 *(22)*. PCOS theca cell cultures also demonstrate increased CYP17 transcription *(23)*. Finally, the mRNA of CYP17 demonstrates increased stability and prolonged half-life because of post-transcriptional mRNA modification *(24)*, suggesting that disordered theca cell regulation in PCOS occurs at multiple sites.

3.2. Abnormal Granulosa Cell Function in PCOS

Impaired granulosa cell function also appears to contribute to hyperandrogenism in PCOS. In the non-PCOS ovary, the vast majority of androstenedione produced by theca cells is converted to estrone and estradiol. The transition to dominant follicle is marked by increased aromatase expression and decreased 5α-reductase activity to nearly undetectable levels. However, the small antral follicles in tissue biopsies of polycystic ovaries express low estradiol levels and decreased aromatase mRNA expression compared with dominant follicles from non-PCOS biopsies. PCOS ovaries demonstrate increased expression of 5α-reductase activity and 1000-fold higher follicular fluid levels of 5α-androstane-3,17-dione, a competitive inhibitor of aromatase activity *(25)*. Overall, these defects likely contribute to decreased aromatase activity, the accumulation of androstenedione, and the failure to develop dominant follicles.

Superimposed upon LH regulation, thecal cell activity may be modulated by the inhibin–follistatin–activin system of the granulosa cells. Inhibins are members of the transforming growth factor-beta peptide family, which acts as negative feedback regulators of follicle-stimulating hormone (FSH) secretion *(26)*. Inhibin-B is the predominant inhibin, produced by small developing follicles in response to FSH. The structurally related activins exert antagonist effects on inhibin action, as does follistatin, an inhibin-binding protein. Inhibin stimulates ovarian androgen production in the ovary *(27)*, whereas activin decreases this effect. Decreased activin effect has been suggested in PCOS patients based on the finding of low activin levels and decreased activin/follistatin ratio *(28)*. Elevated serum inhibin-B responses to FSH stimulation have been demonstrated in PCOS *(29,30)*. However, the increase in inhibin-B may result from the greater cohort of ovarian follicles in PCOS ovaries. Regardless of the cause, excess inhibin-B appears to worsen ovarian AE in PCOS.

4. ADRENOCORTICAL HYPERANDROGENISM

Although the majority of patients with PCOS demonstrate an ovarian source for their high androgen secretion, many also display adrenocortical hyperactivity and adrenal androgen (AA) excess. The measurement of circulating DHEAS is useful as a marker of AA secretion (and excess), as this metabolite is *(1)* 97–99% of adrenocortical origin; *(2)* the most abundant steroid; *(3)* relatively stable throughout the day and the menstrual cycle; and *(4)* easily measured. Previous reports indicated that serum levels of DHEAS were above the normal limit in 40–60% of patients with PCOS *(31–34)*. However, using racial and age normative values, we have determined the prevalence of absolute (i.e. >95th percentile of normal) DHEAS excess to be approximately 25% *(35)*. However, these studies also demonstrated a generalized upward shift in DHEAS values in PCOS women compared with that in controls (Fig. 3), similar to what is observed for ovarian androgen production in response to hCG or GnRH-a stimulation

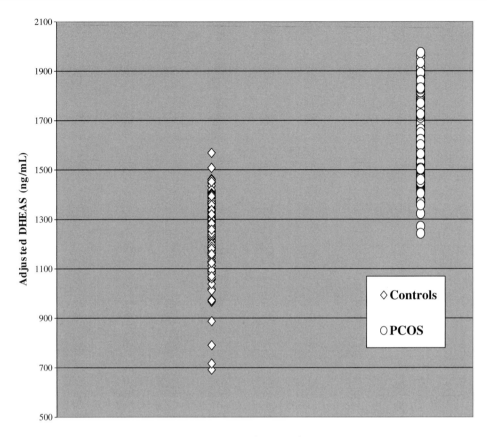

Fig. 3. Circulating dehydroepiandrosterone sulfate (DHEAS) levels, adjusted for body mass index) in 213 polycystic ovary syndrome (PCOS) compared with 185 control women (adapted from ref. *34*).

(36,37). The excess AA production may stem from dysregulation in adrenocortical biosynthesis in response to adrenocorticotropic hormone (ACTH) stimulation or may represent a compensatory response to increased peripheral cortisol (F) metabolism.

4.1. Adrenocortical Hyper-Responsivity in PCOS

Various data support the concept that AA excess, particularly when evident during pubertal development, increases the risk for developing PCOS. For example, patients with premature adrenarche are at higher risk for the development of PCOS than their non-affected peers *(38–41)*. Furthermore, other investigators have suggested that stress resulting in exaggerated AA secretion during the peripuberty increases the risk of developing PCOS *(42)*. Finally, the clearest model illustrating the impact of peripubertal AA excess as a risk factor for PCOS is 21-hydroxylase (21-OH)-deficient non-classic adrenal hyperplasin (NCAH). This disorder is the result of a primary abnormality in adrenocortical dysfunction, namely the excessive production of AA because of a congenital defect in *CYP21*, the gene encoding for the enzyme P450c21, which determines 21-OH activity. NCAH is linked to the development of PCOS-like features, including the development of polycystic-appearing ovaries on ultrasound, elevated LH levels, and ovarian hyperandrogenism *(43–46)*. Overall, data in girls with premature adrenarche and patients with 21-OH-deficient NCAH support the role of AA excess in the development of the PCOS phenotype.

Women with PCOS demonstrate a generalized hypersecretion of adrenocortical products, basally and in response to ACTH, including DHEA and A4, pregnenolone, 17α-hydroxypregnenolone, 17-OHP, 11-deoxycortisol, and Cortisol (F) *(47–51)*. The adrenocortical dysfunction observed does not appear to be the result of NCAH because of rare coding mutations in *CYP21 (52–54)*, *CYP11B1 (55)*, or *HSD3B2 (56,57)*, although it is not yet known whether common polymorphisms in these genes play a role.

Although PCOS patients with DHEAS excess demonstrate an exaggerated secretory response of the adrenal cortex for DHEA and A4 (Fig. 4), they do not demonstrate an altered pituitary response to Corticotropin releasing hormone (CRH) or increased sensitivity (threshold dose) of AAs to ACTH stimulation *(47)*. The single most important steroidogenic difference observed between PCOS women and healthy controls appears to be a greater estimated $\Delta^5$17-hydroxylase activity ($\Delta^5$17-OH) *(54)*, primarily in PCOS patients with supranormal DHEAS levels *(49)*. Although a common polymorphism of *CYP17*, the gene encoding P450c17, did not appear to have an important modulatory role on circulating DHEAS levels *(58)*, more extensive analysis of this gene for other potential variations has not yet been done. Overall, these data indicate that in many PCOS women a generalized adrenocortical hyper-responsivity is present, particularly in those with overt AA excess, similar to the ovarian hyperfunction seen in the disorder.

4.2. Altered Cortisol Metabolism in PCOS

Although the 24-h urine free F concentration in PCOS is increased *(59)*, the total 24-hour F *(60)*, and free F *(61)*, the sensitivity or responsivity of F to ACTH stimulation

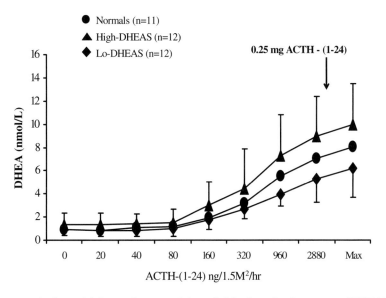

Fig. 4. Adrenocortical sensitivity and responsivity of dehydroepiandrosterone (DHEA) to graded ACTH stimulation in PCOS patients with (high-DHEAS) and without AA excess (Low-DHEAS), and controls (from ref. *46*).

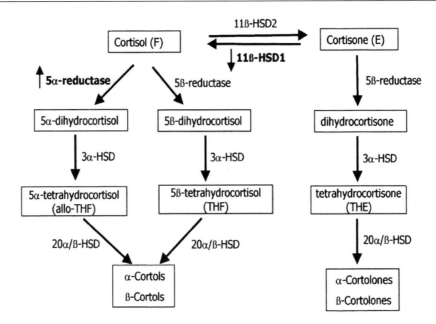

Fig. 5. Principal metabolites of cortisol in urine measured by gas chromatography and mass spectrometry (from ref. *64*).

(46) or the F or ACTH levels across the menstrual cycle *(62)*, are relatively normal in PCOS. This discrepancy between serum measures of F and the urinary excretion of F suggests that the metabolism of this steroid may be accelerated in PCOS. Cortisol metabolism includes irreversible inactivation by 5α- (5α-RA) and 5β-reductase and reversible interconversion with cortisone (E) by 11β-HSD) (Fig. 5). 11β-HSD type 1 (11β-HSD1), an oxoreductase expressed in human liver and adipose tissue, regenerates F from E; 11β-HSD type 2 is a high-affinity dehydrogenase expressed in human mineralocorticoid-target tissues, which inactivates F by converting to E. Most studies in PCOS have observed an increased urinary excretion of AA and F metabolites *(63)*, suggestive of increased peripheral (e.g., hepatic) 5α-RA *(5,46–48)* and decreased 11β-HSD1 activities *(64,65)* (Fig. 5). These alterations have been observed independent of weight, and although insulin appears to enhance 5α-RA, it has no effect on 11β-HSD1 activity in PCOS *(64)*.

Overall, current evidence suggests that PCOS patients, regardless of body weight, demonstrate increased 5α-RA and decreased 11β-HSD1 activities. It is possible that increased metabolism of F in PCOS results in a subtle upregulation of adrenocortical steroidogenesis yielding normal circulating F levels at the expense, at least in part, of AA excess.

4.3. Adrenal AE in PCOS: Acquired Trait?

It is possible that the adrenocortical abnormalities observed in PCOS are secondary to other factors abnormal in the disorder, such as ovarian hyperandrogenism. Some investigators *(66,67)*, but not all *(68,69)*, evaluating the use of ovarian suppression with a long-acting GnRH analogue (GnRH-a) observed a decrease in DHEAS levels, suggesting an ovarian effect on the adrenal in PCOS. However, our studies using exogenous testosterone (T) or estradiol administration *(51,70)* or ovarian suppression with a long-acting GnRH-a *(64)* or oophorectomy *(71)* indicate that although ovarian factors, primarily androgens, may affect the rate of DHEA sulfation (and consequently the circulating levels of DHEAS), the adrenocortical response to ACTH remains relatively unchanged. Likewise, studies in healthy women indicated that, with the exception of a modest increase in A4 secretion, no major differences in adrenal response were observed with simple obesity *(72)*.

In addition, we were unable to detect a significant association between DHEAS and fasting insulin levels among 165 healthy women, whereas, among 186 White PCOS patients, insulin levels were actually negatively associated with DHEAS *(35)*. We also did not observe a relationship between insulin sensitivity (S_i) or acute insulin response to glucose (AIR_g), measured using the frequently sampled intravenous glucose tolerance test (FSIVGTT) and the adrenocortical response to ACTH stimulation in nine PCOS and nine BMI, age, and race-matched controls *(73)*.

Overall, our data indicate that extra-adrenal factors, at least androgens, estrogens, and insulin, and ovarian products, play a limited role in modulating adrenocortical production as assessed by the AA response to ACTH stimulation; a more significant, although still mild, effect on the sulfation of DHEA and on DHEAS levels may be observed. Overall, the modest role of extra-adrenal modulators on the adrenal in PCOS supports the hypothesis of an underlying genetic etiology in the abnormal adrenocortical steroidogenesis and metabolism, and AA excess, of PCOS.

5. INSULIN RESISTANCE AND HYPERANDROGENISM

In 1980, Burghen et al. demonstrated that PCOS women are insulin-resistant, secreting significantly higher baseline and post-glucose-load insulin levels compared with weight-matched, non-PCOS women *(58)*. They noted a positive linear correlation between insulin and androgen levels and proposed a possible etiological significance. The association between PCOS and hyperinsulinemia, independent of body mass index, has been reported by a number of investigators *(59,60)*.

Insulin resistance is a common feature of PCOS and exerts complex effects in the development of hyperandrogenism. Although more than 50% of PCOS patients are in the overweight to obese range, the degree of insulin resistance exceeds that conferred by adiposity alone. Hyperinsulinemic insulin resistance is an important factor mediating the steroidogenic abnormalities. Hyperandrogenemia is a common feature of disorders of insulin receptor number, affinity, or function, many of which result in profound hyperinsulinemia *(61–63)*. In these disorders, the extreme degrees of insulin resistance and subsequent severe hyperinsulinemia appear to stimulate IGF-1 receptor signal transduction in ovarian theca *(43)*. However, the more moderate degrees of hyperinsulinemia seen in PCOS are not high enough to cause activation of the IGF-1 receptor *(64)*. However, even modest degrees of hyperinsulinemia can be associated with increased androgen production in PCOS women and ovulatory controls *(44)*. The beneficial effect of insulin sensitizers, which results in suppression of both circulating insulin and androgen levels *(45,47,51,52,74)*, provides additional supportive evidence of the critical role of hyperinsulinism in the AE of PCOS.

Mechanistically, hyperinsulinemia results in AE in PCOS by suppressing the production of sex hormone-binding globulin (SHBG) and stimulating the theca production of androgens. Hyperinsulinemia may also result in granulosa cell dysfunction, which may favor further the production of ovarian androgens. A number of studies, both in hepatoma cell models and in PCOS women in vivo, have demonstrated the suppressive role of insulin on the hepatic production of SHBG, and, consequently, on the free fraction of SHBG-bound androgens, notably T and DHT *(55,56)*. The stimulatory effect of insulin on ovarian steroidogenesis has been demonstrated in both human and mammalian theca cells in vitro. For example, minced ovarian stroma incubations obtained from a woman with hyperandrogenism, insulin resistance, and acanthosis nigricans, demonstrated increased androstenedione and testosterone accumulation in the presence of insulin *(43)*. Ovarian stroma of hyperandrogenic women also demonstrated increased androstenedione, testosterone, and dihydrotestosterone production in the presence of insulin alone *(48,65)*. The relatively modest degree of hyperinsulinemia observed in PCOS is unlikely to act through IGF-1 receptors but is more likely mediated directly through the insulin receptor.

Insulin has also been shown to have a direct effect on granulosa cell function. At supraphysiologic levels, insulin has been shown to stimulate aromatase activity in human granulosa cells obtained from unstimulated ovarian follicles *(66)*. In granulosa cell cultures of normal and PCOS women, insulin receptor-blocking antibodies disrupted granulosa steroidogenesis; IGF-1 receptor antibodies had no effect on steroidogenesis *(46)*. It is possible that this disruption of granulosa cell function may further enhance androgen production by the PCOS ovary.

REFERENCES

1. Zawadski J, Dunaif A. Diagnostic criteria for polycystic ovary syndrome: towards a rational approach. In: Dunaif A, Given J, Haseltine F, Merriam G, eds. *Polycystic Ovary Syndrome*. Cambridge, MA: Blackwell Scientific Publications, 1992:377.
2. Revised 2003 consensus on diagnostic criteria and long-term health risks related to polycystic ovary syndrome (PCOS). *Hum Reprod* 2004;19:41.
3. Azziz R. Diagnostic criteria for polycystic ovary syndrome: a reappraisal. *Fertil Steril* 2005;83:1343.
4. Rosenfield RL. Ovarian and adrenal function in polycystic ovary syndrome. *Endocrinol Metab Clin North Am* 1999;28:265.
5. Legro RS, Driscoll D, Strauss JF 3rd, Fox J, Dunaif A. Evidence for a genetic basis for hyperandrogenemia in polycystic ovary syndrome. *Proc Natl Acad Sci USA* 1998;95:14956.
6. Azziz R, Sanchez LA, Knochenhauer ES, Moran C, Lazenby J, Stephens KC, Taylor K, Boots LR. Androgen excess in women: experience with over 1000 consecutive patients. *J Clin Endocrinol Metab* 2004;89:453–62.
7. Balen AH, Schachter ME, Montgomery D, Reid RW, Jacobs HS. Polycystic ovaries are a common finding in untreated female to male transsexuals. *Clin Endocrinol (Oxf)* 1993;38:325–9.
8. Abbott DH, Dumesic DA, Eisner JR, Colman RJ, Kemnitz JW. Insights into the development of PCOS from studies of prenatally androgenized female rhesus monkeys. *Trends Endocrinol Metab* 1998;9:62–7.
9. DeVane GW, Czekala NM, Judd HL, Yen SS. Circulating gonadotropins, estrogens, and androgens in polycystic ovarian disease. *Am J Obstet Gynecol* 1975;121:496.
10. Erickson GF, Magoffin DA, Dyer CA, Hofeditz C. The ovarian androgen producing cells: a review of structure/function relationships. *Endocr Rev* 1985;6:371–99.

11. Apter D, Butzow T, Laughlin GA, Yen SS. Accelerated 24-hour luteinizing hormone pulsatile activity in adolescent girls with ovarian hyperandrogenism: relevance to the developmental phase of polycystic ovarian syndrome. *J Clin Endocrinol Metab* 1994;79:119–25.

12. Patton WC, Berger MJ, Thompson IE, Chong AP, Grimes EM, Taymor ML. Pituitary gonadotropin responses to synthetic luteinizing hormone-releasing hormone in patients with typical and atypical polycystic ovary disease. *Am J Obstet Gynecol* 1975;121:382–6.

13. Eagleson CA, Gingrich M, Pastor C, et al. Polycystic ovarian syndrome: evidence that flutamide restores sensitivity of the GnRH pulse generator to inhibition by estradiol and progesterone. *J Clin Endocrinol Metab* 2000;85:4047.

14. Tapanainen JS, Koivunen R, Fauser BC, et al. A new contributing factor to polycystic ovary syndrome: the genetic variant of luteinizing hormone. *J Clin Endocrinol Metab* 1999; 84:1711.

15. Barnes RB, Rosenfield RL, Burstein S, Ehrmann DA. Pituitary-ovarian responses to nafarelin testing in the polycystic ovary syndrome. *N Engl J Med* 1989;320:559–65.

16. Bruning JC, Gautam D, Burks DJ, et al. Role of brain insulin receptor in control of body weight and reproduction. *Science* 2000;289:2122.

17. Rosenfield Rl. Ovarian and adrenal function in polycystic ovary syndrome. *Endocrinol Metab Clin North Am* 1999;28:265.

18. Chang RJ, Laufer LR, Meldrum DR, DeFazio J, Lu JK, Vale WW, Rivier JE, Judd HL. Steroid secretion in polycystic ovarian disease after ovarian suppression by a long-acting gonadotropin-releasing hormone agonist. *J Clin Endocrinol Metab* 1983;56:897–903.

19. Gilling-Smith C, Story H, Rogers V, Franks S. Evidence for a primary abnormality of thecal cell steroidogenesis in the polycystic ovary syndrome. *Clin Endocrinol (Oxf)* 1997;47:93–9.

20. Gilling-Smith C, Willis DS, Beard RW, Franks S. Hypersecretion of androstenedione by isolated thecal cells from polycystic ovaries. *J Clin Endocrinol Metab* 1994;79:1158–65.

21. Mahajan DK. Steroidogenesis in human polycystic ovary. *Endocrinol Metab Clin North Am* 1988;17:751–69.

22. Jakimiuk AJ, Weitsman SR, Navab A, Magoffin DA. Luteinizing hormone receptor, steroidogenesis acute regulatory protein, and steroidogenic enzyme messenger ribonucleic acids are overexpressed in theca and granulosa cells from polycystic ovaries. *J Clin Endocrinol Metab* 2001;8:1318–23.

23. Nelson VL, Legro RS, Strauss JF III, McAllister JM. Augmented androgen production is a stable steroidogenic phenotype of propagated theca cells from polycystic ovaries. *Mol Endocrinol* 1999;13:946–57.

24. Wickenheisser JK, Nelson-Degrave VL, McAllister JM. Dysregulation of cytochrome P450 17alpha-hydroxylase messenger ribonucleic acid stability in theca cells isolated from women with polycystic ovary syndrome. *J Clin Endocrinol Metab* 2005;90:1720–7.

25. Agarwal SK, Judd HL, Magoffin DA. A mechanism for suppression of estrogen production in women with polycystic ovary syndrome. *J Clin Endocrinol Metab* 1996;81:3686–91.

26. Gregory SJ, Kaiser UB. Regulation of gonadotropins by inhibin and activin. *Semin Reprod Med* 2004; 22:253.

27. Hsueh AJ, Dahl KD, Vaughan J, et al. Heterodimers and homodimers of inhibin subunits have different paracrine action in the modulation of luteinizing hormone-stimulated androgen biosynthesis. *Proc Natl Acad Sci USA* 1987;84:5082.

28. Norman RJ, Milner CR, Groome NP, Robertson DM. Circulating follistatin concentrations are higher and activin concentrations are lower in polycystic ovarian syndrome. *Hum Reprod* 2001;16:668.

29. Anderson RA, Groome NP, Baird DT. Inhibin A and inhibin B in women with polycystic ovarian syndrome during treatment with FSH to induce mono-ovulation. *Clin Endocrinol (Oxf)* 1998; 48:577.

30. Elting MW, Kwee J, Schats R, et al. The rise of estradiol and inhibin B after acute stimulation with follicle-stimulating hormone predict the follicle cohort size in women with polycystic ovary

syndrome, regularly menstruating women with polycystic ovaries, and regularly menstruating women with normal ovaries. *J Clin Endocrinol Metab* 2001;86:1589.

31. Wild RA, Umstot ES, Andersen RN, Ranney GB, Givens JR. Androgen parameters and their correlation with body weight in one hundred thirty-eight women thought to have hyperandrogenism. *Am J Obstet Gynecol* 1983;146:602–6.

32. Hoffman DL, Klove K, Lobo RA. The prevalence and significance of elevated dehydroepiandrosterone sulfate levels in anovulatory women. *Fertil Steril* 1984;42:76–81.

33. Steinberger E, Smith KD, Rodriguez-Rigau LJ. Testosterone, dehydroepiandrosterone, and dehydroepiandrosterone sulfate in hyperandrogenic women. *J Clin Endocrinol Metab* 1984;59:471–7.

34. Carmina E, Koyama T, Chang L, Stanczyk FZ, Lobo RA. Does ethnicity influence the prevalence of adrenal hyperandrogenism and insulin resistance in polycystic ovary syndrome? *Am J Obstet Gynecol* 1992;167:1807–12.

35. Kumar A, Woods KS, Bartolucci AA, Azziz R. Prevalence of adrenal androgen excess in patients with the polycystic ovary syndrome (PCOS). *Clin Endocrinol (Oxf)* 2005;62:644–9.

36. Piltonen T, Koivunen R, Perheentupa A, Morin-Papunen L, Ruokonen A, Tapanainen JS. Ovarian age-related responsiveness to human chorionic gonadotropin in women with polycystic ovary syndrome. *J Clin Endocrinol Metab* 2004;89:3769–75.

37. Rosenfield RL, Barnes RB, Ehrmann DA. Studies of the nature of 17-hydroxyprogesterone hyperresponsiveness to gonadotropin-releasing hormone agonist challenge in functional ovarian hyperandrogenism. *J Clin Endocrinol Metab* 1994;79:1686–92.

38. Miller D, Emans SJ, Kohane I. Follow-up study of adolescent girls with a history of premature pubarche. *J Adolesc Health* 1996;18:301–5.

39. Ibanez L, Potau N, Virdis R, Zampolli M, Terzi C, Gussinye M, Carrascosa A, Vicens-Calvet E. Postpubertal outcome in girls diagnosed of premature pubarche during childhood: increased frequency of functional ovarian hyperandrogenism. *J Clin Endocrinol Metab* 1993;76:1599–603.

40. Ibanez L, Potau N, Zampolli M, Street ME, Carrascosa A. Girls diagnosed with premature pubarche show an exaggerated ovarian androgen synthesis from the early stages of puberty: evidence from gonadotropin-releasing hormone agonist testing. *Fertil Steril* 1997;67:849–55.

41. Meas T, Chevenne D, Thibaud E, Leger J, Cabrol S, Czernichow P, Levy-Marchal C. Endocrine consequences of premature pubarche in post-pubertal Caucasian girls. *Clin Endocrinol (Oxf)* 2002;57:101–6.

42. Lobo RA, Goebelsmann U, Horton R. Evidence for the importance of peripheral tissue events in the development of hirsutism in polycystic ovary syndrome. *J Clin Endocrinol Metab* 1983;57:393–7.

43. Levin JH, Carmina E, Lobo RA. Is the inappropriate gonadotropin secretion of patients with polycystic ovary syndrome similar to that of patients with adult-onset congenital adrenal hyperplasia? *Fertil Steril* 1991;56:635–40.

44. Carmina E, Lobo RA. Ovarian suppression reduces clinical and endocrine expression of late-onset congenital adrenal hyperplasia due to 21-hydroxylase deficiency. *Fertil Steril* 1994;62:738–43.

45. Dewailly D, Vantyghem-Haudiquet MC, Sainsard C, Buvat J, Cappoen JP, Ardaens K, Racadot A, Lefebvre J, Fossati P. Clinical and biological phenotypes in late-onset 21-hydroxylase deficiency. *J Clin Endocrinol Metab* 1986;63:418–23.

46. Moran C, Azziz R, Carmina E, Dewailly D, Fruzzetti F, Ibanez L, Knochenhauer ES, Marcondes JA, Mendonca BB, Pignatelli D, Pugeat M, Rohmer V, Speiser PW, Witchel SF. 21-Hydroxylase-deficient nonclassic adrenal hyperplasia is a progressive disorder: a multicenter study. *Am J Obstet Gynecol* 2000;183:1468–74.

47. Azziz R, Black V, Hines GA, Fox LM, Boots LR. Adrenal androgen excess in the polycystic ovary syndrome: sensitivity and responsivity of the hypothalamic-pituitary-adrenal axis. *J Clin Endocrinol Metab* 1998;83:2317–23.

48. Moran C, Potter HD, Reyna R, Boots LR, Azziz R. Prevalence of 3beta-hydroxysteroid dehydrogenase-deficient nonclassic adrenal hyperplasia in hyperandrogenic women with adrenal androgen excess. *Am J Obstet Gynecol* 1999;181:596–600.

49. Moran C, Reyna R, Boots LS, Azziz R. Adrenocortical hyperresponsiveness to corticotropin in polycystic ovary syndrome patients with adrenal androgen excess. *Fertil Steril* 2004;81:126–31.

50. Azziz R, Bradley EL, Jr, Potter HD, Boots LR. 3beta-hydroxysteroid dehydrogenase deficiency in hyperandrogenism. *Am J Obstet Gynecol* 1993;168:889–95.

51. Azziz R, Gay FL, Potter SR, Bradley E Jr, Boots LR. The effects of prolonged hypertestosteronemia on adrenocortical biosynthesis in oophorectomized women. *J Clin Endocrinol Metab* 1991;72:1025–30.

52. Witchel SF, Kahsar-Miller M, Aston CE, White C, Azziz R. Prevalence of CYP21 mutations and IRS1 variant among women with polycystic ovary syndrome and adrenal androgen excess. *Fertil Steril* 2005;83:371–5.

53. Azziz R, Wells G, Zacur HA, Acton RT. Abnormalities of 21-hydroxylase gene ratio and adrenal steroidogenesis in hyperandrogenic women with an exaggerated 17-hydroxyprogesterone response to acute adrenal stimulation. *J Clin Endocrinol Metab* 1991;73:1327–31.

54. Azziz R, Bradley EL Jr, Potter HD, Boots LR. Adrenal androgen excess in women: lack of a role for 17-hydroxylase and 17,20-lyase dysregulation. *J Clin Endocrinol Metab* 1995;80:400–5.

55. Joehrer K, Geley S, Strasser-Wozak EM, Azziz R, Wollmann HA, Schmitt K, Kofler R, White PC. CYP11B1 mutations causing non-classic adrenal hyperplasia due to 11 beta-hydroxylase deficiency. *Hum Mol Genet* 1997;6:1829–34.

56. Lutfallah C, Wang W, Mason JI, Chang YT, Haider A, Rich B, Castro-Magana M, Copeland KC, David R, Pang S. Newly proposed hormonal criteria via genotypic proof for type II 3beta-hydroxysteroid dehydrogenase deficiency. *J Clin Endocrinol Metab* 2002;87:2611–22.

57. Carbunaru G, Prasad P, Scoccia B, Shea P, Hopwood N, Ziai F, Chang YT, Myers SE, Mason JI, Pang S. The hormonal phenotype of nonclassic 3 beta-hydroxysteroid dehydrogenase (HSD3B) deficiency in hyperandrogenic females is associated with insulin-resistant polycystic ovary syndrome and is not a variant of inherited HSD3B2 deficiency. *J Clin Endocrinol Metab* 2004;89:783–94.

58. Kahsar-Miller M, Boots LR, Bartolucci A, Azziz R. Role of a CYP17 polymorphism in the regulation of circulating dehydroepiandrosterone sulfate levels in women with polycystic ovary syndrome. *Fertil Steril* 2004;82:973–5.

59. Invitti C, Pecori Giraldi F, Dubini A, De Martin M, Cavagnini F. Increased urinary free cortisol and decreased serum corticosteroid-binding globulin in polycystic ovary syndrome. *Acta Endocrinol (Copenh)* 1991;125:28–32.

60. Prelevic GM, Wurzburger MI, Balint-Peric L. 24-hour serum cortisol profiles in women with polycystic ovary syndrome. *Gynecol Endocrinol* 1993;7:179–84.

61. Vogeser M, Halser B, Baron A, Jacob K, Demant T. Corticosteroid-binding globulin and unbound serum cortisol in women with polycystic ovary syndrome. *Clin Biochem* 2000;33:157–9.

62. Stewart PM, Penn R, Holder R, Parton A, Ratcliffe JG, London DR. The hypothalamo-pituitary-adrenal axis across the normal menstrual cycle and in polycystic ovary syndrome. *Clin Endocrinol (Oxf)* 1993;38:387–91.

63. Fassnacht M, Schlenz N, Schneider SB, Wudy SA, Allolio B, Arlt W. Beyond adrenal and ovarian androgen generation: increased peripheral 5 alpha-reductase activity in women with polycystic ovary syndrome. *J Clin Endocrinol Metab* 2003;88:2760–6.

64. Tsilchorozidou T, Honour JW, Conway GS. Altered cortisol metabolism in polycystic ovary syndrome: insulin enhances 5alpha-reduction but not the elevated adrenal steroid production rates. *J Clin Endocrinol Metab* 2003;88:5907–13.

65. Rodin A, Thakkar H, Taylor N, Clayton R. Hyperandrogenism in polycystic ovary syndrome. Evidence of dysregulation of 11 beta-hydroxysteroid dehydrogenase. *N Engl J Med* 1994;330:460–5.

66. Azziz R, Rittmaster RS, Fox LM, Bradley EL Jr, Potter HD, Boots LR. Role of the ovary in the adrenal androgen excess of hyperandrogenic women. *Fertil Steril* 1998;69:851–9.

67. Gonzalez F, Hatala DA, Speroff L. Adrenal and ovarian steroid hormone responses to gonadotropin-releasing hormone agonist treatment in polycystic ovary syndrome. *Am J Obstet Gynecol* 1991;165:535–45.

68. Rittmaster RS, Thompson DL. Effect of leuprolide and dexamethasone on hair growth and hormone levels in hirsute women: the relative importance of the ovary and the adrenal in the pathogenesis of hirsutism. *J Clin Endocrinol Metab* 1990;70:1096–102.

69. Cedars MI, Steingold KA, de Ziegler D, Lapolt PS, Chang RJ, Judd HL. Long-term administration of gonadotropin-releasing hormone agonist and dexamethasone: assessment of the adrenal role in ovarian dysfunction. *Fertil Steril* 1992;57:495–500.

70. Slayden SM, Crabbe L, Bae S, Potter HD, Azziz R, Parker CR Jr. The effect of 17beta-estradiol on adrenocortical sensitivity, responsiveness, and steroidogenesis in postmenopausal women. *J Clin Endocrinol Metab* 1998;83:519–24.

71. Chang WY, Stanczyk F, Bartolucci A, Azziz R. Effect of bilateral oophorectomy on basal and adreno-corticotropin (ACTH)-stimulated adrenal androgen (AA) secretion in polycystic ovary syndrome (PCOS). The 86th Annual Meeting of the Endocrine Society New Orleans, LA, 2004, June 16–19.

72. Azziz R, Zacur HA, Parker CR Jr, Bradley EL Jr, Boots LR. Effect of obesity on the response to acute adrenocorticotropin stimulation in eumenorrheic women. *Fertil Steril* 1991;56:427–33.

73. Farah-Eways LA, Reyna R, Knochenhauer ES, Bartolucci A, Azziz R. Glucose action and adreno-cortical biosynthesis in the polycystic ovary syndrome. *Fertil Steril* 2004;81:120–5.

74. Azziz R, Fox LM, Zacur HA, Parker CR Jr, Boots LR. Adrenocortical secretion of dehydroepiandros-terone in healthy women: highly variable response to adrenocorticotropin. *J Clin Endocrinol Metab* 2001;86:2513–7.

18 Recommended Treatment Modalities for Hyperandrogenism

Michel Pugeat, MD, PhD, Nisrin Kaddar, PhD, and Véronique Raverot, PhD

Summary

Improvement in androgenic symptoms generally requires ovarian androgen suppression. Insulin sensitizers may also be effective. Androgen suppression (e.g., oral contraceptives or metformin) alone produces modest decreases in the degree of hirsutism; concomitant antiandrogen therapy improves effectiveness considerably. The use of androgen receptor (AR) competitive inhibitors such as spironolactone, flutamide, or cyproterone acetate is recommended for the treatment of dermatologic hyperandrogenic symptoms, principally hirsutism.

Key Words: Hyperandrogenism; hirsutism; bioavailable testosterone; sex hormone-binding globulin; antiandrogen; spironolactone; cyproterone; flutamide.

1. INTRODUCTION

Hyperandrogenism, according to the Rotterdam Consensus *(1)*, is a basic symptom for the diagnosis of the polycystic ovary syndrome (PCOS), the most frequent endocrine

From: *Contemporary Endocrinology: Polycystic Ovary Syndrome*
Edited by: A. Dunaif, R. J. Chang, S. Franks, and R. S. Legro © Humana Press, Totowa, NJ

disorder in premenopausal women. Excess androgen production in women is generally associated with esthetic prejudice, which is the primary cause for consultation. Hair follicles and their anatomically associated sebaceous glands are the site of 5α reductase activity, transforming testosterone (T) into dihydrotestosterone (DHT), which binds with the highest-affinity androgen receptor (AR) *(2)*. Therefore, hyperandrogenism can be associated with hirsutism—increased hair growth with a male pattern—recurrent acne with increased sebum production and alopecia. In addition, mild androgen excess in women has been associated with increased risk of type 2 diabetes, cardiovascular disease, and endometrial and breast cancer *(3)*.

2. CLINICAL APPROACH TO HYPERANDROGENISM

2.1. Hirsutism

Hirsutism in women is defined medically as excessive terminal hair development with a male pattern (i.e., sexual hair). Hirsutism is to be distinguished from hypertrichosis, a generalized excessive hair growth with a non-sexual pattern, that could be genetic or associated with drugs such as glucocorticoids, phenytoins, minoxidil, or cyclosporine. The Ferriman–Gallwey scale that quantifies the extent of hair growth in the most androgen-sensitive locations is the recommended scoring system, with a score of 8 or more being the most widely accepted definition of hirsutism. Interestingly, 5% of women of reproductive age in the general population fulfill this definition. This scoring system has limitations because of the subjective nature of the evaluation, notably in patients who frequently shave their upper lips or wax their abdomen *(2)*. Moreover, severe hirsutism can be limited to one or two specific areas and thus might be under-scored. Importantly, the severity of hirsutism does not correlate with the circulating levels of androgens.

2.2. Acne

Acne can be isolated or associated with hirsutism and is generally explained by the interaction of androgens with the pilosebaceous units that form sexual-hair follicles. In some skin areas, however, androgens stimulate the sebaceous glands without impact on hair follicles.

2.3. Baldness

Baldness is a severe complication of androgen excess, but one which can be reversed by causal treatment or antiandrogens. In contrast, alopecia is poorly sensitive to antiandrogenic treatment, because its intimate cause is generally only partly associated with increased androgen sensitivity, being more largely a consequence of local inflammatory activity destroying the pilosebaceous unit of the scalp.

2.4. Symptoms of Virilization

Symptoms of virilization with temporal balding, increased muscular mass, clitoromegaly, and/or deepening of the voice are signs of exposure to massive androgen excess and risk indicators for an androgen-secreting tumor, in both premenopausal and postmenopausal women.

2.5. Other Symptoms Related to Androgen Excess

Androgens influence behavior, body composition, and physical functioning in women. The study of women's health across the nation showed a modest correlation of self-reported health with DHEAS, the main adrenal androgen, and of sexual desire with testosterone level (4). In contrast, the sex hormone-binding globulin (SHBG) level was significantly inversely associated with body mass index, body circumference, and the prevalence of metabolic syndrome that was found in 17% of women at baseline.

3. PRINCIPLES OF HYPERANDROGENISM TREATMENT

3.1. Androgen Excess

Androgen excess can be efficiently reduced by administering a combined estrogen–progestin preparation, which tends to suppress gonadotropin secretion and thus ovarian androgen excess, which is the main cause of hyperandrogenism. GnRH analog, although highly effective in suppressing gonadotropin and ovarian steroids, is expensive and generally not used on a long-term basis but can be useful for identifying ovarian androgen-secreting tumors or hyperthecosis (5).

Glucocorticoid therapy to suppress ACTH and adrenal androgen production is recommended in patients with non-classic congenital adrenal hyperplasia but is controversial in other causes of hirsutism (6).

3.2. Increased Testosterone Bioavailability

Increased testosterone bioavailability due to a low SHBG level, associated either with overweight or genetic predisposition (7), benefits from treatment with estrogens, such as ethinyl estradiol, which is present in birth-control pill preparations, and increases SHBG liver secretion, which should in turn limit testosterone biodisposal.

3.3. Increased Sensitivity to Androgens

Increased sensitivity to androgens in hirsute patients with no evidence of androgen excess might benefit from treatment with 5α-reductase inhibitors to lessen the conversion of testosterone into DHT. However, the intimate pathophysiology of patients with the so-called idiopathic hirsutism needs to be elucidated to open up new therapeutic strategies.

3.4. Antiandrogen Prescription

Antiandrogen prescription is, finally, a logical approach in most clinical situations of androgen excess and minimizes the dermatological impact of androgens.

3.5. Cosmetic Measures

Cosmetic measures, including bleaching, shaving and depilation, or eflornithine hydrochloride cream (Vaniqa, approved in the USA for the treatment of facial hirsutism), are important in long-term recovery from hirsutism. This topic, elegantly addressed in a recent review (2), will not be examined in this chapter.

4. COMBINED ESTROGEN–PROGESTIN THERAPY

Combined estrogen–progestin therapy remains the predominant treatment for hirsutism and acne. Its oral contraceptive property suppresses luteinizing hormone and thus, ovarian androgen production. Estrogen also enhances hepatic production of SHBG, thereby reducing the protein-unbound free fraction of circulating testosterone that is passively cleared by most target tissues *(8)*. The choice of progestin is central: progestins such as nor-testosterone derivatives are to be avoided because of their intrinsic androgenic activity, which would reduce their positive impact on hyperandrogenic symptoms: norgestimate and desogestrel, which are virtually non-androgenic progestins, are advised. Recently, drospirenone, an analog of spironolactone *(9)*, has been approved for use in combination with ethinyl estradiol and may be ideal for the treatment of hyperandrogenism *(10)*.

Controversy persists regarding the use of oral contraceptives as first-line therapy in PCOS *(11)*. These agents clearly alleviate hirsutism and acne and protect against unbalanced estrogenic on endometrium hyperplasia, but their potential adverse effects on insulin resistance, glucose tolerance, vascular reactivity, and coagulability are a concern. One study, comparing the effects of associating estrogen and oral contraceptives containing either cyproterone acetate or desogestrel for 12 months, showed decreased insulin sensitivity and, for cyproterone acetate, increased insulin secretion *(12)*.

5. GLUCOCORTICOIDS

Many patients with acne and/or hirsutism have elevated adrenal androgen levels. However, prolonged use of glucocorticoids to suppress adrenal androgens is not advised, particularly because glucocorticoids may induce weight gain and worsen or reveal latent metabolic disorders such as insulin resistance or lipid disorder, notably in patients with PCOS *(2,8)*.

6. ANTIANDROGENS

6.1. Principle

Androgen-responsive genes are activated by ARs bound to either T or DHT. It is believed that ARs are more transcriptionally active when bound to T or DHT. Two classes of antiandrogen are presently available. Steroid-derived antiandrogens are competitive ligands for ARs and inhibit T/DHT binding. They possess mixed agonist and antagonist activities and may have important progestin-like properties, such as antigonadotropic activities (cyproterone acetate) and/or steroidogenesis inhibitory activity (spironolactone). In contrast, the non-steroidal flutamide and its derivatives display exceptionally high relative binding affinity for ARs, without exerting agonistic activity or interacting with other steroid-binding receptors: they are pure non-steroidal antiandrogens without other hormonal activity.

6.2. Spironolactone

Spironolactone is a 17-hydroxyprogesterone derivative that binds ARs with 67% relative DHT-binding affinity (RBA) and shows some inhibitory activity on 17α-hydroxylase and C17,20 lyase activities with weak 5α-reductase inhibitory activity

(13). Its main metabolism canrenone binds SHBG but has no significant antiandrogenic activity. However, the main activity of spironolactone is antimineralocorticoid, with a recommendation for treating hypertension with hypokalemia associated with primary hyperaldosteronism. Spironolactone is also used for treating edema of noninflammatory origin responsible for secondary hyperaldosteronism. Therefore, spironolactone administration has a potential for hyperkalemia that should be checked over the time of treatment.

6.2.1. DOSES OF 50–200 MG

Doses of 50–200 mg daily are usually required for effective alleviation of hirsutism. However, patients should be advised that long-term treatment is generally necessary to obtain such benefit. Spironolactone can restore ovulation in PCOS patients. Although there is no evidence of ambiguous genitalia in exposed male fetuses, birth pill control must be considered during spironolactone administration.

6.2.2. HORMONAL EFFECTS

Hormonal effects are shown in Table 1. In hirsute patients treated with spironolactone (75 mg/day), a slight decrease in testosterone, free testosterone index (testosterone-to-SHBG binding capacity ratio), and androstenedione concentrations with unchanged LH levels is generally observed. Further decrease can be obtained when patients are given a combination of spironolactone and norgesterone (500 mg/day), with some increase in SHBG-binding capacity. Similar results have been reported when patients are given spironolactone with an estrogen–progestin combination *(14)*.

6.2.3. EVIDENCE-BASED EFFICACY

At least seven randomized placebo-controlled studies have shown that 6-month treatment with 100 mg/day spironolactone decreased Ferriman–Gallwey scores *(14)*. The effects of multiple treatment options with spironolactone, alone or associated with an estrogen–progestin combination, have shown a positive trend for the use of

Table 1
Effects of the Administration of Spironolactone (75 mg daily) Alone or Combined with Demegestone, a 19 Nor-Progesterone Derivative, on Hormones in Hirsute Women

	Basal	*Spironolactone (75 mg/day)*	*Spironolactone (75 mg daily) + demegestone (2.5 mg/day)*
Testosterone ng/dl	40 ± 20	31 ± 16[a]	27 ± 10
SHBG mg/dl	0.89 ± 0.41	0.89 ± 0.38	0.94±.47[a]
T/SHBG	58 ± 45	43 ± 32[a]	29±13[b]
Androstenedione ng/dl	181 ± 100	153 ± 83[a]	137 ± 50[b]
DHEAS mg/dl	271 ± 111	291 ± 134	245 ± 91
LH IU/l	9.5 ± 4.9	11.7 ± 8.5	9.0 ± 4.7
LH/FSH	2.3 ± 1.4	2.3 ± 1.4	2.0±1.2

[a]75 mg daily and continuously; $p < 0.05$.
[b]Both associated 21 days per month; $p < 0.01$.

spironolactone in women with PCOS and hirsutism *(15)*. Improved efficacy has been suggested when spironolactone is associated with oral contraceptives. The effectiveness of spironolactone on acne has not been assessed on large series of patients.

6.2.4. SIDE EFFECTS OF SPIRONOLACTONE

Side effects of spironolactone administration include fatigue, nausea, and dyspepsia. However, most studies reported unchanged electrolytes during long-term spirono-lactone treatment. A long-term study reported that, after 200 person-years of exposure to spironolactone and 506 person-years of follow-up over 8 years, no serious side effects could be attributed to spironolactone although diuretic effects and menstrual irregularities were observed in 59% of cases, resulting in cessation of treatment in 15% *(16)*. Weak progestagen activity may be associated with increased menstrual frequency. To overcome this problem, associating spironolactone with oral contraceptives or with nor-progesterone derivatives (demegestone or nomegestrol), which are available in Europe, would be appropriate. Their apparent contraceptive effect, however, has not been definitively validated.

6.3. Cyproterone Acetate

Cyproterone acetate is a 17-OH progesterone derivative with antigonadotropic and some 5α-reductase inhibitory activity. In addition, cyproterone acetate binds ARs with a relative binding affinity close to half that of DHT. Cyproterone acetate has a long biological half-life, storing in fat tissue. Combined administration with ethinyl estradiol (30 µg) at a dose of 2 mg daily or alone at 50 mg/day has been shown to have a contraceptive effect.

6.3.1. DOSES OF CYPROTERONE

Doses of cyproterone ranging from 25 to 50 mg daily have been used in most studies that have reported efficacy in reducing hair growth.

6.3.2. HORMONAL EFFECTS

Although androgen levels are very significantly decreased during cyproterone admin-istration, SHBG has a tendency to decrease, and consequently, the decrease in the free testosterone index might be relatively less than that in the total testosterone or androstenedione level *(17)*. The SHBG decrease might be related to weight gain although the metabolic impact of cyproterone acetate on insulin, insulin resistance, and lipid profile remains unaffected. Therefore, it is recommended to associate oral estrogens to cyproterone acetate for 21 days per month, so as to increase SHBG and normalize free testosterone levels (Table 2).

6.3.3. EVIDENCE-BASED EFFICACY

Seven randomized-controlled trials, comparing cyproterone acetate in association with ethinyl estradiol to placebo, for at least 6 months, have reported subjective alleviation of hirsutism with a significant decrease in Ferriman–Gallwey score *(18)*. A dose of cyproterone acetate ranging from 25 to 50 mg in association with 17β-estradiol (2 mg orally or percutaneously) 21 days per month for at least 6 months, with diet and exercise recommendations, is generally well tolerated and alleviates hirsutism and acne in most patients.

Table 2
Effects of the Administration of Cyproterone Acetate (50 mg daily) Alone or
Combined with 17α-Estradiol (2 mg) on Hormones in Hirsute Women

	Basal	CA (50 mg) + 17α-E₂ (2 mg 21 days/month)
T ng/dl	36 ± 15	23 ± 10^a
SHBG mg/dl	0.98 ± 0.39	1.24 ± 0.54^b
Free T ng/dl	45 ± 0.21	26 ± 0.12^b
Androstenedione ng/dl	185 ± 73	105 ± 59^b
DHEAS mg/dl	337 ± 113	272 ± 106

^{a}$p < 0.05$.
^{b}$p < 0.01$.

6.3.4. Side Effects

Patients receiving cyproterone acetate should be advised of some potential side effects that could limit long-term administration.

Weight Gain. Weight gain during cyproterone acetate treatment should be considered as the main side effect in hirsute patients for a dose of 50 mg/day. Such weight-gain does not exceed a few kilograms, but diet and exercise are recommended—although not proved to overcome this side effect.

Secondary Amenorrhea. Secondary amenorrhea is constantly associated with effective doses of cyproterone acetate. In contrast, severe endometrial atrophy may be associated with uterus bleeding that, in some cases, cannot be compensated by concomitant estrogen administration.

Ambiguous Genitalia in Exposed Male Fetuses. Ambiguous genitalia in exposed male fetuses have been reported only in rare cases, but animal studies strongly suggest that cyproterone acetate should not be administered to pregnant women.

6.4. Effectiveness of Cyproterone Acetate Versus Spironolactone

Several studies have compared the relative benefit and effectiveness of spironolactone and cyproterone acetate. Similar effectiveness on hirsutism has been reported for cyproterone acetate at 50 mg/day and spironolactone at 100 *(19)* or 200 mg/day *(20)*. However, more side effects were reported with cyproterone acetate in one study, with weight gain and increased insulin resistance *(20)*, in contrast to the findings of a previous study by the same group *(21)*. From its antiandrogenic properties, cyproterone acetate may be expected to be more effective in PCOS patients with increased androgen levels than in idiopathic hirsutism with normal androgen levels *(22)*, but this point has not been specifically addressed.

6.5. Flutamide and Derivatives

Flutamide and derivatives are currently the most potent non-steroid or "pure" antiandrogens.

6.5.1. DOSES OF 250 OR 500 MG DAILY

Doses of 250 or 500 mg daily have been shown to be similarly effective in the treatment of hirsutism *(23)*.

6.5.2. HORMONAL CONSEQUENCES

One study reported the effect of a dose of 250 mg twice daily for 1 year in patients with idiopathic hirsutism *(24)*. No effect on LH/FSH pulsatility and unchanged androgen and SHBG levels were reported in flutamide-treated patients who maintained regular and ovulatory menstrual cycles, while disappearance of acne and of seborrhea was observed at 2 months, with a Ferriman–Gallwey score lower than 7 after 12 months. No significant adverse side effects were reported in this study. In another study, flutamide administration (250 mg twice daily) restored ovulation in adolescent PCOS patients *(25)*.

6.5.3. EVIDENCE-BASED EFFICACY

In a prospective study of hirsute patients who failed to respond to oral contraceptives, spironolactone, or dexamethasone, treatment with flutamide (250 mg twice daily) with oral contraceptives resulted in a rapid and marked decrease in hirsutism score, seborrhea, acne, and hair-loss score *(26)*. The clinical efficacy and safety of low-dose flutamide, alone or combined with an oral contraceptive, for the treatment of hirsutism has been shown in non-randomized studies of non-hyperandrogenic (idiopathic) hirsute women *(27–29)*.

6.5.4. THE SIDE EFFECTS OF FLUTAMIDE ADMINISTRATION

The side effects of flutamide administration consist mainly of hepatoxicity. Fulminant liver failure has been reported in flutamide therapy for hirsutism *(30)*. Therefore, serial blood aminotransferase levels should be monitored before and during the first few months of flutamide treatment.

6.6. Comparative Studies of Flutamide

Significant but similar improvement in hirsutism score was reported in a randomized study of idiopathic hirsute patients (*n* = 22) who received flutamide 250 mg twice daily or cyproterone acetate 100 mg for days 5–14 of the menstrual cycle *(31)*. In a 12-month randomized trial, comparing cyproterone acetate (12.5 mg daily for 10 days) associated to ethinyl estradiol (10 μg/day) for 21 days per month (*n* = 20), flutamide 250 mg/day (*n* = 15), finasteride 5 mg/day (*n* = 15), or ketoconazole 300 mg/day (*n* = 16), improved hirsutism scores were observed in each group, cyproterone acetate and flutamide being the most effective *(32)*. In a 6-month randomized trial comparing spironolactone 100 mg/day (*n* = 10), flutamide 250 mg/day (*n* = 10), and finasteride 5 mg/d (*n* = 10) to a placebo group (*n* = 10), each treatment reduced hair diameter and alleviated hirsutism, with no significant differences between groups *(33)*. Comparing administration of combined flutamide and spironolactone to an oral contraceptive containing 35 μg of ethinyl estradiol with 5 mg of cyproterone acetate, a prospective randomized trial showed similar impact on hirsutism score *(34)*.

6.7. Finasteride

Finasteride, an a4-aza steroid and competitive inhibitor of type II 5α-reductase, has been reported in the treatment of hirsutism. A randomized study reported equal efficacy of treatment with finasteride, 5 mg/day (*n* = 20) or cyproterone acetate, 25 mg for 10 days, combined with ethinyl estradiol 20 mg for 20 days, in terms of hirsutism score *(35)*. One study reported that finasteride (5 mg/day) improved the beneficial effect of spironolactone (100 mg/day) on hirsutism score *(36)*.

One study comparing the effectiveness of finasteride, 5 mg/day, cyproterone acetate 12.5 mg/day for the first 10 days of the menstrual cycle, or spironolactone 100 mg/day in idiopathic hirsute patients showed a significant improvement in hirsutism score in each group *(36)*. The prominence of type-I 5α-reductase in the pilosebaceous unit makes it unlikely to be an optimal treatment for the androgen-related cutaneous manifestations associated with the condition *(8)*.

7. INSULIN SENSITIZERS AS TREATMENT OF HYPERANDROGENISM

7.1. Principle

Insulin resistance has been identified in both obese and non-obese patients with PCOS, and there is good evidence that the use of insulin sensitizers such as metformin should be recommended in these patients *(37)*. A few studies have explored the beneficial effect on hirsutism of combining insulin sensitizers with antiandrogenic treatment.

7.2. Metformin or Antiandrogen

A study comparing the effects on hirsutism of 500 mg metformin three times daily versus dinette, a combination of ethinyl estradiol 35 μg/day with cyproterone acetate 2 mg, showed that metformin taken alone was effective on Ferriman–Gallwey score and patient's self-assessment. The authors concluded that hirsutism may be effectively treated by reducing hyperinsulinemia *(38)*.

8. ANTIANDROGENS AND METABOLIC DISORDERS IN HYPERANDROGENIC PATIENTS

8.1. Metabolic Consequences of Antiandrogens

A study reported significant decreases in total cholesterol, low-density lipoprotein (LDL), and TG levels with unchanged liver function test results after a 12-week course of oral flutamide at daily doses of 500 mg *(39)*. A randomized trial of combined flutamide–metformin reported that low doses of flutamide (62.5 mg/day) combined with metformin (850 mg twice daily), in young hyperinsulinemic hyperandrogenic adolescents (*n* = 21) with no oral contraceptive, gave a significant improvement in insulin/glucose ratio, increased SHBG and decreased androgen levels, significant gain in lean mass and loss of total fat, significant decrease in total cholesterol, HDL, LDL and TG, and unchanged liver function test results *(40)*. This study suggested that a minidose of flutamide may considerably enhance metformin reversal of endocrine-metabolic abnormalities.

8.2. *Improved Insulin Resistance*

Improved insulin resistance with antiandrogens was reported in hyperandrogenic women in one study that compared spironolactone ($n = 20$), flutamide ($n = 10$), and the GnRH agonist buserelin ($n = 10$) in 43 hyperandrogenic women, 30 of whom were obese. Increased glucose disposal, measured by hyperinsulinemic–euglycemic clamp, was observed after 3–4 months of each treatment, but no subsequent improvement, the increase being greater in lean than in obese patients *(41)*.

9. CONCLUDING REMARKS

Improvement in androgenic symptoms generally require ovarian androgen suppression, most frequently with an oral contraceptive or high-dose progestin. Insulin sensitizers (metformin and thiazolidinediones) may also be effective. The use of AR competitive inhibitors such as spironolactone, flutamide, or cyproterone acetate is recommended for the treatment of dermatologic hyperandrogenic symptoms, principally hirsutism. Although fewer data are available on the therapeutic benefit of the 5α-reductase inhibitor finasteride in these conditions, this therapy is another potential option and may entail fewer side effects. Androgen suppression (e.g., oral contraceptives or metformin) alone produces modest decreases in the degree of hirsutism; associating antiandrogen therapy improves effectiveness considerably.

A number of future investigations are suggested, including documentation of the response to treatment for hyperandrogenism using longer term studies, determination of the potential beneficial effect of various classes of antiandrogen on metabolic aspects and related morbidity in PCOS, and determination of the optimum antiandrogen doses in the treatment of hyperandrogenic symptoms.

REFERENCES

1. Rotterdam ESHRE/ASRM-Sponsored PCOS Consensus Workshop Group. Revised 2003 consensus on diagnostic criteria and long-term health risks related to polycystic ovary syndrome. *Fertil Steril* 2004;81:19–25.
2. Rosenfield RL. Hirsutism. *N Engl J Med* 2005;353:2578–88.
3. Dahlgren E, Janson PO, Johansson S, Lapidus L, Oden A. Polycystic ovary syndrome and risk for myocardial infarction evaluated from a risk factor model based on a prospective population study of women. *Acta Obstet Gynecol Scand* 1992;71:599–604.
4. Santoro N, Torrens J, Crawford S, Allsworth JE, Finkelstein JS, Gold EB, Korenman S, Lasley WL, Luborsky JL, McConnell D, Sowers MF, Weiss G. Correlates of circulating androgens in mid-life women: the Study of Women's Health Across the Nation (SWAN). *J Clin Endocrinol Metab* 2005;90:4836–45.
5. Pascal MM, Pugeat M, Robert M, Rousset H, Déchaud H, Dutrieux-Berger N, Tourniaire J. Androgen suppressive effect of GnRH agonist in ovarian hyperthecosis and virilizing tumours. *Clin Endocrinol* 1994;41: 571–6.
6. Azziz R, Dewailly D, Owerbach D. Nonclassic adrenal hyperplasia: current concepts. *J Clin Endocrinol Metab* 1994;78:810–5.
7. Cousin P, Calemard-Michel L, Lejeune H, Grenot C, Baret C, Brébant C, Pugeat M Influence of SHBG gene pentanucleotide TAAAA repeat and D327N polymorphism on serum sex hormone-binding globulin concentration in hirsute women. *J Clin Endocrinol Metab* 2004;89: 917–24.

8. Ehrmann DA. Polycystic ovary syndrome. *N Engl J Med* 2005;352:1223–36.

9. Krattenmacher R. Drospirenone: pharmacology and pharmacokinetics of a unique progestogen. *Contraception* 2000;62:29–38.

10. Guido M, Romualdi D, Giuliani M, Suriano R, Selvaggi L, Apa R, Lanzone A. Drospirenone for the treatment of hirsute women with polycystic ovary syndrome: a clinical, endocrinological, metabolic pilot study. *J Clin Endocrinol Metab* 2004;89:2817–23.

11. Diamanti-Kandarakis E, Baillargeon, J-P, Iuorno MJ, Jakubowicz DJ, Nestler JE. A modern medical quandary: polycystic ovary syndrome, insulin resistance, and oral contraceptive pills. *J Clin Endocrinol Metab* 2003;88:1927–32.

12. Mastorakos G, Koliopoulos C, Deligeoroglou E, Diamanti-Kandarakis E, Creastas G. Effects of two forms of combined oral contraceptives on carbohydrate metabolism in adolescents with polycystic ovary syndrome. *Fertil Steril* 2006;85:420–7.

13. Corvol P, Michaud A, Menard J, Freifeld M, Mahoudeau J. Antiandrogenic effect of spironolactones: mechanism of action. *Endocrinology* 1975;97:52–8.

14. Farquhar C, Lee O, Toomath R, Jepson R. Spironolactone versus placebo or in combination with steroids for hirsutism and/or acne. *Cochrane Database Syst Rev* 2003;4:CD000194.

15. Christy NA, Franks AS, Cross LB. Spironolactone for hirsutism in polycystic ovary syndrome. *Ann Pharmacother* 2005;39:1517–21.

16. Shaw JC, White LE. Long-term safety of spironolactone in acne: results of an 8-year follow up study. *J Cut Med Surg* 2002;6:541–5.

17. Vincens M, Mercier-Bodard Ch, Mowszowicz I, Kuttenn F, Mauvais-Jarvis P. Testosterone-estradiol binding globulin (TeBG) under cyproterone acetate (CPA) and percutaneous estradiol treatment of hirsutism. *Gynecologicl Endocrinology* 1988;208, suppl. 2:Abst 260.

18. Vander Spuy ZM, Le Roux PA. Cyproterone acetate for hirsutism. *Cochrane Database System Rev* 2003;4 CD001125.

19. O'Brien RC, Cooper ME, Lamurray RML, Seeman E, Thomas AK, Jerums G. Comparison of sequential cyproterone acetate/estrogen vs. spironolactone/oral contraceptive in the treatment of hirsutism. *J Endocrinol Metab* 1991;72:1008–13.

20. Krotkiewski M, Landin K, Dahlgren E, Janson PO, Holm G. Effect of two modes of antiandrogen treatment on insulin sensitivity and serum leptin in women with PCOS. *Gynecol Obstet Invest* 2003;55:88–95.

21. Dahlgren E, Landin K, Krotkiewski M, Holm G, Janson PO. Effects of two antiandrogen treatments on hirsutism and insulin sensitivity in women with polycystic ovary syndrome. *Hum Reprod* 1998;13:2706–11.

22. Rittmaster RS. Hirsutism. *Lancet* 1997;349:191–5.

23. Muderris II, Bayram F, Sahin Y, Kelestimur F. A comparison between two doses of flutamide (250 mg/d and 500 mg/d) in the treatment of hirsutism. *Fertil Steril* 1997;68:644–7.

24. Couzinet B, Pholsena M, Young J, Schaison G. 1993 The impact of a pure anti-androgen (flutamide) on LH, FSH, androgens and clinical status in idiopathic hirsutism. *Clin Endocrinol (Oxf)* 39: 157–62.

25. De Leo V, Lanzetta D, D'Antona D, la Marca A, Morgante G. Hormonal effects of flutamide in young women with polycystic ovary syndrome. *J Clin Endocrinol Metab* 1998;83:99–102.

26. Cusan L, Dupont A, Belanger A, Tremblay RR, Manhes G, Labrie F. Treatment of hirsutism with the pure antiandrogen flutamide. *J Am Acad Dermatol* 1990;23:462–9.

27. Cusan L, Dupont A, Gomez JL, Tremblay RR, Labrie F. 1994 Comparison of flutamide and spironolactone in the treatment of hirsutism: a randomized controlled trial. *Fertil Steril* 61:281–7.

28. Dodin S, Faure N, Cedrin I, Mechain C, Turcot-Lemay L, Guy J, Lemay A. Clinical efficacy and safety of low-dose flutamide alone and combined with an oral contraceptive for the treatment of idiopathic hirsutism. *Clin Endocrinol (Oxf)* 1995;43:575–82.

29. Venturoli S, Paradisi R, Bagnoli A, Colombo FM, Ravaioli B, Viancllo F, Mancini F, Gualerzi B, Porcu E, Seracchioli R. Low-dose flutamide (125 mg/day) as maintenance therapy in the treatment of hirsutism. *Horm Res* 2001;56:5–31.

30. Andrade RJ, Lucena MI, Fernandez MC, Suarez F, Montero JL, Fraga E, Hidalgo F. Fulminant liver failure associated with flutamide therapy for hirsutism. *Lancet* 1999;353:983.

31. Grigoriou O, Papadias C, Konidaris S, Antoniou G, Karakitsos P, Giannikos L. Comparison of flutamide and cyproterone acetate in the treatment of hirsutism: a randomized controlled trial. *Gynecol Endocrinol* 1996;10:119–23.

32. Venturoli S, Marescalchi O, Colombo FM, Macrelli S, Ravailoli B. Bagnoli A, Paradisi R, Flamigni C. A prospective randomized trial comparing low dose flutamide, finasteride, ketoconazole, and cyproterone acetate – estrogen regimens in the treatment of hirsutism. *J Clin Endocrinol Metab* 1999;84:1304–10.

33. Moghetti P, Tosi F, Tosti A, Negri C, Misciali C, Perrone F, Caputo M, Muggeo M, Castello R. Comparison of spironolactone, flutamide, and finasteride efficacy in the treatment of hirsutism: a randomized, double blind, placebo controlled trial. *J Clin Endocrinol Metab* 2000;85:89–94.

34. Inal MM, Yildirim Y, Taner CE. Comparison of the clinical efficacy of flutamide and spironolactone plus Diane 35 in the treatment of idiopathic hirsutism: a randomized controlled study. *Fertil Steril* 2005;841693–7.

35. Beigi A, Sobhi A, Zarrinkoub F. Finasteride versus cyproterone acetate-estrogen regimens in the treatment of hirsutism. *Int J Gynaecol Obstet* 2004; 87:29–33.

36. Kelestimur F, Everest H, Unluhizarci K, Bayram F, Sahin Y. A comparison between spironolactone and spironolactone plus finasteride in the treatment of hirsutism. *Eur J Endocrinol* 2004;150(3): 351–4.

37. Harborne L, Fleming R, Lyall H, Norman J, Sattar N. Descriptive review of the evidence for the use of metformin in polycystic ovary syndrome. *Lancet* 2003;361:1894–901.

38. Harborne L, Fleming R, Lyall H, Sattar N, Norman J. Metformin or antiandrogen in the treatment of hirsutism in polycystic ovary syndrome. *J Clin Endocrinol Metab* 2003;88:4116–23.

39. Diamanti-Kandarakis E, Mitrakou A, Raptis S, Tolis G, Duleba AJ. The effect of a pure antiandrogen receptor blocker, flutamide, on the lipid profile in the polycystic ovary syndrome. *J Clin Endocrinol Metab* 1998;83:2699–705.

40. Ibanez L, De Zegher F. Flutamide-metformin therapy to reduce fat mass in hyperinsulinemic ovarian hyperandrogenism: effects in adolescents and in women on third-generation oral contraception. *J Clin Endocrinol Metab* 2003;88:4720–4.

41. Moghetti P, Tosi F, Castello R, Magnani CM, Negri C, Brun E, Furlani L, Caputo M, Muggeo M. The insulin resistance in women with hyperandrogenism is partially reversed by antiandrogen treatment: evidence that androgens impair insulin action in women. *J Clin Endocrinol Metab* 1996;81:952–60.

Effective Regimens for Ovulation Induction in Polycystic Ovary Syndrome

Juha S. Tapanainen, MD, PhD, and Laure Morin-Papunen, MD, PhD

CONTENTS

Summary

Several approaches have been used for ovulation induction in women with polycystic ovary syndrome (PCOS). Weight reduction should be recommended for obese women, because even 5% weight loss can be effective. Recent analyses still support the effectiveness of clomiphene citrate (CC) as a first-line medical therapy. Of anovulatory women with PCOS, about 70% will ovulate in response to CC, and the cumulative live birth rate is about 30%. A maximum of 6 CC cycles has been recommended, but some patients may benefit from more cycles, as the cumulative pregnancy rate (PR) continues to rise after 6 cycles. Women who do not respond to a daily dose of 150 mg can be considered CC-resistant. Human gonadotropins can be used as second-line treatment, but depending on the weight and age of the patient and practical clinical circumstances, other treatments may be more effective or easier to carry out. As many women with PCOS are insulin-resistant, it is rational to focus treatment attempts on the improvement of insulin resistance and hyperinsulinemia. Treatment with metformin alone or in combination with CC may be used, and overweight women in particular should be offered this option. Although other insulin-sensitizing agents, i.e. thiazolidinediones, seem to be effective, their safety in the treatment of PCOS is less well documented,

From: *Contemporary Endocrinology: Polycystic Ovary Syndrome*
Edited by: A. Dunaif, R. J. Chang, S. Franks, and R. S. Legro © Humana Press, Totowa, NJ

and they cannot be recommended for women desiring pregnancy. The results of using aromatase inhibitors for ovulation induction have been promising, and they may become a useful alternative for ovulation induction. Laparoscopic ovarian drilling is an effective treatment in CC-resistant women, but being an invasive method, it should be used only for patients resistant to other ovulation induction methods.

Key Words: anovulation, aromatase inhibitors, clomiphene citrate, gonadotropins, metformin, ovulation induction, polycystic ovary syndrome.

1. INTRODUCTION

Polycystic ovary syndrome (PCOS) is the most common cause of anovulatory infertility. Ovulation induction in PCOS needs special attention, as there is a surplus number of small antral follicles and these patients are exposed to the risks of ovarian hyperstimulation syndrome (OHHS) and multiple pregnancy. Therefore, ovulation induction should be aimed at development and ovulation of a single dominant follicle (1). This requires careful monitoring of the treatment cycle, which has not in the past been considered to be as important as it is today. Furthermore, the growing use of in vitro fertilization (IVF), which is effective and relatively straightforward to perform and monitor, has led to some clinicians neglecting traditional ovulation induction methods. In addition, after introduction of elective single embryo transfer (2,3) the risk of multiple pregnancy in IVF has decreased significantly, which allows a controlled and safe treatment option and makes it tempting as first- or second-line treatment of anovulatory PCOS patients. There have been concerns about a possible association between ovarian stimulation and ovarian cancer. The data are conflicting, and it is not clear whether the risk is related to nulliparity or to infertility treatments per se, and at the moment such a link has not been established (4).

Several approaches have been used for ovulation induction in women with PCOS. Clomiphene citrate (CC) has been the drug of choice for decades (5), even though new medical and surgical alternatives have now been developed. Recent advances in the development, however, may significantly change the picture of ovulation induction. It is clear that more attention will be paid to selecting patients and tailoring treatment on an individual basis, taking into account the age, weight, and general health of the patient as well as safety and costs.

2. WEIGHT LOSS AND LIFESTYLE MODIFICATIONS

Women with anovulatory PCOS respond well to lifestyle interventions such as hypocaloric diets, exercise, and group therapy, which should always be the first-line treatment (*see* Chapter 14). Modest weight reduction of only 5% by means of lifestyle modification can restore ovulation in 50% of anovulatory women with PCOS (6–8). Unfortunately, most overweight/obese women with PCOS find it difficult to institute or maintain these lifestyle interventions, and women in the normal weight range may not benefit from weight loss.

3. CLOMIPHENE CITRATE

CC is an anti-estrogen which is a non-steroidal compound resembling an estrogen. It has been in clinical use for ovulation induction for more than 40 years. It competes for receptor binding sites in the hypothalamus and blocks estrogen from its receptors, thus inhibiting the negative feedback effect of estrogens. This induces the release of

GnRH, resulting in increased gonadotropin secretion from the pituitary, stimulating ovarian follicular development and ovulation.

CC is given for 5 days starting on days 2–5. The starting day does not seem to influence the outcome of treatment *(9)*. Usually stimulation is started with a dose of 50 mg daily, and depending on the response the dose can be increased, the highest recommended dose being 150 mg/day. The dose needed to induce ovulation correlates with body weight, and there is an association between increased body mass index (BMI) and ovulation failure *(10–12)*. Therefore, even higher doses can be used, although the existing evidence indicates that there is no advantage in using a dose higher than 150 mg/day *(13)*. About 50% of women will ovulate using a dose of 50 mg *(14)*.

About 70% of anovulatory women (WHO group 2) will ovulate in response to CC, the pregnancy rate (PR) being 30–40% and the cumulative live birth rate about 30% *(15,16)*, but in selected patients these numbers can be higher *(17)*. A maximum of six CC cycles has been recommended, but some patients may benefit from more cycles, as the cumulative PR continues to rise after six cycles *(11,18)*. The majority (70–85%) of pregnancies are achieved within the first three CC cycles *(11,19)*. Women who do not respond to a daily dose of 150 mg can be considered to be CC-resistant. These patients may benefit from alternative and adjunctive treatments.

Human chorionic gonadotropin (hCG, 5000–10000 IU) may be used for triggering ovulation after CC stimulation. It does not normally enhance ovulation induced by CC, but it may be used in cases in which ovulation does not occur despite normal follicular development *(20)*. Furthermore, hCG, given when the follicle(s) are >17 mm in diameter, may be helpful for the timing of intercourse or intra-uterine insemination (IUI) *(16)*.

Careful monitoring of CC cycles is important for the outcome of treatment and for the patient's safety. It is recommended that ultrasound (US) monitoring should be offered, at least during the first cycle of treatment, to assess the number of preovulatory follicles, endometrial thickness, and the time of expected ovulation. To minimize the risk of multiple pregnancy, ultrasonography should be performed in each cycle until ovulation has been confirmed. Mid-luteal assay of serum progesterone is useful for confirming ovulation, although the normalized cycle length alone speaks in favor of ovulation.

The multiple PR after CC stimulation is 6–13% *(11,21–23)* and 0.5% are triplet pregnancies *(22)*. The miscarriage rate varies between 15 and 25% *(11,24)*, which is somewhat higher than the spontaneous miscarriage rate among healthy women. Although this difference has not been observed in all studies *(17,18)*, the possibly lower live birth rate has been attributed to increased serum levels of LH and premature maturation of the oocyte *(16,25)*, and to the anti-estrogenic effect of CC, resulting in endometrial suppression *(26)*.

Up to now, there is no evidence that the malformation rate among children born after CC treatment is higher than after spontaneous pregnancies. In a recent population-based case–control study, CC was not associated with any risk of hypospadias, which has been one of the concerns related to CC *(27)*.

4. GONADOTROPINS

Gonadotropin stimulation has traditionally been the next step in the treatment of women who are resistant to CC, although recently other treatment options such as metformin and its combination with CC or gonadotropins have been used in second-line therapies in PCOS. As ovulation induction with gonadotropins bears risks of OHHS and multiple pregnancy *(28–30)*, several protocols have been developed aiming to achieve maturation and ovulation of a small number of follicles, optimally one, to obtain a singleton pregnancy without complications. The most commonly used protocols are low-dose step-up and step-down regimens. The step-up approach is widely used, and it seems to reduce the risk of multiple follicular growth and needs less monitoring *(31)*, whereas the step-down regimen requires a shorter treatment period *(32)*.

In the classical low-dose step-up protocol, the administration of follicle-stimulating hormone (FSH) is started at any time with a dose of 75 IU/day. After 7–14 days of treatment, the dose is increased by 25–37.5 IU/day at weekly intervals if the diameter of none of the follicles exceeds 11 mm *(16,17,33)*. The chosen dose, not exceeding 225 IU/day, is maintained until the leading follicle is >17 mm in diameter and no other follicles are >14 mm, and hCG is injected to induce ovulation *(34)*. A starting dose of 50 IU/day can be used, but in obese patients, it may often be too low and result in a poor PR *(35)*.

In the step-down approach, stimulation is started with 150 IU/day and continued until the dominant follicle is 10 mm. The dose is then decreased to 112.5 IU/day for 3 days followed by a further decrease to 75 IU/day, which dose is continued until hCG injection *(36)*.

There are no comprehensive controlled studies in which the step-up and step-down protocols have been compared, but existing studies indicate that the clinical outcome is comparable in both regimens. Owing to a shorter duration of stimulation in the step-down protocol, less FSH is needed *(37)*. Monofollicular development can be achieved similarly with both regimens, in 46–70% of cases with the step-up protocol and in 32–88% of cases with the step-down protocol *(16,34)*. The PR per cycle has varied from 13 to 19% in the step-up protocol and from 7 to 31% in the step-down protocol *(34,37)*. The multiple PR after low-dose stimulation has been under 10% in most studies *(16,32,34)*, although higher percentages of up to 25% have also been observed *(38)*. By optimizing the protocol and with patient selection, multiple pregnancies as well as OHHS can practically be avoided *(39,40)*. After 12 months, the cumulative PR in PCOS patients after CC treatment followed by gonadotropins has been as high as 90% *(17)* and the singleton live birth rate was 71% in WHO 2 ovulation induction after 24 months *(23)*.

With regard to the gonadotropin preparation used for ovulation induction, urinary FSH seems to be associated with a reduced risk of OHHS compared with human menopausal gonadotropin (hMG), but otherwise the clinical outcome does not differ *(31)*. Moreover, there is no evidence of a difference in efficacy or safety between urinary and recombinant FSH *(41,42)*. The data on concomitant administration of gonadotropin-releasing (GnRH) agonist with gonadotropins are controversial. It may *(43)* or may not *(44)* reduce the miscarriage rate, but it increases the OHHS rate *(31,45)*, and therefore, it is not recommended for routine use in ovulation induction.

5. INSULIN-LOWERING AGENTS

5.1. Metformin

The most studied insulin-lowering agent in the treatment of ovulation induction in PCOS is metformin, a biguanide anti-hyperglycemic drug. Metformin has been shown to improve abdominal obesity and metabolic abnormalities, e.g., hyperinsulinemia and insulin resistance, to decrease androgen levels in obese and also non-obese women with PCOS, as well as to restore menstrual pattern and ovulatory function in 25–95% of cases *(46–52)*.

Two recent meta-analyses have shown that metformin alone, compared with placebo, increased the ovulation rate 1.5–3.9 times, but it was not significantly better than placebo with regard to achievement of pregnancy (Table 1) *(53,54)*. Ovulation was achieved in 46% of those receiving metformin alone compared with 24% of those receiving placebo *(53)*.

5.2. Metformin and Additive Treatment

5.2.1. Metformin and Clomiphene

The addition of metformin to CC appears to be 2- to 4-fold more effective than CC alone for ovulation induction and achieving pregnancy in women with non-defined CC sensitivity, and even more effective in CC-resistant women (Table 1) *(54,55)*. Ovulation was achieved in 76% of those receiving metformin and CC compared with 42% of those receiving CC only *(53)*. A more recent randomized study in non-obese anovulatory women with PCOS involved comparison of the effectiveness of 6 months of metformin treatment versus six-cycle CC treatment. The ovulation rate did not differ between the two groups (62.9 vs. 67.0%), whereas the miscarriage rate was significantly lower (9.7 vs. 37.5%) and the PR (15.1 vs. 7.2%, $p = 0.009$) and live birth rate (83.9 vs. 56.3%, $p = 0.07$) were higher in the metformin group *(56)*.

However, these results could not be confirmed in two large recent randomized studies, where metformin was significantly less effective than CC, and the combination of the two drugs did not bring any advantages *(57,58,59)*. Thus, CC remains the first line treatment (after lifestyle changes in obese women) in PCOS women with anovulation, and the usefulness of metformin alone or in combination with CC for ovulation induction in PCOS remains controversial.

5.2.2. Metformin and Gonadotropins

The usefulness of the combination of metformin and gonadotropin for ovulation induction is controversial. The addition of metformin to gonadotropins has been shown to improve follicular growth and to decrease the risk of ovarian hyperstimulation in previously CC-resistant PCOS patients *(60)*. It has also been shown to increase the number of mono-ovulatory cycles in a randomized controlled study *(61)*. However, this combination did not significantly improve the rates of ovulation, pregnancy, live birth, multiple pregnancies or OHSS in two placebo-controlled randomized studies *(61,62)*. A recent meta-analysis, including eight randomized controlled trials, demonstrated that the co-administration of metformin and gonadotropin did not significantly improve ovulation (OR = 3.27; 95% CI = 0.31–34.72) or pregnancy (OR = 3.46; 95% CI = 0.98–12.2) rates. However, the authors stated that the results remain inconclusive because of the small number of trials and small sample sizes, limiting the power of the meta-analysis. Further randomized controlled trials are necessary to clarify whether co-administration of metformin and gonadotropin will improve ovulation and PRs *(63)*.

5.2.3. SIDE-EFFECTS OF METFORMIN

Metformin has been administered at doses varying from 1.5 to 2.5 g/day, and it is generally divided into two to three doses. Mild side effects such as gastrointestinal symptoms (nausea, metallic taste in the mouth, and changes in bowel movement frequency) occur in about 5–10% of cases, but the drug is well-tolerated if the dose is increased gradually. Metformin therapy may increase blood lactate levels, and it is very occasionally associated with the development of lactic acidosis, the most feared complication, with a 30–50% mortality risk. However, this is almost always related to coexistent hypoxic conditions, which are contraindications of metformin therapy *(64–66)*.

There are still some unsolved problems with regard to the use of metformin in ovulation induction among women with anovulatory PCOS. Although metformin seems to act in a similar way in obese and non-obese patients, the number of placebo-controlled trials among non-obese patients is few, and these patients should be treated with caution. Moreover, about one-third of women with PCOS do not respond to metformin, and no useful criteria exist to distinguish between responders and non-responders. Whether and for how long metformin should be used during pregnancy is still under debate. Retrospective studies suggest that metformin improves pregnancy outcome by decreasing the risks of early spontaneous miscarriage and gestational diabetes in women with PCOS *(67–69)*. Prospective randomized controlled studies have shown a significant fourfold decrease (9.7 vs. 37.5%) in miscarriage rates compared with CC treatment in non-obese women with PCOS *(56)* and a twofold decrease (15.4 vs. 29.0%) compared with laparoscopic ovarian drilling (LOD) in obese women with PCOS *(70)*. This decrease in miscarriage rates may be due to an increase of endometrial levels of glycodelin or insulin growth factor-binding globulin I, both implicated in implantation *(71)*, to an improvement of endometrial blood flow *(72)*, to a decrease of the plasma levels of plasminogen inhibitor factor I *(73)*, or to some other still unknown effect. One prospective placebo-controlled study showed a reduction of severe pregnancy and post-partum complications in metformin-treated women compared with those receiving placebo *(74)*. Metformin seems to be safe in early pregnancy with respect to congenital abnormalities, growth, and motor-social development in the first 18 months of life *(75)*. However, it has been shown to cross the placenta and to result in fetal serum levels comparable to those in the maternal circulation *(76)*. Therefore, the treatment with metformin should be stopped after a positive pregnancy test result until more consistent data are available.

5.3. True Insulin Sensitizers: Troglitazone, Pioglitazone, Rosiglitazone

Troglitazone is effective in improving ovulation, including ovulation induced by CC *(77)*, but it has been withdrawn from the market in Europe because of hepatotoxicity. Pioglitazone and rosiglitazone seem to be safe with regard to this side effect *(78)*. In a prospective open-label study with rosiglitazone, ovulation occurred in 55% of obese anovulatory women *(79)*, and in a double-blind placebo-controlled study, it enhanced both spontaneous and CC-induced ovulation in overweight and obese women with PCOS *(80)*. However, in a comparative study in non-obese women, metformin was shown to be more effective than rosiglitazone in improving ovulation, and the addition of rosiglitazone to metformin did not add any benefit beyond that of metformin alone *(81)*. Pioglitazone increased the ovulation rate compared with placebo (41 vs. 5.6%) *(82)* and added to metformin it improved menstrual regularity in women with PCOS not optimally responsive to metformin *(83)*. The role of these new agents in the treatment of ovulation in PCOS remains to be established, and because of their possible unfavorable effects on the fetus, they cannot be recommended for women desiring pregnancy and their use should not be continued after conception.

5.4. Others

Acarbose is an α-glucosidase inhibitor that acts by slowing the absorption of carbohydrates from the intestines, thus decreasing the postprandial rise of blood glucose and insulin concentrations *(84)*. In a study in which metformin and acarbose were compared in CC-resistant women, both drugs were equally effective in the treatment of insulin resistance and in improving ovulation rates *(85)*, but there are no data on PRs after acarbose treatment in anovulatory women with PCOS. D-Chiro-inositol has also been shown to improve ovulation compared with placebo *(86)*, but this is not available for routine use, and its safety during pregnancy is not known.

6. AROMATASE INHIBITORS

Aromatase inhibitors (letrozole and anastozole) suppress the biosynthesis of estrogen and, therefore, decrease the estrogenic negative feedback on the hypothalamic pituitary axis, thus increasing FSH secretion and improving ovarian follicle development. These agents do not have the adverse anti-estrogenic effects of CC on the cervical mucus or the endometrium. In CC-resistant women with PCOS, letrozole at doses of 2.5–5 mg daily on days 3–7 of the cycle has been found to induce ovulation in 75% of cases and to result in a PR of 25% *(87,88)*. In combination with FSH, it has improved PR from 11 to 22% *(89)*. In one report, it also improved the ovarian response to FSH in poor responders undergoing ovarian superovulation and IUI *(90)*, and it has been recently found to be more effective than anastazole with regard to ovulation rate (84.4 vs. 60%) and PR per cycle (18.8 vs. 9.7%) in PCOS *(91)*. Aromatase inhibitors are more expensive than CC and their safety during pregnancy remains to be defined, but they may become potential alternatives.

7. OVARIAN DRILLING

LOD is an effective method for ovulation induction in a selected group of PCOS patients. It has been shown to be as effective as gonadotropin treatment in CC-resistant women with PCOS, live-birth and miscarriage rates being similar, but LOD reducing the risk of multiple pregnancy *(92)*. The key question has been who would benefit from LOD. A recent retrospective study analyzing the effect of LOD, LOD combined with CC or rFSH, or rFSH-only demonstrated that marked obesity (BMI = 35), marked hyperandrogenism, and long duration of infertility (>3 years) predict resistance to LOD. In another recent study, the efficacy of laparoscopic ovarian diathermy (LOD) was compared with 6-month treatment with metformin in CC-resistant overweight women with PCOS *(70)*. The total ovulation rate was not statistically different between the groups (metformin 54.8% vs. LOD 55.1%), whereas the miscarriage rate (15.4 vs.

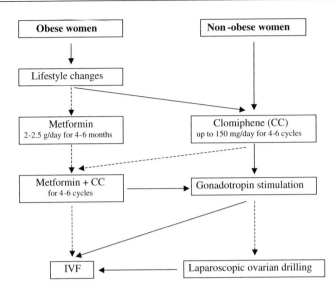

Fig. 1. Algorithm for ovulation induction treatment in anovulatory women with polycystic ovary syndrome (PCOS).

29.0%) was significantly lower and the pregnancy (18.6 vs. 13.4%), and live-birth (82.1 vs. 64.5%) rates were significantly higher in the metformin group. This suggests that the new treatment possibilities among CC-resistant women may reduce the usefulness of LOD. Furthermore, LOD is an invasive method, and there are concerns about long-term effects such as adhesions and premature ovarian failure. Therefore, its use should be restricted to patients resistant to other ovulation induction methods.

8. TREATMENT RECOMMENDATIONS FOR AN ANOVULATORY WOMAN WITH PCOS

In obese anovulatory women with PCOS, lifestyle modification with caloric restriction and exercise should be considered as the first-line therapy before ovulation induction treatments. CC is still considered to be the first-line drug for ovulation induction in these patients *(93)*. The usefulness of metformin alone or in combination with CC for ovulation induction in PCOS remains controversial. The other option, especially in non-obese women, is to use gonadotropin stimulation. The use of laparoscopic drilling should be weighted on the basis that it is an invasive method and may bear long-term side effects that are not known yet. IVF is the last treatment option, but for some patients, it may be the most optimal method relatively early in the treatment chain. In non-obese women, CC remains the first-line therapy, followed by gonadotropin induction and/or laparoscopic drilling, and finally IVF (Fig. 1).

9. CONCLUSIONS

Women with PCOS represent one-third of patients treated for infertility, and they present several problems and risks concerning ovulation induction. CC remains the first-line treatment after lifestyle changes in obese women, but there is increasing evidence that metformin alone or combined with CC may improve ovulation and PRs.

The efficacy of metformin in addition to gonadotropin stimulation, LOD, and/or IVF treatment remains to be defined, and future studies will show whether combination of these treatments brings added efficacy. Other insulin sensitizers may also be effective in ovulation induction in women with PCOS, but their safety during pregnancy is still unknown. Aromatase inhibitors may become potential alternatives to CC for ovulation induction. The most important issue in ovulation induction is to choose the treatment according to individual needs. This means quick decision-making if necessary and, for instance, flexible change-over to IVF at any phase of the treatment if the ovulation induction regimen fails.

REFERENCES

1. ESHRE Capri Workshop Group. Mono-ovulatory cycles: a key goal in profertility programmes. *Hum Reprod Update* 2003;9:263–74.

2. Martikainen H, Tiitinen A, Tomas C, et al. One versus two embryo transfer after IVF and ICSI: a randomized study. *Hum Reprod* 2001;16:1900–3.

3. Thurin A, Hausken J, Hillensjo T, et al. Elective single-embryo transfer versus double-embryo transfer in in vitro fertilization. *N Engl J Med* 2004;351:2392–402.

4. Klip H, Burger CW, Kenemans P, van Leeuwen FE. Cancer risk associated with subfertility and ovulation induction: a review. *Cancer Causes Control* 2000;11:319–44.

5. Greenblatt RB, Barfield WE, Jungck EC, Ray AW. Induction of ovulation with MRL/41. Preliminary report. *JAMA* 1961;178:101–4.

6. Huber-Buchholz MM, Carey DG, Norman RJ. Restoration of reproductive potential by lifestyle modification in obese polycystic ovary syndrome: role of insulin sensitivity and luteinizing hormone. *J Clin Endocrinol Metab* 1999;84:1470–4.

7. Norman RJ, Noakes M, Wu R, Davies MJ, Moran L, Wang JX. Improving reproductive performance in overweight/obese women with effective weight management. *Hum Reprod Update* 2004;10: 267–80.

8. Clark AM, Thornley B, Tomlinson L, Galletley C, Norman RJ. Weight loss in obese infertile women results in improvement in reproductive outcome for all forms of fertility treatment. *Hum Reprod* 1998;13:1502–5.

9. Wu CH, Winkel CA. The effect of therapy initiation day on clomiphene citrate therapy. *Fertil Steril* 1989;52:564–8.

10. Lobo RA, Gysler M, March CM, Goebelsmann U, Mishell DR Jr. Clinical and laboratory predictors of clomiphene response. *Fertil Steril* 1982;37:168–74.

11. Kousta E, White DM, Franks S. Modern use of clomiphene citrate in induction of ovulation. *Hum Reprod Update* 1997;3:359–65.

12. Milsom SR, Gibson G, Buckingham K, Gunn AJ. Factors associated with pregnancy or miscarriage after clomiphene therapy in WHO group II anovulatory women. *Aust N Z J Obstet Gynaecol* 2002;42:170–5.

13. Dickey RP, Taylor SN, Curole DN, Rye PH, Lu PY, Pyrzak R. Relationship of clomiphene dose and patient weight to successful treatment. *Hum Reprod* 1997;12:449–53.

14. Rostami-Hodjegan A, Lennard MS, Tucker GT, Ledger WL. Monitoring plasma concentrations to individualize treatment with clomiphene citrate. *Fertil Steril* 2004;81:1187–93.

15. Messinis IE. Clomiphene citrate. In: Tarzalis B, ed. *Ovulation Induction*. Paris: Elsevier 2002:87–97.

16. Homburg R. Clomiphene citrate–end of an era? a mini-review. *Hum Reprod* 2005;20:2043–51.

17. Messinis IE, Milingos SD. Current and future status of ovulation induction in polycystic ovary syndrome. *Hum Reprod Update* 1997;3:235–53.

18. Hammond MG, Halme JK, Talbert LM. Factors affecting the pregnancy rate in clomiphene citrate induction of ovulation. *Obstet Gynecol* 1983;62(2):196–202.

19. Imani B, Eijkemans MJ, te Velde ER, Habbema JD, Fauser BC. Predictors of patients remaining anovulatory during clomiphene citrate induction of ovulation in normogonadotropic oligoamenorrheic infertility. *J Clin Endocrinol Metab* 1998;83:2361–5.

20. Agarwal SK, Buyalos RP. Corpus luteum function and pregnancy rates with clomiphene citrate therapy: comparison of human chorionic gonadotrophin-induced versus spontaneous ovulation. *Hum Reprod* 1995;10:328–31.

21. Adashi EY. Ovulation induction: clomiphene citrate. In: Adashi EY, Rock JA and Rosenwaks Z, eds. *Reproductive Endocrinology, Surgery and Technology.* Philadelphia/New York, USA: Lippincott-Raven, 1996:1181–206.

22. Wolf LJ. Ovulation induction. *Clin Obstet Gynecol* 2000;43:902–15.

23. Eijkemans MJ, Imani B, Mulders AG, Habbema JD, Fauser BC. High singleton live birth rate following classical ovulation induction in normogonadotrophic anovulatory infertility (WHO 2). *Hum Reprod* 2003;18:2357–62.

24. Dickey RP, Taylor SN, Curole DN, Rye PH, Pyrzak R. Incidence of spontaneous abortion in clomiphene pregnancies. *Hum Reprod* 1996;11:2623–8.

25. Homburg R, Armar NA, Eshel A, Adams J, Jacobs HS. Influence of serum luteinising hormone concentrations on ovulation, conception, and early pregnancy loss in polycystic ovary syndrome. *BMJ* 1988;297:1024–6.

26. Gerli S, Gholami H, Manna C, Di Frega AS, Vitiello C, Unfer V. Use of ethinyl estradiol to reverse the antiestrogenic effects of clomiphene citrate in patients undergoing intrauterine insemination: a comparative, randomized study. *Fertil Steril* 2000;73:85–9.

27. Sorensen HT, Pedersen L, Skriver MV, Norgaard M, Norgard B, Hatch EE. Use of clomifene during early pregnancy and risk of hypospadias: population based case-control study. *BMJ* 2005;330: 126–7.

28. Neyro JL, Barrenetxea G, Montoya F, Rodriguez-Escudero FJ. Pure FSH for ovulation induction in patients with polycystic ovary syndrome and resistant to clomiphene citrate therapy. *Hum Reprod* 1991;6:218–21.

29. Aboulghar MA, Mansour RT. Ovarian hyperstimulation syndrome: classifications and critical analysis of preventive measures. *Hum Reprod Update* 2003;9:275–89.

30. Fauser BC and Macklon NS. Medical approaches to ovarian stimulation for infertility. In: Stauss JF and Barbieri RL, eds. *Yen and Jaffe, Reproductive Endocrinology.* Elsevier Saunders Inc NY, USA 2004;5:965–1012.

31. Nugent D, Vandekerckhove P, Hughes E, Arnot M, Lilford R. Gonadotrophin therapy for ovulation induction in subfertility associated with polycystic ovary syndrome. *Cochrane Database Syst Rev* 2000;4:CD000410.

32. van Santbrink EJ, Eijkemans MJ, Laven JS, Fauser BC. Patient-tailored conventional ovulation induction algorithms in anovulatory infertility. *Trends Endocrinol Metab* 2005;16: 381–9.

33. Polson DW, Mason HD, Saldahna MB, Franks S. Ovulation of a single dominant follicle during treatment with low-dose pulsatile follicle stimulating hormone in women with polycystic ovary syndrome. *Clin Endocrinol (Oxf)* 1987;26:205–12.

34. Messinis IE. Ovulation induction: a mini review. *Hum Reprod* 2005;20(10):2688–97.

35. Franks S, White D. Low-dose gonadotrophin treatment in polycystic ovary syndrome: the step-up protocol. In: Tarlatzis B, ed. *Ovulation Induction.* Paris: Elsevier, 2002:98–107.

36. Macklon NS, Fauser BC. The step-down protocol. In: Tarlatzis B, ed. *Ovulation Induction.* Paris: Elsevier, 2002:108–18.

37. van Santbrink EJ, Donderwinkel PF, van Dessel TJ, Fauser BC. Gonadotrophin induction of ovulation using a step-down dose regimen: single-centre clinical experience in 82 patients. *Hum Reprod* 1995;10:1048–53.

38. Christin-Maitre S, Hugues JN. A comparative randomized multicentric study comparing the step-up versus step-down protocol in polycystic ovary syndrome. *Hum Reprod* 2003;18:1626–31.

39. van Santbrink EJ, Fauser BC. Is there a future for ovulation induction in the current era of assisted reproduction? *Hum Reprod* 2003;18:2499–502.

40. Homburg R, Howles CM. Low-dose FSH therapy for anovulatory infertility associated with polycystic ovary syndrome: rationale, results, reflections and refinements. *Hum Reprod Update* 1999;5:493–9.

41. Bayram N, van Wely M, van Der Veen F. Recombinant FSH versus urinary gonadotrophins or recombinant FSH for ovulation induction in subfertility associated with polycystic ovary syndrome. *Cochrane Database Syst Rev* 2001;2:CD002121.

42. van Wely M, Bayram N, van der Veen F. Recombinant FSH in alternative doses or versus urinary gonadotrophins for ovulation induction in subfertility associated with polycystic ovary syndrome: a systematic review based on a Cochrane review. *Hum Reprod* 2003;18:1143–9.

43. Homburg R, Levy T, Berkovitz D, et al. Gonadotropin-releasing hormone agonist reduces the miscarriage rate for pregnancies achieved in women with polycystic ovarian syndrome. *Fertil Steril* 1993;59:527–31.

44. Clifford K, Rai R, Watson H, Franks S, Regan L. Does suppressing luteinising hormone secretion reduce the miscarriage rate? Results of a randomised controlled trial. *BMJ* 1996;312:1508–11.

45. van der Meer M, Hompes PG, Scheele F, Schoute E, Popp-Snijders C, Schoemaker J. The importance of endogenous feedback for monofollicular growth in low-dose step-up ovulation induction with follicle-stimulating hormone in polycystic ovary syndrome: a randomized study. *Fertil Steril* 1996;66:571–6.

46. Velazquez EM, Mendoza S, Hamer T, Sosa F, Glueck CJ. Metformin therapy in polycystic ovary syndrome reduces hyperinsulinemia, insulin resistance, hyperandrogenemia, and systolic blood pressure, while facilitating normal menses and pregnancy. *Metabolism* 1994;43:647–54.

47. Morin-Papunen LC, Koivunen RM, Ruokonen A, Martikainen HK. Metformin therapy improves the menstrual pattern with minimal endocrine and metabolic effects in women with polycystic ovary syndrome. *Fertil Steril* 1998;69:691–6.

48. Nestler JE, Jakubowicz DJ, Evans WS, Pasquali R. Effects of metformin on spontaneous and clomiphene-induced ovulation in the polycystic ovary syndrome. *N Engl J Med* 1998;338:1876–80.

49. Morin-Papunen LC, Vauhkonen I, Koivunen RM, Ruokonen A, Martikainen HK, Tapanainen JS. Endocrine and metabolic effects of metformin versus ethinyl estradiol-cyproterone acetate in obese women with polycystic ovary syndrome: a randomized study. *J Clin Endocrinol Metab* 2000;85: 3161–8.

50. Pasquali R, Gambineri A, Biscotti D, et al. Effect of long-term treatment with metformin added to hypocaloric diet on body composition, fat distribution, and androgen and insulin levels in abdominally obese women with and without the polycystic ovary syndrome. *J Clin Endocrinol Metab* 2000;85:2767–74.

51. Costello MF, Eden JA. A systematic review of the reproductive system effects of metformin in patients with polycystic ovary syndrome. *Fertil Steril* 2003;79:1–13.

52. Morin-Papunen L, Vauhkonen I, Koivunen R, Ruokonen A, Martikainen H, Tapanainen JS. Metformin versus ethinyl estradiol-cyproterone acetate in the treatment of nonobese women with polycystic ovary syndrome: a randomized study. *J Clin Endocrinol Metab* 2003;88:148–56.

53. Lord JM, Flight IH, Norman RJ. Insulin-sensitising drugs (metformin, troglitazone, rosiglitazone, pioglitazone, D-chiro-inositol) for polycystic ovary syndrome. *Cochrane Database Syst Rev* 2003;3:CD003053.

54. Kashyap S, Wells GA, Rosenwaks Z. Insulin-sensitizing agents as primary therapy for patients with polycystic ovarian syndrome. *Hum Reprod* 2004;19:2474–83.

55. Bruni V, Dei M, Pontello V, et al. The management of polycystic ovary syndrome. *Ann N Y Acad Sci* 2003;997:307–21.

56. Palomba S, Orio F Jr, Falbo A, et al. Prospective parallel randomized, double-blind, double-dummy controlled clinical trial comparing clomiphene citrate and metformin as the first-line treatment for ovulation induction in nonobese anovulatory women with polycystic ovary syndrome. *J Clin Endocrinol Metab* 2005;90:4068–74.

57. Neveu N, Granger L, St-Michel P, Lavoie HB. Comparison of clomiphene citrate, metformin, or the combination of both for first-line ovulation induction and achievement of pregnancy in 154 women with polycystic ovary syndrome. *Fertil Steril* 2006; 27:22.

58. Legro RS, Barnhart HX, Schlaff WD et al. Clomiphene, metformin, or both for infertility in the polycystic ovary syndrome. *NEJM* 2007;356: 551–566.

59. Moll E, Bossuyt PM, Korevaar JC, Lambalk CB, van der Veen F. Effect of clomifene citrate plus metformin and clomifene citrate plus placebo on induction of ovulation in women with newly diagnosed polycystic ovary syndrome: randomized double blind clinical trial. *BMJ* 2006;332:1485.

60. De Leo V, la Marca A, Ditto A, Morgante G, Cianci A. Effects of metformin on gonadotropin-induced ovulation in women with polycystic ovary syndrome. *Fertil Steril* 1999;72:282–5.

61. Palomba S, Falbo A, Orio F Jr, et al. A randomized controlled trial evaluating metformin pre-treatment and co-administration in non-obese insulin-resistant women with polycystic ovary syndrome treated with controlled ovarian stimulation plus timed intercourse or intrauterine insemination. *Hum Reprod* 2005;20:2879–86.

62. Yarali H, Yildiz BO, Demirol A, et al. Co-administration of metformin during rFSH treatment in patients with clomiphene citrate-resistant polycystic ovarian syndrome: a prospective randomized trial. *Hum Reprod* 2002;17:289–94.

63. Costello MF, Chapman M, Conway U. A systematic review and meta-analysis of randomized controlled trials on metformin co-administration during gonadotrophin ovulation induction or IVF in women with polycystic ovary syndrome. *Hum Reprod* 2006;21:1387–99.

64. Bailey CJ, Turner RC. Metformin. *N Engl J Med* 1996;334:574–9.

65. Brown JB, Pedula K, Barzilay J, Herson MK, Latare P. Lactic acidosis rates in type 2 diabetes. *Diabetes Care* 1998;21:1659–63.

66. Kirpichnikov D, McFarlane SI, Sowers JR. Metformin: an update. *Ann Intern Med* 2002;137:25–33.

67. Glueck CJ, Wang P, Kobayashi S, Phillips H, Sieve-Smith L. Metformin therapy throughout pregnancy reduces the development of gestational diabetes in women with polycystic ovary syndrome. *Fertil Steril* 2002;77:520–5.

68. Jakubowicz DJ, Iuorno MJ, Jakubowicz S, Roberts KA, Nestler JE. Effects of metformin on early pregnancy loss in the polycystic ovary syndrome. *J Clin Endocrinol Metab* 2002;87:524–9.

69. Glueck CJ, Goldenberg N, Wang P, Loftspring M, Sherman A. Metformin during pregnancy reduces insulin, insulin resistance, insulin secretion, weight, testosterone and development of gestational diabetes: prospective longitudinal assessment of women with polycystic ovary syndrome from preconception throughout pregnancy. *Hum Reprod* 2004;19:510–21.

70. Palomba S, Orio F Jr, Nardo LG, et al. Metformin administration versus laparoscopic ovarian diathermy in clomiphene citrate-resistant women with polycystic ovary syndrome: a prospective parallel randomized double-blind placebo-controlled trial. *J Clin Endocrinol Metab* 2004;89:4801–9.

71. Jakubowicz DJ, Seppala M, Jakubowicz S, et al. Insulin reduction with metformin increases luteal phase serum glycodelin and insulin-like growth factor-binding protein 1 concentrations and enhances uterine vascularity and blood flow in the polycystic ovary syndrome. *J Clin Endocrinol Metab* 2001;86:1126–33.

72. Palomba S, Russo T, Orio F, et al. Uterine effects of metformin administration in anovulatory women with polycystic ovary syndrome. *Hum Reprod* 2006;21:457–65.

73. Glueck CJ, Phillips H, Cameron D, Sieve-Smith L, Wang P. Continuing metformin throughout pregnancy in women with polycystic ovary syndrome appears to safely reduce first-trimester spontaneous abortion: a pilot study. *Fertil Steril* 2001;75:46–52.

74. Vanky E, Salvesen KA, Heimstad R, Fougner KJ, Romundstad P, Carlsen SM. Metformin reduces pregnancy complications without affecting androgen levels in pregnant polycystic ovary syndrome women: results of a randomized study. *Hum Reprod* 2004;19:1734–40.

75. Glueck CJ, Goldenberg N, Pranikoff J, Loftspring M, Sieve L, Wang P. Height, weight, and motor-social development during the first 18 months of life in 126 infants born to 109 mothers with polycystic ovary syndrome who conceived on and continued metformin through pregnancy. *Hum Reprod* 2004;19:1323–30.

76. Vanky E, Zahlsen K, Spigset O, Carlsen SM. Placental passage of metformin in women with polycystic ovary syndrome. *Fertil Steril* 2005;83:1575–8.

77. Azziz R, Ehrmann D, Legro RS, et al. Troglitazone improves ovulation and hirsutism in the polycystic ovary syndrome: a multicenter, double blind, placebo-controlled trial. *J Clin Endocrinol Metab* 2001;86:1626–32.

78. Fuchtenbusch M, Standl E, Schatz H. Clinical efficacy of new thiazolidinediones and glinides in the treatment of type 2 diabetes mellitus. *Exp Clin Endocrinol Diabetes* 2000;108:151–63.

79. Cataldo NA, Abbasi F, McLaughlin TL, et al. Metabolic and ovarian effects of rosiglitazone treatment for 12 weeks in insulin-resistant women with polycystic ovary syndrome. *Hum Reprod* 2006;21: 109–20.

80. Ghazeeri G, Kutteh WH, Bryer-Ash M, et al. Effect of rosiglitazone on spontaneous and clomiphene citrate-induced ovulation in women with polycystic ovary syndrome. *Fertil Steril* 2003;79:562–6.

81. Baillargeon JP, Jakubowicz DJ, Iuorno MJ, Jakubowicz S, Nestler JE. Effects of metformin and rosiglitazone, alone and in combination, in nonobese women with polycystic ovary syndrome and normal indices of insulin sensitivity. *Fertil Steril* 2004;82:893–902.

82. Brettenthaler N, De Geyter C, Huber PR, Keller U. Effect of the insulin sensitizer pioglitazone on insulin resistance, hyperandrogenism, and ovulatory dysfunction in women with polycystic ovary syndrome. *J Clin Endocrinol Metab* 2004;89:3835–40.

83. Glueck CJ, Moreira A, Goldenberg N, Sieve L, Wang P. Pioglitazone and metformin in obese women with polycystic ovary syndrome not optimally responsive to metformin. *Hum Reprod* 2003;18: 1618–25.

84. Coniff RF, Shapiro JA, Robbins D, et al. Reduction of glycosylated hemoglobin and postprandial hyperglycemia by acarbose in patients with NIDDM. A placebo-controlled dose-comparison study. *Diabetes Care* 1995;18:817–24.

85. Sonmez AS, Yasar L, Savan K, et al. Comparison of the effects of acarbose and metformin use on ovulation rates in clomiphene citrate-resistant polycystic ovary syndrome. *Hum Reprod* 2005;20: 175–9.

86. Nestler JE, Jakubowicz DJ, Reamer P, Gunn RD, Allan G. Ovulatory and metabolic effects of D-chiro-inositol in the polycystic ovary syndrome. *N Engl J Med* 1999;340:1314–20.

87. Mitwally MF, Casper RF. Use of an aromatase inhibitor for induction of ovulation in patients with an inadequate response to clomiphene citrate. *Fertil Steril* 2001;75:305–9.

88. Mitwally MF, Biljan MM, Casper RF. Pregnancy outcome after the use of an aromatase inhibitor for ovarian stimulation. *Am J Obstet Gynecol* 2005;192:381–6.

89. Mitwally MF, Casper RF. Aromatase inhibition reduces gonadotrophin dose required for controlled ovarian stimulation in women with unexplained infertility. *Hum Reprod* 2003;18:1588–97.

90. Mitwally MF, Casper RF. Aromatase inhibition improves ovarian response to follicle-stimulating hormone in poor responders. *Fertil Steril* 2002;77(4):776–80.

91. Al-Omari WR, Sulaiman WR, Al-Hadithi N. Comparison of two aromatase inhibitors in women with clomiphene-resistant polycystic ovary syndrome. *Int J Gynaecol Obstet* 2004;85:289–91.

92. Farquhar C, Lilford RJ, Marjoribanks J, Vandekerckhove P. Laparoscopic "drilling" by diathermy or laser for ovulation induction in anovulatory polycystic ovary syndrome. *Cochrane Database Syst Rev* 2005;3:CD001122.

93. Beck JI, Boothroyd C, Proctor M, Farquhar C, Hughes E. Oral anti-oestrogens and medical adjuncts for subfertility associated with anovulation. *Cochrane Database Syst Rev* 2005;1:CD002249.

20 Pregnancy in Polycystic Ovary Syndrome

Roy Homburg, FRCOG

CONTENTS

Summary

Although many of the pregnancies in women with polycystic ovary syndrome (PCOS) may be uneventful, there are several complications of pregnancy associated with maternal PCOS. These include an increased prevalence of early pregnancy loss (EPL), gestational diabetes (GDM), pregnancy-induced hypertensive disorders (PET/PIH) and the birth of small-for-gestational-age (SGA) babies. Increased risk of EPL has been attributed to obesity, hyperinsulinaemia, elevated luteinizing hormone (LH) concentrations and endometrial dysfunction. Avoiding or managing obesity before pregnancy and treatment with metformin are therapeutic options for these and for the increased prevalence of GDM. Administration of metformin throughout pregnancy is a contentious issue. Screening pregnant women with PCOS for GDM and PET/PIH, especially if obese, is recommended, although data for a firm association between PCOS and PET/PIH is weak. Impaired insulin-mediated growth and fetal programming are possible explanations for a higher prevalence of SGA infants in mothers with PCOS. Prospective studies employing a large cohort of women with well-defined PCOS compared with a control group matched for body mass index (BMI) and parity are needed to solve the remaining questions.

Key Words: PCOS; Early pregnancy loss; gestational diabetes; pregnancy-induced hypertension; small-for-gestational-age; metformin.

1. INTRODUCTION

When compared with healthy mothers with no polycystic ovary syndrome (PCOS), several complications of pregnancy associated with a maternal diagnosis of PCOS have been described. These include an increased prevalence of spontaneous miscarriage,

From: *Contemporary Endocrinology: Polycystic Ovary Syndrome*
Edited by: A. Dunaif, R. J. Chang, S. Franks, and R. S. Legro © Humana Press, Totowa, NJ

gestational diabetes (GDM), pre-eclamptic toxacmia (PET) and pregnancy-induced hypertension (PIH) and the birth of small-for-gestational-age (SGA) babies.

Much of the evidence has been gleaned from retrospective analyses and often the series are small. This makes definitive statements difficult but, nevertheless, provides a basis for further investigation of the true prevalence of these pregnancy complications in mothers with PCOS and their possible prevention. Evidence-based medicine will be quoted here whenever possible and, otherwise, the best available latest research is quoted.

2. PCOS AND MISCARRIAGE

There are three main questions regarding miscarriage in PCOS: Is there really an increased prevalence, if so, why, and what can we do in the way of possible preventative treatment?

2.1. Prevalence

Most probably, women with PCOS have an increased risk of spontaneous miscarriage. This has been difficult to establish for the following reasons:

1. Treatment with ovulation inducing agents to conceive is needed by many women with PCOS and this treatment, whether with anti-estrogens or gonadotrophins, is associated with a higher incidence of spontaneous miscarriage compared with the prevalence in the normally ovulating population who conceive spontaneously.
2. For women with PCOS who conceive spontaneously, the prevalence of spontaneous miscarriage is not known.
3. The majority of published series are based on women attending fertility clinics. They tend to receive closer scrutiny in the very early phase of a pregnancy and, therefore, tend to have a higher quoted prevalence of miscarriage than those who conceive spontaneously.
4. Obesity is often associated with PCOS, and obesity is widely reported to be an important factor associated with spontaneous miscarriage in its own right. Is it the entity of PCOS itself or the obesity that is the important causative factor?
5. The use of various definitions of PCOS, e.g., based on the ultrasound finding of typical polycystic ovaries or including only those who have high LH concentrations, has greatly confused the issue. As PCOS is a very heterogeneous syndrome from both the point of view of clinical symptoms and laboratory manifestations, there may be a particular sub-group (e.g., those with high LH concentrations) that is more prone to miscarriage.

The traditional first-line treatment for anovulatory PCOS is clomiphene citrate (CC), which has a quoted mean miscarriage rate of about 25% (1–3). However, rather than an intrinsic cause associated directly to the presence of PCOS, this may well be due to a high prevalence of obesity in these patients, to the anti-estrogenic action of CC on endometrial estrogen receptors and suppression of pinopode formation (4) and the fact that CC also induces increased release of LH, and not just follicle-stimulating hormone (FSH), which is thought to be detrimental to the successful continuation of the pregnancy (5).

The usual second-line treatment for clomiphene failures is induction of ovulation with a low-dose FSH protocol. This also seems to produce a higher early pregnancy loss (EPL) than in the spontaneously conceiving population *(6)*. Similarly, high rates of EPL were witnessed when using the now defunct conventional gonadotrophin ovulation induction protocols for women with PCOS *(7)*.

Most of the sparse research on the subject of miscarriage in PCOS has involved a retrospective audit of patients with PCOS undergoing in vitro fertilization (IVF). Here, at least, we can gain some insight into the difference in miscarriage rates between PCOS and non-PCOS patients undergoing the same treatment. These are tabulated in Table 1 and indicate a clearly increased prevalence of miscarriage in PCOS *(7–10)*.

Whereas spontaneous miscarriage in non-PCOS women is highly associated with fetal chromosomal abnormalities, the aborted fetuses of women with PCOS and elevated LH levels are more likely to have a normal karyotype *(11)*.

Notwithstanding the constraints mentioned above, the weight of evidence points at an association between the presence of PCOS and an increased prevalence of EPL.

2.2. Etiology

2.2.1. FERTILITY TREATMENT

The apparent increased prevalence of miscarriage in PCOS may be because all series include women with PCOS undergoing some form of ovulation induction or ovarian stimulation, and there is no available comparison with the miscarriage rate of women with PCOS who conceive spontaneously.

2.2.2. OBESITY

Obesity is commonly associated with PCOS and has been conclusively associated with an increased prevalence of miscarriage *(12)*. In an attempt to define whether the increased incidence of miscarriage was due to the presence of PCOS itself or solely to the confounding factor of obesity, Wang et al. *(10)* analysed 1018 women undergoing IVF, 37% of whom had PCOS. The miscarriage rate was 28% in the women with PCOS compared with 18% in the non-PCOS group ($p < 0.01$). However, this significance was lost when a multivariate analysis adjusting for obesity and treatment type was performed, the conclusion being that the higher risk of spontaneous miscarriage in PCOS was due to the higher prevalence of obesity and the type of treatment received.

Table 1
Miscarriage Rate in Women with Polycystic Ovary
Syndrome (PCOS) Undergoing In Vitro Fertilization
(IVF) Compared with Non-PCOS Women
Undergoing the Same Treatment (Controls)

	Miscarriage rate (%)	
	PCOS	Controls
Homburg et al. *(7)*	37	25
Balen et al. *(8)*	36	24
Winter et al. *(9)*	26	15
Wang et al. *(10)*	25	18

2.2.3. HYPERINSULINAEMIA

Hyperinsulinaemia is a common feature of PCOS, particularly in obese patients. Although there is no direct evidence to suggest that hyperinsulinaemia is a direct cause of miscarriage, the risk of pregnancy loss is amplified by obesity and is also strongly associated with elevated concentrations of plasminogen activator inhibitor-1 (PAI-1). Serum concentrations are higher in women with PCOS compared with that in the general population *(13)*. PAI-1 is a potent inhibitor of fibrinolysis and high serum concentrations of genetic origin or acquired in the presence of hyperinsulinaemia could well be a factor in the etiology of EPL *(14)*.

2.2.4. HYPERSECRETION OF LH

High serum concentrations of LH (>10 IU/l) in the early to mid-follicular phase have been associated with an increased EPL in several reports. A field study of 193 normally cycling women planning to become pregnant showed that raised mid-follicular phase serum LH concentrations were associated with a significantly higher miscarriage rate (65%) compared with those in women with normal serum LH concentrations (12%) *(15)*.

In our own study *(16)* of a large group of patients with PCOS undergoing treatment with pulsatile luteinizing hormone-releasing hormone (LHRH) for induction of ovulation, follicular phase serum LH concentrations were significantly higher in those who miscarried (17.9 IU/L) compared with those who delivered successfully (9.6 IU/L). We also found that the miscarriage rate was 33% in women with PCOS compared with 10.6% in those with hypogonadotrophic hypogonadism who were treated in a similar fashion. It was thus very clear from this first study of LH in ovulation induction that in women with PCOS there was a significantly increased risk of miscarriage in those with an elevated follicular phase plasma LH concentration compared with those with PCOS and normal follicular phase LH levels. Furthermore, this study seemed to demonstrate that LH was the true culprit as there were no significant differences of any other hormonal parameter measured (testosterone, dihydroepiandrosterone sulphate, androstendione, FSH and prolactin) between those who delivered and those who miscarried.

In 100 women with PCOS who were treated with low-dose gonadotrophin therapy, the association of raised baseline and/or mid-follicular phase plasma LH concentrations with miscarriage was demonstrated by Hamilton-Fairley et al *(6)* who found that patients with an elevated LH concentration had a higher rate of miscarriage than the women with polycystic ovaries and normal LH levels. In women attending a recurrent miscarriage clinic, 82% had polycystic ovaries, as detected by ultrasound and also had abnormalities of follicular phase LH secretion *(17–18)*.

There is also evidence that GnRH agonist, which reduces the elevated concentrations of LH prevalent in some 40% of women with PCOS, serves to reduce the prevalence of early spontaneous miscarriage. A study from our group *(7)* looked at the performance of women with PCOS undergoing IVF/ET who had high mean LH concentrations, compared with a control group of normally cycling women with mechanical infertility. Pregnancy rates were similar in the two groups but whereas GnRH agonist treatment reduced the miscarriage rate by half compared with gonadotrophin alone in the PCOS group, its administration to the control group had no such effect. In a further study from our centre *(19)*, 239 women with PCOS received hMG with or without GnRH agonist for ovulation induction or superovulation for IVF/embro transfer. Of pregnancies achieved with GnRH agonist, 17.6% miscarried compared with 39% of those achieved with gonadotrophin alone. Cumulative live birth rates after four cycles for GnRH agonist were 64% compared with 26% for gonadotrophin only. Similarly, Balen et al. *(8)* analyzed the outcome of treatment in 182 women with ultrasound detected PCO who conceived after IVF. They found a highly significant reduction in the rate of miscarriage when buserelin was used to achieve pituitary desensitization followed by stimulation with hMG (15/74, 20%) compared with the use of clomiphene and hMG (51/108, 47%).

A marked decrease of serum LH concentrations is the most significant endocrine event following laparoscopic ovarian drilling for the induction of ovulation and pregnancy in women with PCOS. A report on miscarriage rates following laparoscopic ovarian diathermy involved 58 pregnancies with a miscarriage rate of 14%, much lower than that usually experienced in women with PCOS *(20)*.

Taken together, the correlation of high LH concentrations with high rates of miscarriage and the reduction of these rates when LH concentrations are normalized by one means or another, provide compelling evidence of an etiological association between miscarriage and high LH concentrations. Further prospective controlled trials are still needed to confirm this association.

2.2.5. ENDOMETRIAL DYSFUNCTION

The association of PCOS, impaired implantation and EPL has encouraged investigation into the state of the endometrial environment in women with PCOS. Low luteal phase serum glycodelin and insulin-like growth factor-binding protein-1 concentrations in women with PCOS, presumably induced by hyperinsulinaemia, have been demonstrated *(21)*. Plasma endothelin-1 levels are significantly higher in PCOS compared with that in controls *(22)*. Both these latter studies and a further study *(23)* have implicated hyperinsulinism in the etiology of the inadequate endometrial blood flow that was demonstrated, affecting endometrial receptivity. These studies showed a reversal of endometrial dysfunction and, particularly, increased blood flow parameters, following treatment with metformin. However, it is far from clear that endometrial factors play an important role in either subfertility or miscarriage in PCOS.

2.3. *Treatment Modes*

2.3.1. METFORMIN

Metformin, a bi-guanide, oral anti-diabetic drug. is capable of reducing insulin concentrations and consequently PAI-1 concentrations *(13)* without affecting normal glucose levels. In addition, it seems to be capable of enhancing uterine vascularity and blood flow *(21,22)*, reducing plasma endothelin-1 levels *(23,24)*, increasing luteal phase serum glycodelin concentrations *(21)*, lowering androgen and LH concentrations, and even inducing weight loss in some patients *(25)*. These properties would suggest its theoretical clinical usefulness in the prevention of EPL in PCOS, and some trials in the last few years seem to bear out this promise *(26,27)*.

In the largest published series, 328 pregnancies were treated with metformin before and throughout pregnancy and had an EPL rate of 20% compared with 319 pregnancies previously, not treated with metformin, who had an EPL rate of 65% *(27)*. In a further retrospective series *(26)*, 65 women received metformin throughout pregnancy, and the miscarriage rate was 8.8% compared with 42% in a control group of 31 subjects. Although these were retrospective studies in selected patients, not exactly providing Grade A evidence, they demand, at the least, further investigation in properly conducted, randomized prospective trials. Two such trials, conducted by Palomba et al. *(28)* compared, firstly, the use of metformin versus laparoscopic ovarian diathermy of the ovaries for clomiphene-resistant PCOS women who were overweight and then metformin versus clomiphene in non-obese anovulatory PCOS *(29)*. The striking feature of these studies was the fact that metformin yielded superior live birth rates than its 'opponents' because, in both series, despite similar pregnancy rates, the prevalence of EPL was significantly decreased after metformin treatment.

The weight of evidence so far is that metformin is safe when continued throughout pregnancy as there has been no increase in congenital abnormalities, teratogenicity, or adverse effect on infant development *(30)*. The apparent lack of teratogenicity of metformin has earned it a B classification. Preliminary data suggest that this strategy of continuing metformin throughout pregnancy can significantly decrease the high miscarriage rate usually associated with PCOS and even reduce the incidence of GDM, pre-eclampsia and fetal macrosomia *(27,31)*. However, as far as EPL is concerned, it would seem that the same effect may well be achieved when metformin is discontinued when pregnancy is confirmed *(28,29)*. Once again, however, there is, at the time of writing, a lack of large randomized controlled trials to support these encouraging but preliminary findings.

2.3.2. WEIGHT LOSS

Overweight and frank obesity, amplifiers of insulin resistance in women with PCOS, have a profound influence on miscarriage rates *(10,32)*. Loss of weight by change of life style before pregnancy is capable of reversing the deleterious effects of obesity on fertility potential. In a study examining the effect of a change in lifestyle programme on 67 anovulatory, obese [body mass index (BMI) > 30] women who had failed to conceive with conventional treatment for 2 years or more, the mean weight loss was 10.2 kg after 6 months *(33)*. Following the loss of weight, 60 of the 67 resumed ovulation and 52 achieved a pregnancy, 18 of them spontaneously. Most importantly, only 18% of these pregnancies miscarried compared with a 75% miscarriage rate in pregnancies achieved before the weight loss.

2.3.3. REDUCTION OF LH CONCENTRATIONS

Gonadotrophin-releasing hormone (GnRH) agonists suppress LH concentrations before and during ovarian stimulation, avoiding premature LH surges, and this has earned them an undisputed place in IVF treatment protocols. They also neutralize any possible deleterious effect of high LH concentrations in women with PCOS. Their application during ovulation induction should also be particularly relevant in the presence of the chronic, tonic, high serum concentrations of LH observed in a high proportion of women with PCOS. By suppressing LH concentrations, GnRH agonists not only eliminate premature luteinization but improve the high miscarriage rates witnessed in this group of patients *(7)*. However, GnRH agonist has not become standard treatment for ovulation induction in PCOS, although our experience and that of others has shown a lower miscarriage rate in women receiving combination treatment of agonist and gonadotrophins when tonic LH concentrations are high. The reasons are that co-treatment with GnRH agonist and low-dose gonadotrophin therapy is more cumbersome, longer, requires more gonadotrophins to achieve ovulation, has a greater prevalence of multiple follicle development and consequently more ovarian hyper-stimulation syndrome (OHSS) and multiple pregnancies. Combining GnRH agonist with gonadotrophin stimulation will exacerbate the problem of multiple follicular development and therefore increase rates of cycle cancellation, OHSS and multiple pregnancy *(34,35)*. The loss of the endogenous feedback mechanism when using GnRH agonist and greater stimulation of follicles by the larger amounts of gonadotrophins needed are the reasons why GnRH agonists are not an appropriate solution to the problem of EPL as a result of gonadotrophin induction of ovulation for PCOS. The combination of a GnRH agonist with low-dose gonadotrophins should probably be reserved for women with high serum concentrations of LH who have repeated premature luteinization, stubbornly do not conceive on gonadotrophin therapy alone, or who have conceived and had early miscarriages on more than one occasion.

The use of a GnRH antagonist to suppress high LH concentrations during gonadotrophin ovulation induction for PCOS could avoid several of the drawbacks of using an agonist. However, no evidence has yet been forthcoming to suggest that it could be beneficial in the prevention of EPL in these patients.

A summary of our present state of knowledge of possible therapeutic strategies to decrease EPL in PCOS would suggest that, in addition to the avoidance of overweight and obesity before pregnancy, treatment with metformin has the most potential. More data confirming the lack of not just short, but long-term effects on the offspring, would be reassuring.

3. GESTATIONAL DIABETES

A higher than normal incidence of GDM in PCOS women would be expected considering the high prevalence of obesity and of insulin resistance among these women. A number of studies have suggested that this is indeed the case *(36–40)*.

The prevalence of women with PCOS among those with GDM *(41–44)* was much higher compared with controls even when subjects and controls were weight-matched *(44)*. The problems involved in examining this question have been the variation in the definitions of both PCOS and GDM and particularly the confounding factor of obesity. Indeed, some series suggested that BMI was a better predictor of GDM than PCOS *(38,45)*. When PCOS women were weight matched with controls, one series with 66 women with PCOS had the same incidence of GDM as controls *(46)*, whereas a smaller series *(40)* reported a higher prevalence of impaired glucose tolerance and GDM in the PCOS group.

The clinical conclusion from this data is that it is advisable to screen pregnant women with PCOS for GDM if they are overweight or obese.

As mentioned above, the administration of metformin throughout pregnancy is a contentious issue. However, the reported reduction in the prevalence of GDM and fetal macrosomia by administering metformin *(31)* is logical enough to prompt further research into whether this strategy is a feasible option in our present state of knowledge.

4. PREGNANCY-RELATED HYPERTENSION

Polycystic ovary syndrome appears to be a significant risk factor for hypertension, especially in women over the age of 40 years and in those who are obese and insulin resistant. The trigger of pregnancy might be expected to produce an increased incidence of PIH and PET. Certainly, in the studies with fairly small cohorts (n = 22–47) this would seem to be true. For example, two series consisting of cohorts of 22 in each *(40,47)* found that the incidence of PIH and PET, respectively, was increased in women with PCOS, very similar to the findings of an earlier series *(48)* (n = 33). Similar results were reported by Urman et al. *(36)* who found an increased incidence of PIH in women with PCOS, independent of BMI and Bjercke et al. *(37)* who also reported an increased incidence of PIH in PCOS but of PET only in PCOS associated with insulin resistance. A further series *(49)* compared blood pressure measurements throughout pregnancy in PCOS (n = 33) and controls (n = 66) and found no difference until the third trimester in which the incidence of hypertensive disorders was significantly higher in women with PCOS. In contrast, the two large series *(38,46)* that examined cohorts of 66 and 99, respectively, found no relation between PCOS and PIH and weight-matched controls *(46)* nor between PCOS and PET, although the PCOS subjects had a higher mean BMI and an increased prevalence of nulliparity compared with controls *(38)*.

This confusing body of evidence cannot yet convincingly point to a firm association between PCOS and hypertensive disorders of pregnancy. The only way to solve this question is to perform a prospective study employing a large cohort of women with well-defined PCOS compared with a control group matched for BMI and nulliparity.

5. SMALL FOR GESTATIONAL AGE BABIES

It has been suggested, controversially, that women, later diagnosed to have PCOS, were more likely to have been born SGA and that an SGA baby is more prone to develop the symptoms of PCOS later in life. Whereas some have found a relationship between these two conditions *(50,51)*, others found no association *(52)*. Less concern has been paid to the birth weight of offspring born to mothers with PCOS. Whereas the probable association of higher maternal body weight, increased weight gain during pregnancy and increased prevalence of GDM in women with PCOS would be expected to produce higher than mean birth weights, the prevalence of SGA offspring seems to be increased in women with PCOS. A comparison of the birth weights of 47 infants born from singleton pregnancies in women with PCOS with 180 infants born from singleton pregnancies in healthy controls demonstrated a significantly higher incidence of SGA infants in women with PCOS (12.8%) compared with controls (2.8%) with a similar prevalence of large for gestational age infants in the two groups *(53)*. Insulin resistance resulting in impaired insulin-mediated growth *(54)* and the fetal programming hypothesis *(55)* are the possible explanations for this higher prevalence of SGA infants in mothers with PCOS suggested by the authors.

6. SUMMARY

The complications of pregnancy that have been associated with maternal PCOS are increased prevalence of EPL, GDM, pregnancy-induced hypertensive disorders (PET/PIH) and the birth of SGA babies. The increased risk of EPL has variously been attributed to obesity, hyperinsulinaemia and raised PAI-1 levels, elevated LH concentrations and endometrial dysfunction. In addition to the avoidance of overweight and obesity before pregnancy, on present evidence, treatment with metformin seems to be a viable therapeutic option, which, even when discontinued at the diagnosis of pregnancy, seems to decrease EPL to acceptable rates. Metformin has also been proposed to counteract the increased prevalence of GDM, although its administration throughout pregnancy is still a contentious issue awaiting ratification of the absence of long-term effects on the infants. Screening pregnant women with PCOS for GDM and PET/PIH, especially if obese, is recommended although data for a firm association between PCOS and PET/PIH are weak. Insulin resistance and impaired insulin-mediated growth and the fetal programming hypothesis are possible explanations for a higher prevalence of SGA infants in mothers with PCOS. Prospective studies employing a large cohort of pregnant women with well-defined PCOS and compared with a control group matched for BMI and parity are needed to confirm these findings, to answer the remaining questions and verify the viability of the treatment options that have been proposed.

REFERENCES

1. Kousta E, White DM & Franks S. Modern use of clomiphene citrate in induction of ovulation. *Hum Reprod Update* 1997;3: 359–365.
2. Dickey RP, Taylor SN, Curole DN, et al. Incidence of spontaneous abortion in clomiphene pregnancies. *Hum Reprod* 1996;11: 2623–2628.
3. Macgregor AH, Johnson JE & Bunde CA (1968) Further clinical experience with clomiphene citrate. *Fertil Steril* 1968;19: 616–622.
4. Creus M, Ordi J, Fabregues F, et al. The effect of different hormone therapies on integrin expression and pinopode formation in the human endometrium: a controlled study. *Hum Reprod* 2003;18: 683–693.
5. Shoham Z, Borenstein R, Lunenfeld B & Pariente C. Hormonal profiles following clomiphene citrate therapy in conception and nonconception cycles. *Clin Endocrinol (Oxf)* 1990;33: 271–278.
6. Hamilton-Fairley D, Kiddy D, Watson H, et al. Association of moderate obesity with a poor pregnancy outcome in women with polycystic ovary syndrome treated with low dose gonadotrophin. *Br J Obstet Gynaecol* 1992;99: 128–131.
7. Homburg R, Levy T, Berkovitz D, et al. Gonadotropin-releasing hormone agonist reduces the miscarriage rate for pregnancies achieved in women with polycystic ovary syndrome. *Fertil Steril* 1993;59: 527–531.
8. Balen AH, Tan SL, MacDougall J & Jacobs HS. Miscarriage rates following in-vitro fertilisation are increased in women with polycystic ovaries and reduced by pituitary desensitisation with buserelin. *Hum Reprod* 1993;8: 959–964.
9. Winter E, Wang J, Davies MJ & Norman R. Early pregnancy loss following assisted reproductive technology treatment. *Hum Reprod* 2002;17: 3220–3223.
10. Wang JX, Davies MJ & Norman RJ. Polycystic ovarian syndrome and the risk of spontaneous abortion following assisted reproductive technology treatment. *Hum Reprod* 2001;16: 2606–2609.
11. Hasegawa I, Tanaka K, Sanada H, et al. Studies on the cytogenetic and endocrinologic background of spontaneous abortion. *Fertil Steril* 1996;65: 52–54.
12. Wang JX, Davies MJ, Norman RJ. Obesity increases the risk of spontaneous abortion during infertility treatment. *Obes Res* 2002;10: 551–554.
13. Palomba S, Orio F Jr, Falbo A, et al. Plasminogen activator inhibitor 1 and miscarriage after metformin treatment and laparoscopic ovarian drilling in patients with polycystic ovarian syndrome. *Fertil Steril* 2005;84: 761–765.

14. Glueck CJ, Wang P, Fontaine RN, et al. Plasmonogen inhibitor activity: an independent risk factor for the high miscarriage rate during pregnancy in women with polycystic ovary syndrome. *Metabolism* 1999;48: 1589–1595.

15. Regan L, Owen EJ & Jacobs HS. Hypersecretion of luteinising hormone, infertility and miscarriage. *Lancet* 1990;336: 1141–1144.

16. Homburg R, Armar NA, Eshel A, Adams J & Jacobs HS. Influence of serum luteinising hormone concentrations on ovulation, conception and early pregnancy loss in polycystic ovary syndrome. *BMJ* 1988;297: 1024–1026.

17. Sagle M, Bishop K, Alexander FM, et al. Recurrent early miscarriage and polycystic ovaries. *BMJ* 1988;297: 1027–1028.

18. Watson H, Hamilton-Fairley D, Kiddy D, et al. Abnormalities of follicular phase luteinising hormone secretion in women with recurrent early miscarriage. *J Endocrinol* 1989;123 Suppl, Abstract 25.

19. Homburg R, Berkovitz D, Levy T, et al. In-vitro fertilization and embryo transfer for the treatment of infertility associated with polycystic ovary syndrome. *Fertil Steril* 1993;60: 858–863.

20. Armar NA & Lachelin GCL. Laparoscopic ovarian diathermy: an effective treatment for anti-oestrogen resistant anovulatory infertility in women with the polycystic ovary syndrome. *British J Obstet Gynaecol* 1993;100: 161–164.

21. Jakubowicz DJ, Seppala M, Jakubowicz S, et al. Insulin reduction with metformin increases luteal phase serum glycodelin and insulin-like growth factor-binding protein 1 concentrations and enhances uterine vacularity and blood flow in the polycystic ovary syndrome. *J Clin Endocrinol Metab* 2001;86; 1126–1133.

22. Palomba S, Russo T, Orio F Jr, et al. Uterine effects of metformin administration in anovulatory women with polycystic ovary syndrome. Hum Reprod 2006;21:457–465.

23. Diamantis-Kandarakis E, Alexandraki K, Protogerou A, et al. Metformin administration improves endothelial function in women with polycystic ovary syndrome. *Eur J Endocrinol* 2005;152: 749–756.

24. Orio F Jr, Palomba S, Cascella T, et al. Improvement in endothelial structure and function after metformin treatment in young normal-weight women with polycystic ovary syndrome: results of a 6-month study. *J Clin Endocrinol Metab* 2005;90: 6072–6076.

25. Fleming R, Hopkinson ZE, Wallace AM, et al. Ovarian function and metabolic factors in women with oligomenorrhea treated with metformin in a randomized double blind placebo-controlled trial. *J Clin Endocrinol Metab* 2002;87: 569–574.

26. Jakubowicz DJ, Iuorno MJ, Jakubowicz S, et al. Effects of metformin on early pregnancy loss in the polycystic ovary syndrome. *J Clin Endocrinol Metab* 2002; 87: 524–529.

27. Glueck CJ, Wang P, Goldenberg N & Sieve-Smith L. Pregnancy outcomes among women with polycystic ovary syndrome treated with metformin. *Hum Reprod* 2002; 17:2858–2864.

28. Palomba S, Orio F, Nardo LG, et al. Metformin administration versus laparoscopic ovarian diathermy in clomiphene citrate resistant women with polycystic ovary syndrome: A prospective parallel randomized double-blind placebo-controlled trial. *J Endocrinol Metab* 2004;89: 4801–4809.

29. Palomba S, Orio F, Falbo A, et al. Prospective parallel randomized, double-blind, double-dummy controlled clinical trial comparing clomiphene citrate and metformin as first-line treatment for ovulation induction in nonobese anovulatory women with polycystic ovary syndrome. *J Clin Endocrinol Metab* 2005;90: 4068–4074.

30. Glueck CJ, Goldenberg N, Pranikoff J, et al. Height, weight, and motor-social development during the first 18 months of life in 126 infants born to 109 mothers with polycystic ovary syndrome who conceived on and continued metformin through pregnancy. *Hum Reprod* 2004;19: 1323–1230.

31. Glueck CJ, Wang P, Kobayashi S, et al. Metformin therapy throughout pregnancy reduces the development of gestational diabetes in women with polycystic ovary syndrome. *Fertil Steril* 2002;77: 520–525.

32. Clark AM, Thornley B, Tomlinson L. et al. Weight loss results in significant improvement in reproductive outcome for all forms of fertility treatment. *Hum Reprod* 1998;13: 1502–1505.

33. Homburg R. Adverse effect of luteinizing hormone on fertility: fact or fantasy. *Bailliere's Clin Obstet Gynaecol* 1996;12: 555–563.

34. Van der Meer M, Hompes PGA, Scheele F, et al. The importance of endogenous feedback for monofollicular growth in low-dose step-up ovulation induction with FSH in PCOS, a randomized study. *Fertil Steril* 1996; 66:571–575.

35. Homburg R, Eshel A, Kilborn J, et al. Combined luteinizing hormone releasing hormone analogue and exogenous gonadotrophins for the treatment of infertility associated with polycystic ovaries. *Hum Reprod* 1990;5: 32–37.

36. Urman B, Sarac E, Dogan L & Gurgan T. Pregnancy in infertile PCOD patients. Complications and outcome. *J Repod Med* 1997;42: 501–505.

37. Bjercke S, Dale PO, Tanbo T, et al. Impact of insulin resistance on pregnancy complications and outcome in women with polycystic ovary syndrome. *Gynecol Obstet Invest* 2002;54: 94–98.

38. Mikola M, Hiilesman V, Halttunen M, et al. Obstetric outcome in women with polycystic ovary syndrome. *Hum Reprod* 2001;16: 226–229.

39. Weerakiet S, Srisombut C, Rojanasakul A, et al. Prevalence of gestational diabetes mellitus and pregnancy outcomes in Asian women with polycystic ovary syndrome. *Gynecol Endocrinol* 2004;19: 134–140.

40. Radon PA, McMahon MJ & Meyer WR. Impaired glucose tolerance in pregnant women with polycystic ovary syndrome. *Obstet Gynecol* 1999;94: 194–197.

41. Holte J, Gennarelli G, Wide L, et al. High prevalence of polycystic ovaries and associated clinical, endocrine and metabolic features in women with previous gestational diabetes mellitus. *J Clin Endocrinol Metab* 1998;83: 1143–1150.

42. Kousta E, Cela E, Lawrence N, et al. The prevalence of polycystic ovaries in women with a history of gestational diabetes. *Clin Endocrinol* 2000;53: 501–507.

43. Koivunen RM, Juutinen J, Vauhkonen I, et al. Metabolic and steroidogenic alterations related to increased frequency of polycystic ovaries in women with a history of gestational diabetes. *J Clin Endocrinol Metab* 2001;86: 2591–2599.

44. Anttila L, Karjala K, Pentilla RA, et al. Polycystic ovaries in women with geatational diabetes. *Obstet Gynecol* 1998;92: 13–16.

45. Turhan NO, Seckin NC, Aybar F & Inegol I. Assessment of glucose tolerance and pregnancy outcome of polycystic ovary patients. *Int J Gynaecol Obstet* 2003;81: 163–168.

46. Haakova L, Cibula D, Rezabek K, et al. Pregnancy outcome in women with PCOS and in controls matched by age and weight. *Hum Reprod* 2003;18: 1438–1441.

47. Kashyap S & Claman P. Polycystic ovary disease and the risk of pregnancy-induced hypertension. *J Reprod Med* 2000;45: 991–994.

48. Diamant YZ, Rimon E & Evron S. High incidence of preeclamptic toxemia in patients with polycystic ovarian disease. *Eur J Obstet Gynecol Reprod Biol* 1982;14: 199–204.

49. Fridstrom M, Nisell H, Sjoblom P & Hillensjo T. Are women with polycystic ovary syndrome at an increased risk of pregnancy-induced hypertension and/or preeclampsia. *Hypertens Preg* 1999;18: 73–80.

50. Ibanez L, Potau N, Francois I & de Zegher F. Precocious pubarche, hyperinsulinism and ovarian hyperandrogenism in girls: relation to reduced fetal growth. *J Clin Endocrinol Metab* 1998;83: 3558–3562.

51. Benitez R, Sir-Petermann T, Palomino A, et al. Prevalence of metaboli c disorders among family members of patients with polycystic ovary syndrome. *Rev Med Chil* 2001;129: 707–712.

52. Laitinen J, Taponen S, Martikainen H, et al. Body size from birth to adulthood as a predictor of self-reported polycystic ovary syndrome symptoms. *Int J Obs Relat Metab Disord* 2003;27: 710–715.

53. Sir-Petermann T, Hitchsfeld C, Maliqueo M, et al. Birth weight in offspring of mothers with polycystic ovarian syndrome. *Hum Reprod* 2005;20: 2122–2126.

54. Hattersley AT & Tooke JE. The fetal insulin hypothesis: an alternative explanation of the association of low birth weight with diabetes and vascular diseases. *Lancet* 1999; 353: 1789–1792.

55. Barker DPJ & Osmond C. Infant mortality, chidhood nutrition and ischaemic heart disease in England and Wales. *Lancet* 1986;i: 1077–1081.

21

Impact of Diagnostic Criteria
NICHD Versus Rotterdam

Bulent O. Yildiz, MD

CONTENTS

1 INTRODUCTION
2 DEFINITION OF PCOS: 1990 NIH VERSUS 2003 ROTTERDAM
3 COMMON CRITERIA SHARED BY BOTH 1990 NIH AND 2003 ROTTERDAM
4 DIFFERENCES BETWEEN 1990 NIH AND 2003 ROTTERDAM
5 CONCLUSION

Summary

Polycystic ovary syndrome (PCOS) is the most common endocrine disorder of the reproductive-aged women with considerable metabolic and reproductive morbidity. There has been an ongoing debate regarding definition and diagnostic criteria of PCOS since its first description by Stein and Leventhal in 1935. The most widely used diagnostic criteria (so-called 1990 NIH criteria) define PCOS as the presence of hyperandrogenism and oligo-ovulation after exclusion of the other known disorders. Alternatively, a recently convened international workshop sponsored by European Society of Human Reproduction and Embryology (ESHRE)/American Society for Reproductive Medicine (ASRM) suggested that PCOS should be defined by the presence of two of the following three criteria: (1) oligo- or anovulation; (2) clinical and/or biochemical signs of hyperandrogenism; and (3) polycystic ovaries (PCO). The Rotterdam conference provided clear guidelines for determination of clinical, hormonal, and biochemical features of PCOS, and acknowledged the limitations and difficulties in assessment of clinical hyperandrogenism, hyperandrogenemia, and PCO. Essentially, all patients diagnosed by 1990 NIH criteria would also be defined as having PCOS according to 2003 Rotterdam criteria. However, Rotterdam conference introduced two new phenotypes: *(1)* hyperandrogenism with PCO and normal ovulation, and *(2)* PCO and oligo-anovulation without hyperandrogenism. Hyperandrogenic ovulatory women with PCO appear to have similar metabolic and reproductive features, albeit at a modest level, compared with classic PCOS patients with hyperandrogenic chronic anovulation. However, data are scarce regarding phenotypic features of normoandrogenic oligo-ovulatory women with PCO. The 2003 Rotterdam criteria will potentially increase the number of individuals identified as having PCOS, as it will capture the phenotypes that appear to represent the milder forms of the syndrome. Studies assessing the metabolic and reproductive

From: *Contemporary Endocrinology: Polycystic Ovary Syndrome*
Edited by: A. Dunaif, R. J. Chang, S. Franks, and R. S. Legro © Humana Press, Totowa, NJ

characteristics of the different subgroups of PCOS patients diagnosed by Rotterdam criteria are urgently needed. It is of utmost importance that the applied diagnostic criteria in clinical studies of PCOS are thoroughly documented for the interpretation and comparability of the results.

Key Words: Androgen excess; hyperandrogenism; hyperandrogenemia; polycystic ovary; oligo-ovulation; anovulation.

1. INTRODUCTION

Initial descriptions of the polycystic ovary morphology (PCO) date back to 18th *(1)* and 19th centuries *(2)*. Later on, Stein and Leventhal *(3)* identified the association of particular symptoms and signs with polycystic ovaries (PCO) in 1935. This seminal paper described the classic form of polycystic ovary syndrome (PCOS) documenting the clustering of bilateral enlarged PCO, oligo-amenorrhea, and clinical findings of androgen excess and obesity *(3)*. In this series of seven women who had both oligo-amenorrhea and PCO, four were hirsute and three were obese, suggesting that clinical features might vary considerably between the patients. Further studies in the second half of the 20th century identified the association of certain hormonal and biochemical abnormalities with oligo-anovulation and PCO. These features included elevated levels of circulating luteinizing hormone (LH), and androgens, but they were not consistently noted in all PCOS patients. Thus, it became clear that there is a considerable heterogeneity of clinical, hormonal, and biochemical features of the syndrome.

There has been an ongoing debate regarding definition and diagnostic criteria of PCOS *(4,5)*. In 1990, an international conference was sponsored by the National Institute of Child Health and Human Development (NICHD) with a major goal of establishing specific criteria for definition and diagnosis of PCOS. A questionnaire distributed at that conference led to the major research criteria (so-called 1990 NIH diagnostic criteria) for PCOS (Table 1). These most widely used diagnostic criteria appeared in the proceedings of the conference in 1992 include *(1)* hyperandrogenism and/or hyperandrogenemia, *(2)* oligo-ovulation, and *(3)* exclusion of other known disorders such as Cushing's syndrome, hyperprolactinemia, and non-classic adrenal

Table 1
Current Diagnostic Criteria for the Definition of Polycystic Ovary Syndrome (PCOS)

1990 NIH Criteria[a]
   1) Clinical and/or biochemical signs of hyperandrogenism
   2) Oligo-ovulation and exclusion of other known disorders[b]
2003 Rotterdam Criteria[c]
   1) Oligo- or anovulation
   2) Clinical and or biochemical signs of hyperandrogenism
   3) Polycystic ovaries and exclusion of other known disorders[b]

   [a]Both 1 and 2 are required for the diagnosis.
   [b]These include but not limited to Cushing's syndrome, hyperpro-lactinemia, and non-classic congenital adrenal hyperplasia.
   [c]2 of 3 are required for the diagnosis.

hyperplasia *(6)*. The 1990 NIH criteria was an important step for standardization of PCOS diagnosis and led to increased awareness and interest in the field. Using the 1990 NIH criteria, prevalence studies conducted in different populations consistently documented that PCOS is the most common endocrine disorder of reproductive-aged women with an estimated prevalence of 5–10% *(7–10)*. A recent Medline search using the keyword "PCOS" identified only 2608 citations in 56 years between 1935 and 1991, whereas this number was 3502 between 1992 and 2006. Of interest, review articles summarizing and evaluating recently published work and providing specific perceptions and opinions about PCOS comprise almost one of four papers in the field within the last 15 years, suggesting that expert opinion remains dominating in diagnosis and management of PCOS.

More recently, an expert meeting sponsored by European Society of Human Reproduction and Embryology (ESHRE)/American Society for Reproductive Medicine (ASRM) expanded the definition of PCOS, suggesting that it should include two of the following three criteria: *(1)* oligo- and/or anovulation, *(2)* clinical and/or biochemical signs of hyperandrogenism, and *(3)* PCO on ultrasonography (US) and exclusion of related disorders *(11,12)* (Table 1). In this chapter, we will briefly overview the impact of suggested diagnostic criteria for PCOS.

2. DEFINITION OF PCOS: 1990 NIH VERSUS 2003 ROTTERDAM

A syndrome is defined as "a combination of signs and/or symptoms that forms a distinct clinical picture indicative of a particular disorder" (from Oxford Concise Medical Dictionary). It is now well recognized that PCOS represents a common and complex syndrome of unknown etiology and that both genetic and environmental factors play a role in the development of this disorder. What is not universally accepted however are the diagnostic criteria of the syndrome, making PCOS a real challenge for both practicing physician and clinical investigator. Heterogeneity of the symptoms and signs, and changing phenotype of a patient over time are some of the other difficulties in the diagnosis of PCOS.

During the 1990 NIH conference, participants were queried about nomenclature and diagnostic criteria for PCOS to reach a uniform and precise definition of the syndrome *(6)*. Regarding nomenclature, 88% of the participants felt that PCOS is a manifestation of disease rather than a disease entity or specific diagnosis, whereas 60% agreed that PCOS is a diagnosis of exclusion. The conference concluded that PCOS can be diagnosed by the presence of hyperandrogenism and oligo-ovulation after exclusion of related disorders, and suggested that PCO on US is not necessary for PCOS diagnosis *(6)*. Although this was a useful statement that provided guidance for the controversy over the diagnostic options of the syndrome and 1990 NIH criteria has been widely used by investigators from the USA, most of the investigators from the United Kingdom and continental Europe defined PCOS in their studies as the presence of PCO on US combined with hyperandrogenism and/or ovulatory dysfunction.

Heterogeneity of the clinical presentation of the PCOS itself and of the different diagnostic criteria used by different investigators in the literature along with the ongoing debate about the definition and diagnosis of the syndrome brought the necessity of an international consensus meeting to establish the criteria both for research and for clinical use. Accordingly, a representative group of experts in the field of PCOS assembled at a consensus workshop jointly sponsored by ESHRE and ASRM in 2003. The workshop proposed that PCOS can be diagnosed, after exclusion of the related disorders, by determination of the two of the following three criteria: *(1)* oligo- or anovulation, *(2)* clinical and/or biochemical signs of hyperandrogenism, and *(3)* PCO *(11,12)*.

Medical consensus is a public statement on a particular aspect of medical knowledge available at the time it was written, and that is generally agreed upon as the evidence-based, state-of-the-art knowledge by a representative group of experts in that area. Its main objective is to counsel physicians on the best possible and acceptable way to diagnose and treat certain disorders. The most usual way to produce a medical consensus is to convene an independent panel of experts usually by a medical association. In cases where there is little controversy regarding the subject under study, establishing what the consensus is can be quite straightforward. Obviously, this has not been the case for PCOS, and the debate regarding definition and diagnosis of the syndrome continues after the 2003 Rotterdam meeting *(13–18)*.

At the 1990 NIH conference, it was noted that the major goal of establishing specific diagnostic criteria for PCOS was precisely specifying a phenotype to further understand the pathogenesis of the disorder *(6)*. It was also emphasized at that meeting that a classification system may need to change over time as the understanding of the disorder changes *(6)*. Although we now have remarkable progress in our understanding of this evolving syndrome, the etiology, genetic and mechanistic basis of PCOS remains largely unknown, suggesting that the revised 2003 Rotterdam criteria is potentially subject to changes/modifications in the forthcoming years. Indeed, consensus statements in general provide a "snapshot in time" of the state of knowledge in a particular topic, and they must be periodically revisited as the new evidence accumulates.

A patient with a diagnosis of PCOS based on the 1990 NIH criteria will automatically have the same diagnosis when the 2003 Rotterdam criteria are applied. In other words, androgen excess and chronic anovulation are the common features shared by both 1990 NIH and 2003 Rotterdam criteria, and make the classical form of PCOS when they present with or without PCO. Alternatively, the 2003 Rotterdam conference proposed that PCO on US should be one of the three criteria for the diagnosis of PCOS and introduced two new phenotypes: *(1)* hyperandrogenism with PCO and normal ovulation, and *(2)* PCO and oligo-anovulation without hyperandrogenism *(11,12)* (Fig. 1). Following,

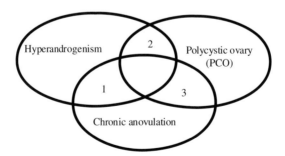

Fig. 1. Venn diagram of polycystic ovary syndrome (PCOS) phenotypes: Area 1 (hyperandrogenism and chronic anovulation) represents the classic form of PCOS. Area 2 (hyperandrogenism and PCO) and Area 3 (PCO and chronic anovulation) represent the new additional phenotypes suggested by the revised Rotterdam 2003 diagnostic criteria.

we will first discuss the common diagnostic criteria suggested by both conferences (hyperandrogenism and chronic anovulation). Then, we will overview the available evidence regarding PCO and the two newly introduced phenotypes.

3. COMMON CRITERIA SHARED BY BOTH 1990 NIH AND 2003 ROTTERDAM

3.1. Androgen Excess

In the original series of Stein and Leventhal (3), four of seven patients were hirsute and one was acneic. Early studies reported that an average of 69% (between 17 and 83%) of PCOS patients had hirsutism (19,20). In three large studies evaluating patients with PCO in the United Kingdom, the prevalence of hirsutism and acne ranged from 61 to 66% and from 24 to 35%, respectively (21–23). These studies also showed that some anovulatory non-hirsute patients have hyperandrogenemia, whereas some anovulatory hirsute women might have normal serum androgen concentrations (21–23). Apparently, clinical manifestations of hyperandrogenism including hirsutism, acne, and androgenic alopecia can be observed in the absence of biochemical hyperandrogenemia. Alternatively, biochemical hyperandrogenemia may present in some PCOS patients, particularly in Asian women, without obvious peripheral manifestations of hyperandrogenism (24). Thus, both the 1990 NIH (6) and 2003 Rotterdam (11,12) criteria for the diagnosis of PCOS include determination of clinical and/or biochemical hyperandrogenism.

During the NIH conference in 1990, 64% of the participants agreed on that hyperandrogenemia is a definite/probable criterion for the definition of PCOS whereas 48 and 52% suggested clinical hyperandrogenism as a definite/probable and possible diagnostic criterion respectively (6). The 1990 NIH criteria did not make any specific suggestions for the definition of clinical or biochemical hyperandrogenism, although the questionnaire distributed at the conference included hirsutism, alopecia, and acne as the clinical signs of hyperandrogenism, and increased concentrations of testosterone, free testosterone, androstenedione, and dehydroepiandrosterone sulfate (DHEAS) for defining biochemical hyperandrogenism. The conference also acknowledged that hyperandrogenemia is not precisely reproducible and that measurement of androgens may considerably vary (6).

Alternatively, the 2003 Rotterdam conference concluded that hirsutism is the primary clinical marker for androgen excess provided that it has certain limitations including inter-observer variability and lack of normative population data (11,12). Acne and androgenic alopecia are other common androgenic skin changes and might be observed without hirsutism in some hyperandrogenic women. However, isolated presence of any of these manifestations was not suggested to be used as an indicator of androgen excess (11,12).

There is a wide variability of circulating androgens in women, and it is critical to note that there is no clear distinction between normal and abnormal in interpreting androgen levels (25). Nevertheless, evaluation of excessive androgen production is usually performed by the measurement of androgenic hormones in the circulation. Again, different from the 1990 NIH conference, the 2003 Rotterdam conference clearly acknowledged the limitations of defining androgen excess by the measurement of circulating androgen levels and suggested that the measurement of free testosterone, or the free androgen index, notwithstanding certain limitations, is the sensitive method for determination of biochemical hyperandrogenemia *(11,12)*. Recommended methods for the assessment of free testosterone include equilibrium dialysis, ammonium sulfate precipitation, or calculation of free testosterone from total testosterone, and sex hormone-binding globulin levels *(11,12,26)*.

A few PCOS patients may have "isolated" elevations in DHEAS. Thus, measurement of DHEAS could be of limited value in the hormonal evaluation of women with PCOS. Normative and clinical data for androstenedione are lacking, and there is little data available about the value of androstenedione in evaluation of androgen excess in women. Regarding measurement of these androgenic steroids, the 2003 Rotterdam conference recommended that isolated elevations of DHEAS or androstenedione should not routinely be used for the assessment of biochemical hyperandrogenism *(11,12)*.

Finally, we should make it very clear that metabolic characteristics might differ in PCOS patients depending on whether they have clinical hyperandrogenism, biochemical hyperandrogenemia, or both. For example, we have previously documented in a group of PCOS patients who all have hirsutism, oligo-anovulation, and PCO on US that women with hyperandrogenemia were more insulin resistant than women with normo-androgenemia *(27)*. Similarly, in a large group of PCOS patients diagnosed by 1990 NIH criteria, it was shown that women with hyperandrogenemia and hirsutism had a greater degree of metabolic dysfunction (insulin resistance and beta-cell dysfunction) compared with women with hirsutism, and normo-androgenemia. Women with hyperandrogenemia but without hirsutism demonstrated intermediate degree of metabolic dysfunction in that study *(28)*.

3.2. Oligo-Anovulation

The classic PCOS paper by Stein and Leventhal *(3)* reported oligo-amenorrhea in all of the seven patients in this series. Earlier studies of PCOS suggest that the average prevalence of oligo-amenorrhea is around 80% *(19,20)*. Between 71 and 80% of patients with PCO on US have oligo-amenorrhea *(21–23)*. Accordingly, both 1990 NIH *(6)* and 2003 Rotterdam *(11,12)* conferences include oligo-anovulation as a diagnostic criterion for PCOS.

The questionnaire distributed at the 1990 NICHD conference included menstrual dysfunction (≤6 menses/year) as a potential diagnostic criterion for PCOS, and 52% of the participants listed it as a definite/probable criterion whereas 45% thought it was a possible diagnostic criterion. The conference concluded that oligo-ovulation was the second major research criterion of PCOS after hyperandrogenism *(6)*. Rotterdam 2003 conference also included oligo-anovulation in revised diagnostic criteria of PCOS *(11,12)*.

Chronic anovulation in PCOS usually presents as oligomenorrhea, amenorrhea, or dysfunctional uterine bleeding. The 1990 NIH conference specifically defined chronic anovulation as six or fewer menses per year *(6)*, whereas the 2003 Rotterdam conference did not make any specific recommendations for the definition of oligo-anovulation in PCOS *(11,12)*. There is a considerable heterogeneity in the literature regarding the definition and evaluation of ovulatory function in PCOS patients. We should also emphasize that up to 20% of PCOS patients report regular vaginal bleeding

(11,12,29,30), and ovulatory dysfunction could be confirmed in these patients by obtaining a luteal phase progesterone level on days 20–22 (i.e. 20–22 days after the start of menstruation) with or without basal body temperature monitoring *(30)*.

4. DIFFERENCES BETWEEN 1990 NIH AND 2003 ROTTERDAM

4.1. Polycystic Ovaries

Available evidence suggests that PCO on US might be a component of the heterogeneous spectrum of PCOS rather than being a normal morphological variant of the ovarian appearance. PCO on US was observed in 50–87% of patients with hirsutism and regular menses *(21,30–32)*. Women with PCO have higher androgen levels and a higher prevalence of irregular menstrual cycles than women with normal ovaries *(33,34)*. Normal weight women with PCO develop typical phenotypic features of PCOS when they become overweight or obese *(35)*. The prevalence of PCO among ovulatory women with infertility is higher than among healthy controls *(36)*. Finally, women with regular menses and PCO respond to ovarian stimulation similar to PCOS patients and have an increased risk of ovarian hyperstimulation syndrome *(37)*, and US evaluation of ovaries in anovulatory infertility might be helpful to predict the response to ovarian stimulation *(38)*.

PCO on US has been most commonly diagnosed by Adams criteria that defined PCO as the presence of 10 or more peripheral cysts (2–8 mm) around a dense core of stroma in enlarged ($\geq$8 ml) ovaries *(39)*. Alternatively, Rotterdam conference concluded that PCO should be defined as the presence of 12 or more follicles in each ovary measuring 2–9 mm in diameter, and/or increased ovarian volume ($\geq$10 ml) *(11,12)*. Only one ovary fitting this definition would be sufficient for the PCO diagnosis. Whether the clinical, hormonal, and biochemical phenotypes of patients diagnosed having PCOS based on Rotterdam criteria differ from those diagnosed by Adams criteria remain to be determined in future studies.

The results of the US evaluation of the ovaries correlate well with the appearance of the ovaries at the time of surgery, and ovarian histological findings *(40,41)*. However, a recent study evaluating the variability in the detection of PCO and normal ovaries on transvaginal US by experienced practitioners reported a mean intra- and inter-observer agreements about 69 and 51%, respectively *(42)*. These results suggested that the assessment of ovaries by US shows significant variability and might not be a reliable and reproducible diagnostic tool for PCOS *(42)*. It is important to note that transabdominal and transvaginal US are not equally sensitive for detection of PCO *(43,44)* and that transvaginal approach should be preferred whenever possible *(11,12)*.

Rotterdam conference clearly provided the recommendations for the use of the US in defining PCO, and acknowledged the advantages and limitations *(11,12)*. For example, ovarian volume might be reduced in women taking oral contraceptive pills *(45)*, and the PCO definition by Rotterdam criteria does not apply to these women. PCO on US can be detected in postmenopausal women, although there is no threshold available for ovarian volume or follicle number *(46)*. Furthermore, multicystic ovaries usually observed in adolescent girls could not be easily discriminated from PCO *(47)*. We should also note that PCO on US can be observed in up to 30% of healthy women *(34,43,48–50)*, and it could be associated with other disorders including hyper-prolactinemia, non-classical congenital adrenal hyperplasia, functional hypothalamic amenorrhea *(50)*, and Cushing's syndrome *(51)*. Finally, some of the anovulatory women with hyperandrogenism do not appear to have PCO on US *(52)*. Nevertheless, using the 2003 Rotterdam criteria for definition of PCO on US, Legro and colleagues *(53)* recently reported that 95% of obese patients who had diagnosis of PCOS based on 1990 NIH criteria, and 48% of healthy women had PCO. However, PCO on US neither predicts the metabolic or reproductive phenotype *(53)* nor does it affect cardiovascular risk profile in PCOS patients defined by 1990 NIH criteria *(54)*.

4.2. Two Newly Introduced PCOS Phenotypes by the 2003 Rotterdam Criteria

Hyperandrogenism and chronic anovulation with or without PCO are the phenotypes defined as PCOS both by the 1990 NIH and by 2003 Rotterdam criteria *(6,11,12)*. However, the 2003 Rotterdam conference introduced two new phenotypes expanding the definition of the syndrome. These are *(1)* hyperandrogenism and PCO with normal ovulatory function and *(2)* PCO and chronic anovulation without hyperandrogenism *(11,12)*. A key question needs to be answered is whether these new phenotypes truly represent PCOS and share the same metabolic and reproductive morbidity with the classic form of PCOS defined by the 1990 NIH criteria. There are a few studies that partially address these issues.

The results of the earlier studies where the diagnosis was based on US criteria are highly concordant with those in which the 1990 NIH criteria were used *(23,55,56)*. Indeed, the prevalence of clinical hyperandrogenism or chronic anovulation are both over 70% in women with PCO on US *(22,23,55)*. Among PCOS patients diagnosed by the presence of hyperandrogenism and PCO, those with irregular menstrual cycles show insulin resistance and hyperinsulinemia whereas the patients with regular cycles and healthy women appear to have similar insulin resistance parameters *(57)*. Ovulatory women with hyperandrogenism and PCO might have some subtle metabolic and reproductive abnormalities similar to classic PCOS patients with hyperandrogenism and chronic anovulation *(58)* although not all agree *(59)*.

Recently, it was reported in a retrospective study that about 21% of the PCOS patients who were examined for clinical hyperandrogenism at a single center between 1980 and 2004 were ovulatory *(60)*. A subgroup analysis of the patients from the same cohort regarding cardiovascular and metabolic risk showed that ovulatory PCOS patients had a risk profile that is lower than classic PCOS patients but higher than hyperandrogenic ovulatory women who had normal ovaries on US *(60)*.

Available data are scarce regarding PCO and chronic anovulation without hirsutism. Women with PCO on US have a higher incidence of menstrual irregularities compared with those with normal ovarian morphology *(34)*. It was reported earlier that among patients with PCO on US, 30% had chronic oligo-anovulation without hirsutism *(22)*. More recently, PCO on US was detected in about 48% of women who self-reported oligomenorrhea *(61)*. Women with PCO on US, but without hyperandrogenism, showed similar disturbances in insulin resistance and lipid parameters compared with patients with PCO on US and hyperandrogenism *(62)*. In this study, menstrual irregularity was associated with higher insulin resistance in both groups *(62)*.

5. CONCLUSION

The definition and diagnosis of PCOS remains as a bone of contention. There is no universally accepted clinical definition of PCOS and no single clinical, hormonal, or biochemical parameter appears to be a sine qua non of the syndrome. The 2003 Rotterdam conference addressed both clinical and research needs in the field of PCOS and provided specific guidelines for definition of the components of the syndrome including clinical hyperandrogenism, hyperandrogenemia, and PCO on US *(11,12)*. This consensus conference brings in the use of PCO on US as a diagnostic criterion of PCOS and introduces two new combinations for the diagnosis of the syndrome that would not meet 1990 NIH criteria *(11,12)*. Adoption of widespread use of 2003 Rotterdam criteria will potentially increase the number of subjects diagnosed as having PCOS, as it will capture a spectrum of clinical expressions that might be the milder forms of the same disorder.

PCOS is a heterogeneous disorder, and even though the prevalence of the syndrome is similar and consistently high in different populations worldwide when similar diagnostic criteria are used, we are beginning to understand that the phenotype and clinical outcomes might significantly differ between different populations *(24,63,64)* and even within the same population *(28)*. Obviously, population-specific characteristics could have a potential impact on the definition of the syndrome. Recognition of these factors emphasizes the unexplained residue, whose understanding will be a task for the future. Meanwhile, urgent studies are needed for a detailed examination of the different PCOS phenotypes and determination of associated metabolic and reproductive outcome. In clinical studies of PCOS, documentation of the applied diagnostic criteria in detail is critical for the interpretation and comparability of the results. More research may lead to improvement in our understanding of the fundamental biology and etiology of PCOS that has proved to be a challenging scientific problem of enormous clinical relevance. Consequently, we might ultimately reach to a universally agreed definition and diagnostic criteria for the syndrome.

REFERENCES

1. Vallisneri A. Storia della generazione dell'uomo e dell'animale; 1721. Cited in Cooke ID, Lunenfeld B. *Res Clin Forums* 1989; 11:109–113.
2. Chereau A. Mémories pour servir a l'étude des maladies des ovaries. Masson & Cie 1844:Paris: Fortin.
3. Stein IF, Leventhal, M.L. Amenorrhea associated with bilateral polycystic ovaries. *Am J Obstet Gynecol* 1935; 29:181–91.
4. Balen A, Michelmore K. What is polycystic ovary syndrome? Are national views important? *Hum Reprod* 2002; 17:2219–27.
5. Homburg R. What is polycystic ovarian syndrome? A proposal for a consensus on the definition and diagnosis of polycystic ovarian syndrome. *Hum Reprod* 2002; 17:2495–9.
6. Zawadzki JK, Dunaif A. Diagnostic criteria for polycystic ovary syndrome. In: Dunaif A, Givens J, Haseltine F, Merriam GR, eds. *Polycystic Ovary Syndrome*. Boston: Blackwell Scientific Publications, 1992:377–84.
7. Knochenhauer ES, Key TJ, Kahsar-Miller M, Waggoner W, Boots LR, Azziz R. Prevalence of the polycystic ovary syndrome in unselected black and white women of the southeastern United States: a prospective study. *J Clin Endocrinol Metab* 1998; 83:3078–82.

8. Diamanti-Kandarakis E, Kouli CR, Bergiele AT, et al. A survey of the polycystic ovary syndrome in the Greek island of Lesbos: hormonal and metabolic profile. *J Clin Endocrinol Metab* 1999; 84:4006–11.

9. Asuncion M, Calvo RM, San Millan JL, Sancho J, Avila S, Escobar-Morreale HF. A prospective study of the prevalence of the polycystic ovary syndrome in unselected Caucasian women from Spain. *J Clin Endocrinol Metab* 2000; 85:2434–8.

10. Azziz R, Woods KS, Reyna R, Key TJ, Knochenhauer ES, Yildiz BO. The prevalence and features of the polycystic ovary syndrome in an unselected population. *J Clin Endocrinol Metab* 2004; 89:2745–9.

11. Rotterdam ESHRE/ASRM-sponsored PCOS Consensus Workshop Group. Revised 2003 consensus on diagnostic criteria and long-term health risks related to polycystic ovary syndrome. *Fertil Steril* 2004; 81:19–25.

12. Rotterdam ESHRE/ASRM-sponsored PCOS Consensus Workshop Group. Revised 2003 consensus on diagnostic criteria and long-term health risks related to polycystic ovary syndrome (PCOS). *Hum Reprod* 2004; 19:41–7.

13. Carmina E. Diagnosis of polycystic ovary syndrome: from NIH criteria to ESHRE-ASRM guidelines. *Minerva Ginecol* 2004; 56:1–6.

14. Dunaif A. Hyperandrogenemia is necessary but not sufficient for polycystic ovary syndrome. *Fertil Steril* 2003; 80:262–3.

15. Azziz R. Androgen excess is the key element in polycystic ovary syndrome. *Fertil Steril* 2003; 80:252–4.

16. Azziz R. Diagnostic criteria for polycystic ovary syndrome: a reappraisal. *Fertil Steril* 2005; 83: 1343–6.

17. Azziz R. Diagnosis of polycystic ovarian syndrome: the rotterdam criteria are premature. *J Clin Endocrinol Metab* 2006; 91:781–5.

18. Franks S. Diagnosis of polycystic ovarian syndrome: in defense of the rotterdam criteria. *J Clin Endocrinol Metab* 2006; 91:786–9.

19. Goldzieher JW, Axelrod LR. Clinical and biochemical features of polycystic ovarian disease. *Fertil Steril* 1963; 14:631–53.

20. Smith KD, Steinberger E, Perloff WH. Polycystic ovarian disease. A report of 301 patients. *Am J Obstet Gynecol* 1965; 93:994–1001.

21. Franks S. Polycystic ovary syndrome: a changing perspective. *Clin Endocrinol (Oxf)* 1989; 31: 87–120.

22. Conway GS, Honour JW, Jacobs HS. Heterogeneity of the polycystic ovary syndrome: clinical, endocrine and ultrasound features in 556 patients. *Clin Endocrinol (Oxf)* 1989; 30:459–70.

23. Balen AH, Conway GS, Kaltsas G, et al. Polycystic ovary syndrome: the spectrum of the disorder in 1741 patients. *Hum Reprod* 1995; 10:2107–11.

24. Carmina E, Koyama T, Chang L, Stanczyk FZ, Lobo RA. Does ethnicity influence the prevalence of adrenal hyperandrogenism and insulin resistance in polycystic ovary syndrome? *Am J Obstet Gynecol* 1992; 167:1807–12.

25. The evaluation and treatment of androgen excess. *Fertil Steril* 2004; 82 Suppl 1:S173–80.

26. Rosner W. Errors in the measurement of plasma free testosterone. *J Clin Endocrinol Metab* 1997; 82:2014–5.

27. Yildiz BO, Gedik O. Insulin resistance in polycystic ovary syndrome: hyperandrogenemia versus normoandrogenemia. *Eur J Obstet Gynecol Reprod Biol* 2001; 100:62–6.

28. Chang WY, Knochenhauer ES, Bartolucci AA, Azziz R. Phenotypic spectrum of polycystic ovary syndrome: clinical and biochemical characterization of the three major clinical subgroups. *Fertil Steril* 2005; 83:1717–23.

29. Azziz R, Sanchez LA, Knochenhauer ES, et al. Androgen excess in women: experience with over 1000 consecutive patients. *J Clin Endocrinol Metab* 2004; 89:453–62.

30. Carmina E, Lobo RA. Do hyperandrogenic women with normal menses have polycystic ovary syndrome? *Fertil Steril* 1999; 71:319–22.

31. O'Driscoll JB, Mamtora H, Higginson J, Pollock A, Kane J, Anderson DC. A prospective study of the prevalence of clear-cut endocrine disorders and polycystic ovaries in 350 patients presenting with hirsutism or androgenic alopecia. *Clin Endocrinol (Oxf)* 1994; 41:231–6.

32. Dewailly D, Robert Y, Helin I, et al. Ovarian stromal hypertrophy in hyperandrogenic women. *Clin Endocrinol (Oxf)* 1994; 41:557–62.

33. Clayton RN, Ogden V, Hodgkinson J, et al. How common are polycystic ovaries in normal women and what is their significance for the fertility of the population? *Clin Endocrinol (Oxf)* 1992; 37:127–34.

34. Michelmore KF, Balen AH, Dunger DB, Vessey MP. Polycystic ovaries and associated clinical and biochemical features in young women. *Clin Endocrinol (Oxf)* 1999; 51:779–86.

35. Kiddy DS, Sharp PS, White DM, et al. Differences in clinical and endocrine features between obese and non-obese subjects with polycystic ovary syndrome: an analysis of 263 consecutive cases. *Clin Endocrinol (Oxf)* 1990; 32:213–20.

36. Kousta E, White DM, Cela E, McCarthy MI, Franks S. The prevalence of polycystic ovaries in women with infertility. *Hum Reprod* 1999; 14:2720–3.

37. Homburg R. Polycystic ovary syndrome - from gynaecological curiosity to multisystem endocrinopathy. *Hum Reprod* 1996; 11:29–39.

38. Enskog A, Henriksson M, Unander M, Nilsson L, Brannstrom M. Prospective study of the clinical and laboratory parameters of patients in whom ovarian hyperstimulation syndrome developed during controlled ovarian hyperstimulation for in vitro fertilization. *Fertil Steril* 1999; 71:808–14.

39. Adams J, Franks S, Polson DW, et al. Multifollicular ovaries: clinical and endocrine features and response to pulsatile gonadotropin releasing hormone. *Lancet* 1985; 2:1375–9.

40. Eden JA. Which is the best test to detect the polycystic ovary? *Aust N Z J Obstet Gynaecol* 1988; 28:221–4.

41. Saxton DW, Farquhar CM, Rae T, Beard RW, Anderson MC, Wadsworth J. Accuracy of ultrasound measurements of female pelvic organs. *Br J Obstet Gynaecol* 1990; 97:695–9.

42. Amer SA, Li TC, Bygrave C, Sprigg A, Saravelos H, Cooke ID. An evaluation of the inter-observer and intra-observer variability of the ultrasound diagnosis of polycystic ovaries. *Hum Reprod* 2002; 17:1616–22.

43. Farquhar CM, Birdsall M, Manning P, Mitchell JM, France JT. The prevalence of polycystic ovaries on ultrasound scanning in a population of randomly selected women. *Aust N Z J Obstet Gynaecol* 1994; 34:67–72.

44. Ardaens Y, Robert Y, Lemaitre L, Fossati P, Dewailly D. Polycystic ovarian disease: contribution of vaginal endosonography and reassessment of ultrasonic diagnosis. *Fertil Steril* 1991; 55:1062–8.

45. Franks S, Adams J, Mason H, Polson D. Ovulatory disorders in women with polycystic ovary syndrome. *Clin Obstet Gynaecol* 1985; 12:605–32.

46. Birdsall MA, Farquhar CM. Polycystic ovaries in pre and post-menopausal women. *Clin Endocrinol (Oxf)* 1996; 44:269–76.

47. Herter LD, Magalhaes JA, Spritzer PM. Relevance of the determination of ovarian volume in adolescent girls with menstrual disorders. *J Clin Ultrasound* 1996; 24:243–8.

48. Polson DW, Adams J, Wadsworth J, Franks S. Polycystic ovaries–a common finding in normal women. *Lancet* 1988; 1:870–2.

49. Koivunen R, Laatikainen T, Tomas C, Huhtaniemi I, Tapanainen J, Martikainen H. The prevalence of polycystic ovaries in healthy women. *Acta Obstet Gynecol Scand* 1999; 78:137–41.

50. Abdel Gadir A, Khatim MS, Mowafi RS, Alnaser HM, Muharib NS, Shaw RW. Implications of ultrasonically diagnosed polycystic ovaries. I. Correlations with basal hormonal profiles. *Hum Reprod* 1992; 7:453–7.

51. Kaltsas GA, Korbonits M, Isidori AM, et al. How common are polycystic ovaries and the polycystic ovarian syndrome in women with Cushing's syndrome? *Clin Endocrinol (Oxf)* 2000; 53:493–500.

52. Ehrmann DA, Rosenfield RL, Barnes RB, Brigell DF, Sheikh Z. Detection of functional ovarian hyperandrogenism in women with androgen excess. *N Engl J Med* 1992; 327:157–62.

53. Legro RS, Chiu P, Kunselman AR, Bentley CM, Dodson WC, Dunaif A. Polycystic ovaries are common in women with hyperandrogenic chronic anovulation but do not predict metabolic or reproductive phenotype. *J Clin Endocrinol Metab* 2005; 90:2571–9.

54. Loucks TL, Talbott EO, McHugh KP, Keelan M, Berga SL, Guzick DS. Do polycystic-appearing ovaries affect the risk of cardiovascular disease among women with polycystic ovary syndrome? *Fertil Steril* 2000; 74:547–52.

55. Franks S. Polycystic ovary syndrome. *N Engl J Med* 1995; 333:853–61.

56. Carmina E, Lobo RA. Polycystic ovaries in Hirsute women with normal menses. *Am J Med* 2001; 111:602–6.

57. Robinson S, Kiddy D, Gelding SV, et al. The relationship of insulin insensitivity to menstrual pattern in women with hyperandrogenism and polycystic ovaries. *Clin Endocrinol (Oxf)* 1993; 39:351–5.

58. Chang PL, Lindheim SR, Lowre C, et al. Normal ovulatory women with polycystic ovaries have hyperandrogenic pituitary-ovarian responses to gonadotropin-releasing hormone-agonist testing. *J Clin Endocrinol Metab* 2000; 85:995–1000.

59. Vanky E, Kjotrod S, Salvesen KA, Romundstad P, Moen MH, Carlsen SM. Clinical, biochemical and ultrasonographic characteristics of Scandinavian women with PCOS. *Acta Obstet Gynecol Scand* 2004; 83:482–6.

60. Carmina E, Rosato F, Janni A, Rizzo M, Longo RA. Extensive clinical experience: relative prevalence of different androgen excess disorders in 950 women referred because of clinical hyperandrogenism. *J Clin Endocrinol Metab* 2006; 91:2–6.

61. Taponen S, Ahonkallio S, Martikainen H, et al. Prevalence of polycystic ovaries in women with self-reported symptoms of oligomenorrhoea and/or hirsutism: Northern Finland Birth Cohort 1966 Study. *Hum Reprod* 2004; 19:1083–8.

62. Norman RJ, Hague WM, Masters SC, Wang XJ. Subjects with polycystic ovaries without hyperandrogenaemia exhibit similar disturbances in insulin and lipid profiles as those with polycystic ovary syndrome. *Hum Reprod* 1995; 10:2258–61.

63. Wijeyaratne CN, Balen AH, Barth JH, Belchetz PE. Clinical manifestations and insulin resistance (IR) in polycystic ovary syndrome (PCOS) among South Asians and Caucasians: is there a difference? *Clin Endocrinol (Oxf)* 2002; 57:343–50.

64. Carmina E, Legro RS, Stamets K, Lowell J, Lobo RA. Difference in body weight between American and Italian women with polycystic ovary syndrome: influence of the diet. *Hum Reprod* 2003; 18: 2289–93.

Subject Index